T0221050

Nutritional Management of Hospitalized Small Animals

This title is also available as an e-book.
For more details, please see
www.wiley.com/buy/9781444336474
or scan this QR code:

Nutritional Management of Hospitalized Small Animals

EDITED BY

Daniel L. Chan, DVM, DACVECC, DECVECC, DACVN, FHEA, MRCVS

Professor of Veterinary Emergency and Critical Care
Clinical Nutritionist, Head of Nutritional Support Service
Section Head of Emergency and Critical Care
Department of Veterinary Clinical Science and Services
The Royal Veterinary College, University of London, UK

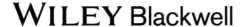

Registered Office
John Wiley & Sons, Ltd, The Atrium, Southern Gate, Chichester, West Sussex, PO19 8SQ, UK

Editorial Offices
9600 Garsington Road, Oxford, OX4 2DQ, UK
The Atrium, Southern Gate, Chichester, West Sussex, PO19 8SQ, UK
1606 Golden Aspen Drive, Suites 103 and 104, Ames, Iowa 50010, USA

For details of our global editorial offices, for customer services and for information about how to apply for permission to reuse the copyright material in this book please see our website at www.wiley.com/wiley-blackwell.

Library of Congress Cataloging-in-Publication Data
Nutritional management of hospitalized small animals / edited by Daniel L. Chan.
    p. ; cm.
  Includes bibliographical references and index.
  ISBN 978-1-4443-3647-4 (cloth)
1. Animal nutrition.   2. Veterinary nursing.   3. Animal feeding.   4. Veterinary diet therapy.
I. Chan, Daniel L., 1973– , editor.
  [DNLM: 1. Animal Nutritional Physiological Phenomena.   2. Nutritional Support–veterinary.
3. Nutritional Requirements.   4. Nutritional Status.   5. Veterinary Medicine–methods.   SF 95]
  SF95.N888 2015
  636.08'52–dc23
                                    2015007221

A catalogue record for this book is available from the British Library.

Set in 9.5/12pt Meridien by SPi Global, Pondicherry, India

1   2015

Contents

Contributors

Sophie Adamantos, BVSc, DACVECC, DECVECC, MRCVS, FHEA
Langford Veterinary Services, University of Bristol, UK

Karin Allenspach, Dr.med.vet., FVH, DECVIM-CA, PhD, FHEA, MRCVS
Professor of Internal Medicine, Department of Clinical Science and Services, The Royal Veterinary College, University of London, UK

Robert C. Backus, MS, DVM, PhD, DACVN
Associate Professor, Department of Veterinary Medicine and Surgery, College of Veterinary Medicine, University of Missouri, USA

Matthew W. Beal, DVM Diplomate ACVECC
Associate Professor, Emergency and Critical Care Medicine, Director of Interventional Radiology Services, College of Veterinary Medicine, Michigan State University, USA

Iveta Becvarova, DVM, MS, Diplomate ACVN
Director, Academic Affairs, Hill's Pet Nutrition Manufacturing, Czech Republic

Ross Bond, BVMS, PhD, DVD, DECVD, MRCVS
Professor of Dermatology, Department of Clinical Sciences and Services, The Royal Veterinary College, University of London, UK

Jeleen A. Briscoe, VMD, DABVP (Avian)
Animal Care Program, United States Department of Agriculture Animal and Plant Health Service, Riverdale, MD, USA

Daniel L. Chan, DVM, DACVECC, DECVECC, DACVN, FHEA, MRCVS
Professor, Veterinary Emergency and Critical Care, Clinical Nutritionist, Department of Veterinary Clinical Sciences and Services, The Royal Veterinary College, University of London, UK

Laura Eirmann, DVM, DACVN
Oradell Animal Hospital; Nestle Purina PetCare, Ringwood, NJ, USA

Denise A. Elliott, BVSc (Hons) PhD, DACVIM, DACVN
Head of Research, Waltham Centre for Pet Nutrition, Waltham on the Wolds, Leicestershire, UK

Lisa M. Freeman, PhD, DVM, DACVN
Professor of Nutrition, Department of Clinical Sciences, Tufts Cummings School of Veterinary Medicine, North Grafton, MA, USA

Jason W. Gagne, DVM, DACVN
Nestle Purina Incorporated, St Louis, MO, USA

Isuru Gajanayake, BVSc, CertSAM, DACVIM, MRCVS
Willows Veterinary Centre and Referral Service, Shirley, Solihull, West Midlands, UK

Cailin R. Heinze, VMD, MS, DACVN
Assistant Professor, Department of Clinical Sciences, Tufts Cummings School of
Veterinary Medicine, North Grafton, MA, USA

Marta Hervera, BVSc, PhD, DECVCN
Servei de Dietètica i Nutrició, Fundació Hospital Clínic Veterinari, Universitat Autònoma
de Barcelona, Bellaterra, Spain

Kristine B. Jensen, DVM, MVetMed, DACVIM, MRCVS
Djursjukhuset Malmö, Cypressvägen Malmö, Sweden

La'Toya Latney, DVM
Exotic Companion Animal Medicine and Surgery, University of Pennsylvania School of
Veterinary Medicine, Philadelphia, PA, USA

F. A. (Tony) Mann, DVM, MS, DACVS, DACVECC
Professor, Veterinary Medical Teaching Hospital, College of Veterinary Medicine,
University of Missouri, Columbia, MO, USA

Kathryn E. Michel, DVM, MS, DACVN
Professor, Department of Clinical Studies, School of Veterinary Medicine, University of
Pennsylvania, Philadelphia, PA, USA

Sally Perea, DVM, MS, DACVN
Mars Pet Care, Mason, OH, USA

Renee M. Streeter, DVM
Liverpool, NY, USA

Cecilia Villaverde, BVSc, PhD, DACVN, DECVCN
Servei de Dietètica i Nutrició, Fundació Hospital Clínic Veterinari, Universitat Autònoma
de Barcelona, Bellaterra, Spain

Andrea V. Volk, DVM, Dr med.vet, MVetMed, DipECVD, MRCVS
Dermatology Service, Department of Clinical Sciences and Services, The Royal
Veterinary College, University of London, UK

Joseph J. Wakshlag, DVM, PhD, DACVN, DACVSMR
Cornell University College of Veterinary Medicine, Ithaca, NY, USA

Lisa P. Weeth, DVM, DACVN
Weeth Nutrition Services, Edinburgh, Scotland, UK

Preface

After many years of nutritional support in many veterinary hospitals amounting to "too little and too late" there is finally concrete recognition that nutritional support is a key aspect of successful patient recovery. The application, techniques and strategies of nutritional support in small animals have gone through many changes in the past several years and effective nutritional support is a hallmark of high quality standard of care. Perhaps it is the close interface between nutrition and all other aspects of care that ensures that the art and science of nutrition remains dynamic as it evolves with advances in patient care. This is what makes nutritional support a very exciting and challenging field in which to practice. In the management of many ill animals, clinicians face numerous challenges of providing optimal nutritional care. In formulating the best plans, clinicians must not only possess a keen understanding of nutritional principles, techniques and strategies, but also have a strong foundation in physiology, pathophysiology and therapeutics.

It is worth emphasizing that no single nutritional therapeutic plan will be applicable to all patient populations. Medical treatments and interventions, including nutritional therapies, vary significantly among different patient populations and veterinary facilities. With various disease states, there may be significant alterations in the physiologic and metabolic pathways that can impact the nutritional plan. The goals of this book are to provide a comprehensive reference on the principles and practice of nutritional support in small animals that require hospitalization. The primary target for this book includes general practitioners, advanced practitioners, specialists, veterinary nurses, technicians, support staff and those studying and researching the science of nutritional support.

The first section of the book comprises chapters exploring techniques for assessing the nutritional status and energy needs of small animal patients, routes of nutritional support, the various options for feeding tubes, the techniques for placing these feeding tubes, and the formulation and use of parenteral nutrition. The second section of the book deals with the issues and the strategies for providing nutritional support in various conditions affecting hospitalized small animals. There are chapters that discuss the pathophysiology of malnutrition, appropriate use of appetite stimulants, common conditions requiring specific nutritional alterations, such as kidney disease, hepatic failure, acute pancreatitis, and less common situations where nutritional recommendations are sparse and largely untested, such as sepsis, short-bowel syndrome, respiratory failure, refeeding syndrome and patients with gastrointestinal motility disorders. The final chapter is devoted to the nutritional management of hospitalized small exotic species, which are becoming more popular in practice and present particular challenges in terms of nutritional support.

Chapters have been written by a prominent group of authors, who have committed their careers to their area of interest and in many cases currently practise in the subject area about which they wrote. It is hoped that this should allow them to share some greater insight of the nuances of the practice of nutritional support for the hospitalized small animal patient. The vision for this book is that it becomes an indispensable nutritional resource for small animal practitioners and the reference book of choice as a practical and useful guide for the nutritional support of hospitalized small animal patients.

It is also the intent of the book to describe clinically applicable techniques that can be incorporated in most practice environments. The scientific evidence behind these recommendations is briefly explored, providing the reader with references for further reading if desired. Many of the contributors are practising nutritionists who are providing practical solutions for their patients. Others contributors are specialists in their fields and show how nutritional support can be effectively used to manage problems they encounter in their practice. In summary, it is an exciting time for the continued development of nutritional care in veterinary patients and this book attempts to capture this excitement.

It is our sincere hope that this book becomes a valuable resource in a wide range of practice settings from small practices to large multi-disciplinary referral centers and that optimal nutritional support becomes the standard of care for every patient.

Daniel L. Chan
DVM, DACVECC, DECVECC, DACVN, MRCVS

Acknowledgements

Needless to say, a project such as this doesn't just happen. It takes a tremendous amount of work, dedication, perseverance and, perhaps most of all, patience. I would first like to thank the team at Wiley for their total support of this project and particularly for their patience. I would also like to thank a group of people whose invaluable guidance has gotten me to where I am today – no one gets to where they are alone. I have been extremely fortunate to have a number of people who I am proud to call my mentors. Lisa Freeman, John Rush and Liz Rozanski have had a great influence on my career and I hope I can impart some of their wisdom to my residents, interns and students. There are many people that can teach, but few that can inspire. Last but not least, I would especially like to thank my wife Liz and my family for all of their love and support over the years, their sacrifice, endless patience, understanding and inspiration.

CHAPTER 1

Nutritional assessment in small animals

Kathryn E. Michel

Department of Clinical Studies, School of Veterinary Medicine, University of Pennsylvania, Philadelphia, PA, USA

Introduction

It is generally believed that hospitalized patients experiencing malnutrition are at greater risk of morbidity and mortality. There is ample evidence in human patients that this is the case, and while this association has not been clearly established in small animal patients, caloric intake has been found to be positively associated with hospital discharge (Mullen et al., 1979, Brunetto et al., 2010). Despite the lack of a proven direct causal relationship between impaired nutritional status and poor clinical outcome, the assumption is that the prevention or correction of nutritional deficiencies should minimize or eliminate the risk of nutritionally associated morbidity and mortality.

Inadequate food intake is a very common presenting complaint in small animal practice and only a minority of dogs and cats achieve adequate voluntary food intake during hospitalization (Remillard et al., 2001). The task of identifying and determining the magnitude of malnutrition in a patient and deciding whether steps need to be taken to address the problem is complicated by several factors. First, the degree of malnutrition and its impact on a patient's body composition, metabolism and functional status varies considerably with the extent of insufficiency of calorie and nutrient intake, the patient's illness and other physiological demands (See Chapter 11). Furthermore, as many of the parameters used to assess the nutritional status of patients are substantially affected by illness and injury, it is therefore difficult, if not impossible, to gauge the extent to which malnutrition, as opposed to the underlying disease, has contributed to changes in any given parameter. Alterations in visceral proteins (e.g., albumin, transferrin), markers of immune function (e.g., total lymphocyte counts, intradermal skin testing), and body composition (e.g., weight loss, skin fold thickness, body condition scoring) have all been explored as markers of nutritional status in both human and small animal patients (Mullen et al., 1979, Otto et al., 1992, Michel 1993). Additionally, functional tests such as grip strength and peak expiratory flow rate and sophisticated body composition analysis using dual X-ray absorptiometry, bioelectrical impedance and other modalities have been investigated in human patients (Hill, 1992). Ultimately,

Nutritional Management of Hospitalized Small Animals, First Edition. Edited by Daniel L. Chan.
© 2015 John Wiley & Sons, Ltd. Published 2015 by John Wiley & Sons, Ltd.

however, the diagnostic accuracy of these tests remains unknown because there is still no universally accepted "gold standard" of malnutrition with which these tests can be compared.

The recognition that a true "diagnostic test" for malnutrition might not be forthcoming caused a shift in perspective on nutritional assessment. Many of the parameters used to assess malnutrition have been found to be associated with clinical outcome. While they might not be specific markers of nutritional status (many could be deranged for reasons other than malnutrition), they could be used as prognostic indicators. Thus nutritional assessment has evolved into a prognostic, rather than a diagnostic instrument. The techniques that are used to assess nutritional status are those known to be associated with malnutrition, and these have proven to be useful in predicting which patients are more likely to suffer complications. Patients are selected for nutritional support not simply because they are malnourished but rather on the basis of whether nutritional support might have an impact on their clinical outcome. The corollary is that there are malnourished patients for whom providing nutritional support, with its inherent risks and cost, will confer no benefit.

Indications for nutritional assessment

The importance of nutritional assessment is receiving growing recognition in small animal medicine (Freeman et al., 2011). All hospitalized patients should undergo nutritional assessment as part of their initial work up. Given the likelihood that the majority of patients will have inadequate voluntary food intake throughout their hospitalization, the task of nutritional assessment will allow early identification of that subset of patients who are truly at risk, and thus enable prioritization of time and resources for addressing the needs of those patients. The process of nutritional assessment can also facilitate decision-making with regard to selecting an appropriate diet for the patient, deciding whether assisted feeding is indicated and, if it is indicated, determining the best route of assisted feeding for that patient. Furthermore, a properly done nutritional assessment will permit the clinician to anticipate potential complications and develop a feeding plan that will monitor for and minimize the risk of those complications.

Methods of nutritional assessment

There have been only limited investigations of prognostic markers of nutritional status in small animal patients. Admission serum albumin concentration has been shown to correlate with risk of mortality in critically ill dogs (Michel, 1993). In the same population, admission body condition score and lymphocyte count did not correlate with outcome. Intradermal skin testing has been shown to be a feasible means of evaluating cell-mediated immunity in cats but whether this test is associated with nutritional status or is predictive of clinical outcome has not yet been investigated (Otto et al., 1992). Also noted in feline patients is an association between elevation of serum creatinine kinase activity and anorexia which resolves upon reintroduction of food (Fascetti, Mauldin and Mauldin, 1997).

For human patients a rapid, simple, 'bedside' prognostic tool for nutritional assessment called *subjective global assessment* (SGA) has been in use for approximately 3 decades (Baker et al., 1982). The technique was designed to utilize readily available historical and physical parameters to identify malnourished patients who are at increased risk for complications and who will presumably benefit from nutritional intervention. The assessment involves determining whether nutrient assimilation has been restricted because of decreased food intake, maldigestion or malabsorption, whether any effects of malnutrition on organ function and body composition are evident, and whether the patient's disease process influences its nutrient requirements. The findings of the historical and physical assessment are used to categorize the patient as A: well nourished, B: moderately malnourished or at risk of becoming malnourished, and C: severely malnourished. SGA has been investigated for its ability to identify patients at risk of medical complications in diverse patient populations, and has been shown to have excellent inter-observer agreement and better predictive accuracy than traditional markers of nutritional status (Keith, 2008).

The SGA can easily be adapted to veterinary patients. The patient history should be assessed for indications of malnutrition, including evidence of weight loss and the time frame in which it has occurred, sufficiency of dietary intake including the nutritional adequacy of the diet, the presence of persistent gastrointestinal signs, the patient's functional capacity (e.g., evidence of weakness, exercise intolerance) and the metabolic demands of the patient's underlying disease state. The physical exam should focus on changes in body composition, presence of edema or ascites, and appearance of the patient's hair coat. With regard to assessing changes in body composition, it is important to recognize that while metabolically stressed patients experience catabolism of lean tissue, these changes may not be noted using standard body condition scoring systems if the patient has normal or excessive body fat (Figure 1.1). Since catabolism of lean tissue can have deleterious consequences for outcome, it is important that along with evaluation of body fat, patients undergo evaluation of muscle mass to assess lean tissue status (Freeman et al., 2011). A muscle mass scoring system that has been used in dogs and cats is outlined in Table 1.1 (Michel, Sorenmo and Shofer, 2004, Michel et al., 2011).

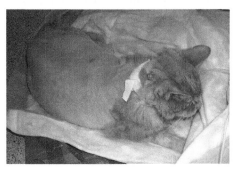

Figure 1.1 An example of a patient exhibiting significant wasting of the epaxial musculature despite having excessive body fat.

Table 1.1 Description of a muscle mass scoring system for dogs and cats.

Score	Muscle Mass
0	On palpation over the spine, muscle mass is severely wasted
1	On palpation over the spine, mass is moderately wasted
2	On palpation over the spine, muscle mass is mildly wasted
3	On palpation over the spine, muscle mass is normal

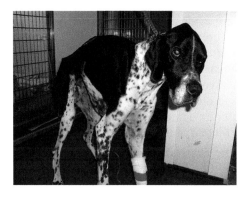

Figure 1.2 A dog with advanced malnutrition in which nutritional support is indicated.

The next step of nutritional assessment is to determine whether or not the patient's voluntary food intake is sufficient. To do this one must have a caloric goal, select an appropriate food and formulate a feeding recommendation for the patient. This will permit an accurate accounting of how much food is offered to the patient and will allow evaluation of the patient's intake based on how much of the food is consumed. A reasonable initial caloric goal for hospitalized dogs and cats is based on an estimate of resting energy requirement (see Chapter 2).

Clearly patients that are already significantly malnourished at the time of presentation (Figure 1.2) should receive nutritional support. However, given the catabolic stress associated with critical illness, patients who have experienced or are anticipated to experience substantially reduced food intake for longer than 3 days also deserve attention (Figure 1.3). Furthermore, as the clinical course of a hospitalized patient may change rapidly, it is important that nutritional assessment is viewed as an ongoing process so that the feeding plan can be adjusted in a timely fashion.

If a patient is deemed a candidate for assisted feeding, the nutritional assessment will encompass several additional steps. If enteral feeding is being contemplated, gastrointestinal tract function must be evaluated (e.g., presence of vomiting, ileus, ischemia) as well as the patient's ability to tolerate the feeding tube and tube placement (e.g., anesthesia required, abnormal hemostasis). A critical step is to assess the patient's level of consciousness and gag reflex. One of the most serious complications of enteral feeding is aspiration pneumonia, which can be a fatal complication in critically ill patients. If parenteral nutrition

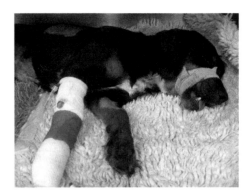

Figure 1.3 A dog with severe trauma to oral and nasal cavity that places this dog at high risk of becoming malnourished if a route of nutrition is not identified.

is under consideration, it is necessary to assess the patient's fluid tolerance, determine whether dedicated venous access is possible and whether that access will be central or peripheral. Furthermore, patients receiving parenteral nutrition require close monitoring for technical and metabolic complications and should be cared for in a facility that has 24 h nursing care and the ability to perform point of care serum biochemistry.

Summary

In conclusion, nutritional assessment of veterinary patients is a largely subjective process that should identify those patients at risk of malnutrition-associated complications, rather than just malnourished patients. All hospitalized patients should undergo nutritional assessment with the goal to identify those patients for whom nutritional intervention is likely to improve clinical outcome. Furthermore, a nutritional assessment will facilitate decision-making with regard to selecting appropriate diet, deciding whether assisted feeding is indicated and, when it is indicated, determining the best route of assisted feeding. It will also permit optimization of a feeding plan that will maximize the benefits to the patient while minimizing the risks of complications.

KEY POINTS

- All hospitalized patients should undergo nutritional assessment with the goal to identify those patients for whom nutritional intervention is likely to improve clinical outcome.

- Through subjective evaluation of historical and physical data, a patient's degree of malnutrition and the need for nutritional intervention can be determined.

- Nutritional assessment will also aid in development of the feeding plan including determining a route of assisted feeding, selecting a diet and optimizing the plan to minimize complications.

- Nutritional assessment should be viewed as an ongoing process so that the feeding plan can be adjusted in a timely fashion in the event that the condition of the patient changes.

References

Baker, J.P., Detsky, A.S., Wesson, D.E. et al. (1982) Nutritional assessment: A comparison of clinical judgment and objective measurements. *New England Journal of Medicine*, **306**, 969–972.

Brunetto, M.A., Gomes, M.O.S., Andre, M.R. et al. (2010) Effects of nutritional support on hospital outcome in dogs and cats. *Journal of Veterinary Emergency and Critical Care*, **20**, 224–231.

Fascetti, A.J., Mauldin, G.E. and Mauldin, G.N. (1997) Correlation between serum creatinine kinase activities and anorexia in cats. *Journal of Veterinary Internal Medicine*, **11**, 9–13.

Freeman, L., Becvarova, I., Cave, N. et al. (2011) WSAVA Nutritional Assessment Guidelines. *Journal of Small Animal Practice*, **52**, 385–396.

Hill, G.L. (1992) Body composition research: Implications for the practice of clinical nutrition. *JPEN: Journal of Parenteral and Enteral Nutrition*, **16**, 197–218.

Keith, J.N. (2008) Bedside nutrition assessment-past, present, and future: A review of the subjective global assessment. *Nutrition in Clinical Practice*, **23**, 410–116.

Michel, K.E. (1993) Prognostic value of clinical nutritional assessment in canine patients. *Journal of Veterinary Emergency and Critical Care*, **3**, 96–104.

Michel, K.E., Sorenmo, K. and Shofer, F.S. (2004) Evaluation of body condition and weight loss in dogs presenting to a veterinary oncology service. *Journal of Veterinary Internal Medicine*, **18**, 692–695.

Michel, K. E., Anderson, W., Cupp, C. et al. (2011) Correlation of a feline muscle mass score with body composition determined by DXA. *British Journal of Nutrition*, **106**, S57–S59.

Mullen, J.L., Gertner, M.H., Buzby, G. P. et al. (1979) Implications of malnutrition in the surgical patient. *Archives of Surgery*, **114**, 121–125.

Otto, C. M., Brown, K. A., Lindl, P. A. et al. (1992) Clinical evaluation of cell-mediated immunity in the cat. Proceedings of the International Veterinary Emergency and Critical Care Symposium September 20–23, San Antonio, USA, p. 838.

Remillard, R.L., Darden, D.E., Michel, K.E. et al. (2001) An investigation of the relationship between caloric intake and outcome in hospitalized dogs. *Veterinary Therapeutics*, **2**, 301–310.

CHAPTER 2

Estimating energy requirements of small animal patients

Daniel L. Chan

Department of Veterinary Clinical Sciences and Services, The Royal Veterinary College, University of London, UK

Introduction

One of the main objectives of initiating nutritional support in hospitalized patients is to minimize catabolism and maintain lean muscle mass without overly stressing the patient's metabolic system with excess nutrients. Ideally, nutritional support should provide ample substrates for gluconeogenesis, protein synthesis and the energy necessary to maintain homeostasis. Estimating the energy requirements of hospitalized patients is a considerable challenge in clinical practice. Ensuring that sufficient calories are being provided to sustain critical physiologic processes necessitates measuring an individual patient's total energy expenditure. However, precise measurements of energy expenditure in clinical veterinary patients are seldom performed. While a few studies have measured energy expenditure in select populations of clinical veterinary patients, the technique, the equipment, and expertise required for this technique is not feasible in clinical practice. As such, the use of mathematical formulas remains the only practical means for estimating the energy needs of patients. It is, however, important to appreciate the limitations of relying on mathematical equations of energy requirements and to understand the issues that make accurate assessment of energy needs in clinical patients challenging. This chapter will cover the basics relating to measurement of energy expenditure in animals and the use of mathematical formulas to estimate energy needs, and will discuss the recommended procedure for devising appropriate nutritional plans.

Assessing energy requirements

The prevailing view is that nutritional support plays a key role in the management of hospitalized animals. Malnutrition has been well documented to result in lean muscle loss, poor wound healing, immunosuppression, compromised organ function, and increased morbidity and mortality (Barton, 1994; Biolo et al., 1997;

Nutritional Management of Hospitalized Small Animals, First Edition. Edited by Daniel L. Chan.
© 2015 John Wiley & Sons, Ltd. Published 2015 by John Wiley & Sons, Ltd.

Biffl et al., 2002). Unfortunately, providing either excessive or insufficient calories appears to adversely impact patient outcome (Krishnan et al., 2003; Stappleton, Jones and Hayland, 2007; Dickerson, 2011; Heyland et al., 2014). Although a relationship between increasing energy delivery and positive outcomes has been demonstrated in critically ill animals (Brunetto et al., 2010), overfeeding may contribute to additional complications, such as hyperglycemia, volume overload, excessive nitrogenous waste production (e.g, increased blood urea nitrogen) and vomiting or regurgitation (Chan, 2014). A mismatch between predicted energy expenditure and actual energy requirements remains a challenge in the care of critically ill human patients and this also appears to hold true in veterinary medicine (Walton et al., 1996; Krishman et al., 2003; O'Toole et al., 2004; Stappleton et al., 2007; Dickerson, 2011). Therefore, in the delivery of nutritional support to critically ill and hospitalized animals, it is imperative that estimation of energy needs should be as accurate as possible with an emphasis on avoiding overfeeding patients.

Methods for determining energy needs

Direct calorimetry is one method of determining energy expenditure. This method measures heat production by the animal and extrapolates energy expenditure. The major assumption with direct calorimetry is that during the maintenance phase, total energy consumed is expended and released solely as heat (no net gain in body energy) and that there is no energy or heat storage in the animal. Direct calorimeters typically take the form of chambers that precisely measure heat within the chamber. These calorimetry systems are accurate but not feasible for clinical patients.

Indirect calorimetry is a more manageable method for assessing energy expenditure in animals and has been used in both dogs and cats. The method of measuring energy expenditure is also called 'indirect respiratory calorimetry' and requires accurate measurement of oxygen consumption and carbon dioxide production (Figure 2.1). These measurements are usually made via a face mask, a hood, canopy, helmet or within a chamber. A major limitation, however, is that use of face masks, hoods or helmets can be stressful to dogs and cats and measurements are likely to be higher than the true energy expenditure of the animal. Acclimatizing procedures are needed to minimize this effect, however, this process can take weeks although some studies only allowed 15 minutes for animals to acclimatize to the device and this may have adversely impacted the results (Hill, 2006; Ramsey, 2012). The principle of calculating energy from oxygen consumption and carbon dioxide production is based on the fact that heat released during oxidation of a substrate is constant. The ratio of carbon dioxide production to oxygen consumption (CO_2/O_2) is termed the respiratory quotient (RQ) and is indicative of the predominant substrate being oxidized. For example, a RQ of 0.7 indicates that lipids are being metabolized, a RQ of 0.8 indicates that proteins are being metabolized and a RQ of 1.0 indicates that carbohydrates are predominantly being used for energy (Blaxter, 1989). With the derivation of RQ what is also known is the amount of heat released per liter of oxygen consumed

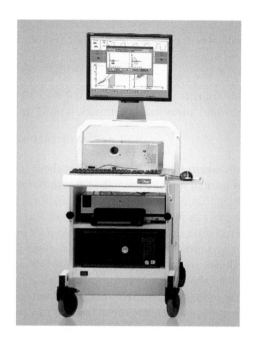

Figure 2.1 An example of a modern indirect respiratory calorimeter that can be used to estimate energy expenditures in animals.

and liter of carbon dioxide produced. If a reasonable estimate of the expected RQ of an animal can be made (e.g., RQ = 0.8), the energy expenditure can be calculated from the consumption of O_2 or production of CO_2. With the addition of urea nitrogen, energy expenditure can be calculated via the Weir equation (Weir, 1949):

$$\text{Energy expenditure (kcal)} = 3.94(LO_2) + 1.11(LCO_2) - 2.17(\text{g urinary nitrogen})$$

Although the reliability of indirect calorimeters has improved and equipment has become more streamlined (Sion-Sarid et al., 2013) it is unlikely that it will become standard practice in every hospital, human or veterinary. Nevertheless, indirect calorimetry studies are important as they can be used to assess the utility of predictive energy equations. (O'Toole et al., 2001, Walton et al., 1996)

Predictive equations of energy needs

Because of the impracticalities associated with measurement of indirect calorimetry in clinical patients, the use of mathematical predictive equations is the most feasible method for estimating their energy needs (Walker and Heuberger, 2009). By using the body weight (the author uses the current body weight in hospitalized animals rather than ideal body weight), one is able to predict energy expenditure by use of a number of proposed equations. The equation that is most commonly cited for energy estimation in animals was proposed by Kleiber (1961) and is used to predict the resting energy requirement (RER) of both dogs and cats. The RER is generally defined as the number of calories required for maintaining homeostasis at rest in a thermoneutral environment while the animal is in a postabsorptive state (Gross et al., 2010) and is calculated as follows:

$$RER = 70 \times (\text{current body weight in kg})^{0.75}$$

For animals weighing between 2 and 30 kg, there is also a linear formula that provides a reasonable estimation of RER:

$$RER = (30 \times \text{current body weight in kg}) + 70$$

It is worth noting, however, that these formulas were determined from studies in normal healthy animals. Disease states can change the energy requirements dramatically and extensive thermal burns are an example where energy requirements can more than double (Chan and Chan, 2009). Until recently, there was a recommendation to multiply the RER by an illness factor between 1.1 and 2.3 to account for increases in metabolism associated with different diseases and injuries. (Donoghue, 1989). However, less emphasis is now being placed on such subjective and extrapolated factors and the current recommendation is to use more conservative energy estimates, that is, start with the animal's RER, to avoid overfeeding. Overfeeding can result in metabolic and gastrointestinal complications, hepatic dysfunction and increased carbon dioxide production. (Ramsey, 2012). Although controversial, results of indirect calorimetry studies in dogs support the recent trend of formulating nutritional support to meet RER rather than more generous illness energy requirements. The reason that overall energy requirements of ill patients may be closer to RER despite the presence of pathological processes that increase energy expenditure (Figure 2.2) (e.g., pyrexia, inflammation, oxidative stress) may be negated by the decrease in physical activity because of illness, confinement during hospitalization and even the use of sedatives.

Although there were some methodological concerns in the studies by Walton et al. (1996), and O'Toole et al. (2004), both of these studies demonstrated that energy expenditure as measured by indirect respiratory calorimetry in ill dogs more closely matched the calculated RER without the use of illness factors. When studies evaluating parenteral nutritional support in animals are compared, those that applied an illness factor in the calculation of energy needs

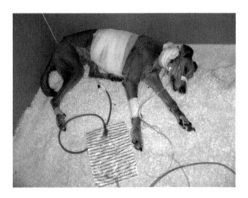

Figure 2.2 Studies using indirect calorimetry have shown that the energy requirements of critically ill patients are closer to resting energy requirement and do not require application of illness factors. The increase in energy needs associated with disease processes are counterbalanced by the decreased physical activity experienced by hospitalized ill animals.

demonstrated higher complication rates than studies with more conservative energy estimates (Lippert, Fulton and Parr, 1993, Reuter et al., 1998, Chan et al., 2002, Pyle et al., 2004, Crabb et al., 2006). Given the probable increased risk of complications when ill animals are overfed, combined with the lack of any evidence that feeding above energy requirements is beneficial, the current recommendation for calculating the energy needs of ill cats and dogs is to start at RER and to increase or decrease the amount fed only depending on the animal's tolerance and response to feeding (Hill, 2006, Chan, 2014). However, determining the energy requirements of ill dogs and cats remains an area that requires further investigation.

Summary

Despite the current limitations in the knowledge of energy requirements of critically ill dogs and cats, there are certain points that can serve to guide nutritional support of critically ill animals. The preservation of lean body mass should be a primary goal of nutritional support and, as such, close monitoring of the patient's body weight, fluid distribution, response or tolerance to feedings, and changes in the underlying condition should dictate whether to increase the number of calories provided in the nutritional plan. Typically, if an animal continues to lose weight on nutritional support, the number of calories provided should be increased by 25% and the plan should be reassessed in a few days. The nutritional plan should also be flexible enough to meet the changing needs of the patient and so regular reassessment is paramount in the successful nutritional management of critically ill patients. Until new findings can better discern the nutritional and energy requirements of hospitalized patients, provision of nutritional support must continue to be guided by sound clinical judgment and continual reassessment of the patient.

KEY POINTS

- Estimating the energy requirements of hospitalized patients continues to be a considerable challenge in clinical practice.

- Precise measurements of energy expenditure in clinical veterinary patients (e.g., via indirect calorimetry) are seldom performed.

- The technique, the equipment and expertise required to use indirect calorimetry in clinical patients is rarely available.

- The use of mathematical formulas remains the only practical means for estimating energy needs of patients.

- The resting energy requirement for hospitalized dogs and cats is predicted using the equation RER (kcal/day) = $70 \times$ kg $BW^{0.75}$ or ($30 \times$ kg BW) + 70 if patients weigh between 2 and 30 kg.

- The use of illness factors as multipliers of RER for energy estimation requirements for hospitalized animals is not recommended.

References

Barton, R.G. Nutrition support in critical illness. (1994) *Nutrition Clinical Practice*, **9**,127–139.

Biffl, W.L., Moore, E.E., Haenel, J.B. et al. (2002) Nutritional support of the trauma patient. *Nutrition*, **18**,960–965.

Biolo G., Toigo G., Ciocchi B. et al. (1997) Metabolic response to injury and sepsis: Changes in protein metabolism. *Nutrition*, **13**,52S–57S.

Blaxter, K. (1989) *Energy Metabolism in Animals and Man*, Cambridge University Press, Cambridge.

Brunetto, M.A., Gomes, M.O.S., Andre, M.R. et al. (2010) Effects of nutritional support on hospital outcome in dogs and cats. *Journal of Veterinary Emergency and Critical Care*, **20**, 224–231.

Chan, D.L. (2014) Nutrition in critical care, in Kirk's Current Veterinary Therapy XV, (eds J.D. Bonagura and D.C. Twedt), Elsevier Saunders, St Louis, pp. 38–43.

Chan, D.L., Freeman, L.M., Labato, M.A. et al. (2002) Retrospective evaluation of partial parenteral nutrition in dogs and cats. *Journal of Veterinary Internal Medicine*, **16**, 440–445.

Chan, M.M. and Chan, G.M. (2009) Nutritional therapy for burns in children and adults. *Nutrition*, **25**, 261–269.

Crabb, S.E., Chan, D.L., Freeman, L.M. et al. (2006) Retrospective evaluation of total parenteral nutrition in cats: 40 cases (1991–2003). *Journal of Veterinary Emergency and Critical Care*, **16**, S21–26.

Dickerson, R.N. (2011) Optimal caloric intake for critically ill patients: First, do no harm. *Nutrition in Clinical Practice*, **26**, 48–54.

Donoghue, S. (1989) Nutritional support of hospitalized patients. *Veterinary Clinics of North America: Small Animal Practice*, **19**, 475–95.

Gross, K.L., Yamka, R. M., Khoo, C. et al. (2010) Macronutrients, in *Small Animal Clinical Nutrition*, 5th edn (eds M.S. Hand, C.D. Thatcher, R.L. Remillard, P. Roudebush, and B.J. Novotny) Mark Morris Institute, Topeka, KS, pp. 49–105.

Heyland, D.K., Dhaliwal, R., Wang, M. et al. (2014) The prevalence of iatrogenic underfeeding in the nutritionally 'at-risk' critically ill patient: Results of an international, multicenter, prospective study. *Clinical Nutrition*, doi: 10.1016/j.clnu.2014.07.008.

Hill, R.C. (2006) Challenges in measuring energy expenditure in companion animals: A clinician's perspective. *Journal of Nutrition*, **136**, 1967S–1972S.

Kleiber, M. (1961) The Fire of Life, John Wiley & Sons, Inc., New York.

Krishnan, J.A., Parce, P.B., Martinez, A. et al. (2003) Caloric intake in medical intensive care unit patients: Consistency of care with guidelines and relationship to clinical outcomes. *Chest*, **124**, 297–305.

Lippert, A.C., Fulton, R.B. and Parr, A.M. (1993) A retrospective study of the use of total parenteral nutrition in dogs and cats. *Journal of Veterinary Internal Medicine*, **7**, 52–64.

O'Toole, E., Miller, C.W., Wilson, B.A. et al. (2004) Comparison of the standard predictive equation for calculation of resting energy expenditure with indirect calorimetry in hospitalized and healthy dogs. *Journal of American Veterinary Medical Association*, **225**, 58–64.

O'Toole, E., McDonell, W.N., Wilson, B.A. et al. (2001) Evaluation of accuracy and reliability of indirect calorimetry for the measurement of resting energy expenditure in healthy dogs. *American Journal of Veterinary Research*, **62**, 1761–67.

Pyle, S.C., Marks, S.L., Kass, P.H. et al. (2004) Evaluation of complication and prognostic factors associated with administration of parenteral nutrition in cats: 75 cases (1994–2001). *Journal of the American Veterinary Medical Association*, **225**, 242–250.

Ramsey, J.J. (2012) Determining energy requirements, in *Applied Veterinary Clinical Nutrition*, 1st edn (eds A.J. Fascetti and S. J. Delaney) Wiley-Blackwell Chichester, pp. 23–45.

Reuter, J.D., Marks, S.L., Rogers, Q. R. et al. (1998) Use of total parenteral nutrition in dogs: 209 cases (1988–1995) *Journal of Veterinary Emergency and Critical Care*, **8**, 201–213.

Sion-Sarid, R., Cohen, J., Houri, Z. et al. (2013) Indirect calorimetry: a guide for optimizing nutrition support in the critically ill child. *Nutrition*, **29**, 1094–1099.

Stappleton, R.D., Jones, N. and Heyland, D.K. (2007) Feeding critically ill patients: What is the optimal amount of energy? *Critical Care Medicine*, **35**, S535–540.

Walker, R.N. and Heuberger, R.A. (2009) Predictive equations for energy needs for the critically ill. *Respiratory Care*, **54**, 509–520.

Walton, R.S., Wingfield, W.E., Ogilvie, G.K. et al. (1996) Energy expenditure in 104 postoperative and traumatically injured dogs with indirect calorimetry. *Journal of Veterinary Emergency and Critical Care*, **6**, 71–79.

Weir, J.B. de V. (1949) New methods of calculating metabolic rate with special reference to protein metabolism. *Journal of Physiology*, **109**, 1–9.

CHAPTER 3

Routes of nutritional support in small animals

Sally Perea

Mars Pet Care, Mason, OH, USA

Introduction

Determination of the route of nutritional support is an important step in the assessment and management of critical care patients. Routes of nutritional support are broadly categorized into enteral and parenteral routes. Enteral routes to be considered include nasoesophageal, esophagostomy, gastrostomy and jejunostomy feeding tubes, while parenteral routes include peripheral and central venous catheters. The route or combination of routes selected for each patient will be influenced by the patient's medical and nutritional status, the anticipated length of required nutritional support, and the nutritional needs and diet limitation and advantages presented by each route.

Enteral routes of nutritional support

Nasoesophageal tube feeding

Nasoesophageal feeding is a relatively easy and convenient method of nutritional delivery for patients who require short-term (fewer than 5 days) nutritional support, and/or for patients who are not candidates for general anesthesia (see Chapter 4). Nasoesophageal feeding tubes provide the advantages of being relatively easy to place and being inexpensive. However, because of the risk of aspiration, nasoesophageal feeding should not be implemented in patients with vomiting or who lack a gag reflex. The major disadvantage of nasoesophageal feeding tubes is their smaller diameter (typically 3.5–5 French in cats and 6–8 French in dogs), which limits diet selection to liquid enteral formulas. Liquid formulations may be delivered via continuous or intermittent bolus feedings. Although continuous feeding can be helpful in pets in which high feeding volumes may not be tolerated, a recent study demonstrated that gastric residual volumes and clinical outcome did not differ between the two feeding methods (Holahan et al., 2010).

Common complications of nasoesophageal feeding include epistaxis, rhinitis, and tracheal intubation with secondary pneumonia (Marks, 1998). An Elizabethan

Nutritional Management of Hospitalized Small Animals, First Edition. Edited by Daniel L. Chan.
© 2015 John Wiley & Sons, Ltd. Published 2015 by John Wiley & Sons, Ltd.

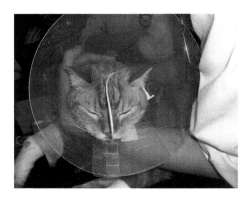

Figure 3.1 Elizabethan collars are often necessary to prevent premature removal of feeding tubes.

collar should be placed to prevent the patient from physically removing the tube (Figure 3.1). Removal of the feeding tube secondary to sneezing, coughing or vomiting, despite the continuous use of Elizabethan collars, is also a common complication with nasoesophageal feeding in cats (Abood and Buffington, 1992). Radiographic confirmation of nasoesophageal tube placement is recommended to minimize risks associated with inappropriate placement of the feeding tube prior to implementation of feeding.

Esophagostomy tube feeding

Placement of an esophagostomy feeding tube requires general anesthesia for placement, but is still a relatively quick and simple procedure (see Chapter 5). Compared to nasoesophageal feeding tubes, esophagostomy tubes can be used for an extended period of time with a feeding period of ~23 days (1 to 557 days) (Crowe and Devey, 1997a; Levine, Smallwood and Buback, 1997). Other advantages include increased comfort for the animal and an increased tube diameter (12–14 French), allowing a wider selection of diets that may be fed through the tube. The most common complication associated with esophagostomy tubes is wound infection at the ostomy site where the tube exits the skin (Crowe and Deveya, 1997; Devitt and Seim, 1997). To help prevent infection, daily care and cleaning of the ostomy site is recommended. Other reported complications include kinking or obstruction of the tube, tracheal intubation, vomiting, displacement of the tube, and swelling of the head (Crowe and Devey, 1997a; Devitt and Seim, 1997). In general, the complications associated with esophagostomy tubes are easily managed, and minor compared with more severe complications that can be associated with gastrostomy tubes (Ireland et al., 2003).

Gastrostomy tube feeding

Gastrostomy tubes require general anesthesia, and can be placed via laparotomy or by using a percutaneous technique (Figure 3.2) (see Chapter 6). Although gastrostomy tubes require longer anesthesia and procedure duration, they provide the advantage of bypassing the esophagus for animals with esophageal disease. Similar to the step-up from nasoesophageal to esophagostomy tube, the gastrostomy tube allows for a longer period of placement for patients where assisted feeding is expected to be prolonged.

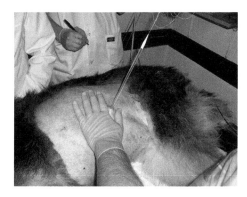

Figure 3.2 A dog undergoing percutaneous endoscopic-guided gastrostomy tube placement.

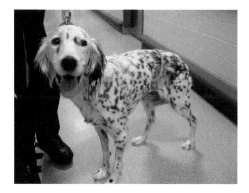

Figure 3.3 A dog with a gastrostomy tube in place.

One retrospective study comparing the use of esophagostomy to gastrostomy tubes in cats found that the gastrostomy tubes remained in place for a significantly longer period of time with a median duration of 43 days versus 26 days (Ireland et al., 2003). Because of their anatomical location, gastrostomy tubes may be less susceptible to premature removal or stoma site infection secondary due to the patient scratching or pawing at the tube (Figure 3.3). However, as previously mentioned, oesophagostomy tubes have been used clinically for periods of greater than one year. Therefore, both methods are suitable for extended periods of feeding. Another advantage of gastrostomy tubes is their larger diameter (18–20 French), which may allow for an increased selection of foods that can be fed through the tube. The larger diameter also requires less water dilution for blenderization of canned foods, which can help to increase the energy density of the slurry.

Complications associated with gastrostomy tubes include cellulites around the ostomy site, gastric pressure necrosis, tube migration, pyloric outflow obstruction, inadvertent tube removal, leaking of food around the ostomy site (Figure 3.4), and vomiting with secondary aspiration pneumonia (Levine et al., 1997; Glaus et al., 1998; Marks, 1998). Although tube migration or premature removal are not very common, if these complications occur prior to adequate healing at the fistula (< 14 days) they can lead to more serious consequences such as life-threatening peritonitis.

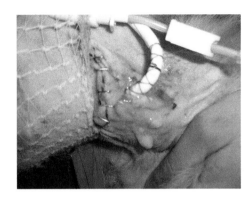

Figure 3.4 A dog with an infected and leaking gastrostomy site that requires tube removal and surgical management.

Jejunostomy tube feeding

Placement of jejunostomy tubes require general anesthesia and they are general placed by surgical methods (Crowe and Devey, 1997b; Daye, Huber and Henderson, 1999) (see Chapter 7). However, endoscopic techniques are being improved, and successful management of endoscopically placed nasojejunal and gastrojejunostomy tubes have been reported in dogs and cats (Jennings et al., 2001; Jergens et al., 2007; Pápa et al., 2009) (see Chapter 8). Placement of a nasojejunal feeding tube using fluoroscopic guidance has also been described in the dog (Wohl, 2006; Beal and Brown, 2011). Jejunostomy tubes are indicated for patients with gastric outlet obstruction, recurrent aspiration, gastroparesis and pancreatitis (Marks, 1998). In general, jejunostomy tubes are used for a shorter time period than oesophagostomy or gastrostomy feeding tubes, with reported feeding periods ranging from 9 to 14 days (Daye et al., 1999; Swann, Sweet and Michel, 2002).

Complications of jejunostomy tubes include cellulites at the ostomy site, leaking of food around the ostomy site, dehiscence, tube migration, vomiting, diarrhoea, abdominal discomfort, retrograde movement of tube, tube obstruction, and inadvertent tube removal with subsequent peritonitis (Daye et al., 1999; Swann et al., 2002).

Parenteral nutrition

For patients that cannot tolerate enteral feeding, parenteral nutrition may be an appropriate feeding route alternative (Figure 3.5) (Chapter 11). Indications for parenteral nutrition include intractable vomiting or diarrhea; anesthesia or lack of a gag reflex; recovery from severe gastric or intestinal resection; poor anesthetic candidate for proper feeding tube placement; or inability to meet full energy requirements via the enteral route. Parenteral nutrition has commonly been employed for pets suffering from pancreatitis; however, a recent pilot study demonstrated that early enteral nutrition via an esophagostomy tube was well tolerated and resulted in fewer complications than parenteral nutrition in a group of 10 dogs with pancreatitis (Mansfield et al., 2011).

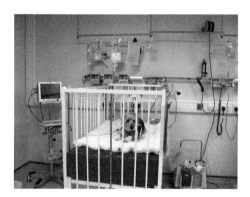

Figure 3.5 A dog whose gastrointestinal tract is severely dysfunctional and is receiving parenteral nutritional support.

Parenteral nutrition may be administered via a central or peripheral venous catheter (see Chapter 10). While peripheral venous access is easier to establish, peripheral solutions are limited to a lower osmolarity (< 750 mOsmol/L) to reduce risk of thrombophlebitis. When central venous access is obtainable, central parenteral nutrition (CPN) is generally preferred due to fewer restrictions in solution formulation, easier ability to meet full energy requirements and reduced incidence of thrombophlebitis. However, successful administration of peripheral parenteral nutrition (PPN) in dogs and cats has been described, and may be a more practical tool for practitioners who do not routinely place central catheters (Zsombor-Murray and Freeman, 1999; Chan et al., 2002). Shorter durations of administration and the use of lipid-containing admixtures can also help to reduce the incidence of thrombophlebitis (Chandler, Guilford and Payne-James, 2000; Griffiths and Bongers, 2005).

Mechanical complications associated with parenteral nutrition include catheter dislodgement, thrombophlebitis, catheter occlusion, chewed lines, and kinking of catheter (Chan et al., 2002; Pyle, Marks and Kass, 2004). Metabolic complications of parenteral and enteral nutrition are discussed in detail in subsequent chapters (see Chapters 9 and 10).

Combined enteral and parenteral approach

Although most patients who are initially started on parenteral nutrition are not candidates for enteral nutrition, many may tolerate a slow weaning onto enteral nutrition, or a proportion of their energy and nutrient needs simultaneously administered by the enteral route (Figure 3.6) (Griffiths and Bongers, 2005). One retrospective study evaluating PPN in dogs and cats demonstrated improved survival in patients receiving concurrent enteral nutrition (Chan et al., 2002). Concurrent administration of enteral feeding may help to maintain intestinal integrity, immune and gut-barrier functions (Heidegger et al., 2007).

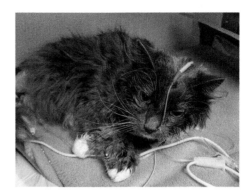

Figure 3.6 Cat being managed with a combination of parenteral and enteral nutritional support.

Summary

Implementing a nutritional support plan is a key component to the successful management of hospitalized canine and feline patients. The variety of routes in which nutritional support can be delivered provide multiple options that can be tailored to the patient's specific needs and limitations. The subsequent chapters provide further detail for each route of nutritional support, indications, placement technique, and proper monitoring.

KEY POINTS

- Determining the route of nutritional support is an important step in the assessment and management of critical care patients.

- Enteral routes to be considered include nasoesophageal, esophagostomy, gastrostomy and jejunostomy feeding tubes.

- For patients that cannot tolerate enteral feeding, parenteral nutrition may be an appropriate feeding route alternative.

- Indications for parenteral nutrition include intractable vomiting, diarrhea or lack of gag reflex, recovery from severe gastric or intestinal resection, poor anesthetic candidate for proper feeding tube placement or inability to meet energy requirements via enteral route alone.

- The variety of routes in which nutritional support can be delivered provides multiple options that can be tailored to the patient's specific needs and limitations.

References

Abood, S.K. and Buffington, C.A.T. (1992) Enteral feeding of dogs and cats: 51 cases (1989–1991). *Journal of the American Veterinary Medical Association*, **4**, 619–622.

Beal, M.W. and Brown, A. J. (2011) Clinical experience utilizing a novel fluoroscopic technique for wire-guided nasojejunal tube placement in the dog: 26 cases (2006–2010). *Journal of Veterinary Emergency and Critical Care*, **21**,151–157.

Chan, D.L., Freeman, L.M., Labato, M.A. et al. (2002) Retrospective evaluation of partial parenteral nutrition in dogs and cats. *Journal of Veterinary Internal Medicine*, **16**, 440–445.

Chandler, M.L. Guilford, W.G. and Payne-James, J. (2000) Use of peripheral parenteral nutritional support in dogs and cats. *Journal of the American Veterinary Medical Association*, **216** (5), 669–673.

Chandler, M.L. and Payne-James, J. (2006) Prospective evaluation of a peripherally administered three-in-one parenteral nutrition product in dogs. *Journal of Small Animal Practice*, **47**, 518–523.

Crowe, D.T. and Devey, J.J. (1997a) Esophagostomy tubes for feeding and decompression: Clinical experience in 29 small animal patients. *Journal of the American Animal Hospital Association*, **33**, 393–403.

Crowe , D.T. and Devey, J.J. (1997b) Clinical experience with jejunostomy feeding tubes in 47 small animal patients. *Journal of Veterinary Emergency and Critical Care*, **7**, 7–19.

Daye, R.M., Huber, M.L. and Henderson, R.A. (1999) Interlocking box jejunostomy: A new technique for enteral feeding. *Journal of the American Animal Hospital Association*, **35**, 129–134.

Devitt, C.M. and Seim, H.B. (1997) Clinical evaluation of tube esophagostomy in small animals. *Journal of the American Veterinary Medical Association*, **33**, 55–60.

Glaus, T.M., Cornelius, L.M., Bartges, J.W. et al. (1998) Complications with non-endoscopic percutaneous gastrostomy in 31 cats and 10 dogs: a retrospective study. *Journal of Small Animal Practice*, **39**, 218–222.

Griffiths, R.D. and Bongers, T. (2005) Nutrition support for patients in the intensive care unit. *Postgraduate Medical Journal*, **81**(960), 629–636.

Heidegger, C.P., Romand, J.A., Treggiari, M.M. et al. (2007) Is it now time to promote mixed enteral and parenteral nutrition for the critically ill patient? *Intensive Care Medicine*, **33**, 963–969.

Holahan, M., Abood, S., Hautman, J. et al. (2010) Intermittent and continues enteral nutrition in critically ill dogs: A prospective randomized trial. *Journal of Veterinary Internal Medicine*, **24**, 520–536.

Ireland, L.A., Hohenhaus, A.E., Broussard, J.D. et al. (2003) A comparison of owner management and complications with 67 cats with esophagostomy and percutaneous endoscopic gastrostomy feeding tubes. *Journal of the American Animal Hospital Association*, **39**, 241–246.

Jergens, A.E., Morrison, J.A., Miles, K.G. et al. (2007) Percutaneous endoscopic gastrojejunostomy tube placement in healthy dogs and cats. *Journal of Veterinary Internal Medicine*, **21**, 18–24.

Jennings M., Center S.A., Barr S.C. et al. (2001) Successful treatment of feline pancreatitis using an endoscopically placed gastrojejunostomy tube. *Journal of the American Animal Hospital Association*, **37**,145–152.

Levine, P.B., Smallwood, L.J. and Buback, J.L. (1997) Esophagostomy tubes as a method of nutritional management in cats: A retrospective study. *Journal of the American Animal Hospital Association*, **33**, 405–410.

Marks, S.L. (1998) The principles and practical application of enteral nutrition. *Veterinary Clinics of North America (Small Animal)*, **28**, 677–708.

Mansfield, C.S., James, F.E., Steiner, J.M. et al. (2011) A pilot study to assess tolerability of early enteral nutrition via esophagostomy tube feeding in dogs with severe acute pancreatitis. *Journal of Veterinary Internal Medicine*, **25**, 419–425.

Pápa, K., Psáder, R., Sterczer, A. et al. (2009) Endoscopically guided nasojejunal tube placement in dogs for short-term postduodenal feeding. *Journal of Veterinary Emergency and Critical Care*, **19**(6), 554–563.

Pyle, S.C., Marks, S.L. and Kass, P.H. (2004) Evaluation of complications and prognostic factors associated with administration of total parenteral nutrition in cats: 75 cases (1994–2001). *Journal of the American Veterinary Medical Association*, **225**(2), 242–250.

Swann, H.M., Sweet, D.C. and Michel. K. (2002) Complications associated with use of jejunostomy tubes in dogs and cats: 40 cases (1989–1994). *Journal of the American Veterinary Medical Association*, **12**, 1764–1767.

Wohl, J.S. (2006) Nasojejunal feeding tube placement using fluoroscopic guidance: technique and clinical experience in dogs. *Journal of Veterinary Emergency and Critical Care*, **16**, S27–S33.

Zsombor-Murray, E. and Freeman, L.M. (1999) Peripheral Parenteral Nutrition. *Compendium on Continual Education for the Practicing Veterinarian*, **21**(6), 1–11.

CHAPTER 4

Nasoesophageal feeding tubes in dogs and cats

Isuru Gajanayake

Willows Veterinary Centre and Referral Service, Shirley, Solihull, West Midlands, UK

Introduction

Indications, contraindications and patient selection

Nasoesophageal feeding tubes are placed into the distal esophagus via the nares. This can be a very useful feeding technique in clinical cases where a relatively short-term nutritional intervention (e.g., for about 3 to 5 days) is required (Figure 4.1). This type of feeding tube does not require any specialized equipment or expertise for placement and thus can be a very useful tool in general practice. In addition, nasoesophageal feeding tubes can be placed without the need for general anesthesia (or heavy sedation) and, as such, they can act as a temporary intervention in patients where anesthesia may be contraindicated.

Nasoesophageal feeding tubes are unlikely to be tolerated for extended periods of time and thus are not suitable for long-term or home feeding. Furthermore, patients with nasal pathology (e.g., rhinitis, neoplasia, maxillary fractures) or those with esophageal disease (e.g., esophagitis or megaesophagus) may not tolerate these tubes, as they are likely to augment discomfort or worsen clinical signs. Patients with a poor gag reflex, protracted vomiting or with reduced mentation would be at high risk of aspiration with this feeding technique and as such this should be avoided. Nasoesophageal feeding tubes may also not be an appropriate technique in overly aggressive patients, as feeding and management of the tube will require handling of the head. Finally, as there are limited choices of diets that can be administered via nasoesophageal feeding tubes, the characteristics of these diets can be quite limiting (i.e., high fat and protein content) and may lead to this technique not being suitable for certain patients.

Procedure for tube placement and confirmation of correct positioning

Materials required for nasoesophageal feeding tube placement:
1 A nasoesophageal feeding tube of the appropriate size
2 Sedative agent (e.g., butorphanol) may be useful but is not required

Nutritional Management of Hospitalized Small Animals, First Edition. Edited by Daniel L. Chan.
© 2015 John Wiley & Sons, Ltd. Published 2015 by John Wiley & Sons, Ltd.

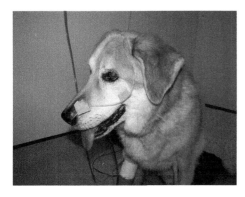

Figure 4.1 A dog with a nasoesophageal feeding tube in place.

3 Topical local anesthetic agent (e.g., proparacaine, proxymetacaine)
4 Adhesive tape
5 Lubricating gel (with or without topical anesthetic)
6 Suture material (non-absorbable suture) or tissue glue
7 Syringe and saline
8 Radiography, fluouroscopy or end-tidal carbon dioxide monitor.

Choosing feeding tube type and size

Nasoesophageal feeding tubes can be made of different materials, including polyurethane, polyvinylchloride, silicone and red rubber. Polyurethane tubes are stronger while silicone tubes are more biocompatible. Polyvinylchloride tubes can lead to mucosal irritation with prolonged use but this may not be a concern with nasoesophageal tubes as they are intended for short-term use. The external diameter of these tubes range from 4 French (1.3 mm) to 10 French (3.3 mm). Tube choice is thus dependent on the size of the patient (the size of the nares being the limiting factor) but in general tubes sizes between 3.5 and 5 French are adequate for most cats, whereas tubes with sizes >6 French may be appropriate for a medium to large dog. In brachycephalic dogs and cats it may be necessary to place a smaller tube due to the smaller external nares.

Tube placement technique

1 Position the conscious or sedated patient in sternal recumbency.
2 Apply 1–2 drops of local anesthetic (e.g., proxymetacaine) into one nostril with the head held up so that the anesthetic agent flows caudally into the nasal cavity (Figure 4.2).
3 While waiting for the local anesthetic to take effect (usually 1 or 2 minutes), measure the tube from the nares to the 7th or 8th intercostal space – mark this position on the tube with some adhesive tape.
4 Lubricate the tube with gel.
5 Hold the head at a normal angle and direct the tube ventrally and medially (i.e., toward the opposite ear) for passage into the ventral nasal meatus (Figure 4.3); in dogs it may be necessary to pass the tube dorsally initially (for about 1 cm) over the ventral ridge and then in a ventral and medial direction while holding the external nares in a dorsal position (Abood and Buffington, 1991).

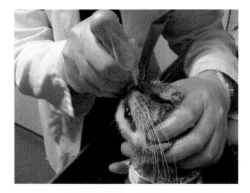

Figure 4.2 A cat being prepared for nasoesophageal tube placement by the application of a local anesthetic (e.g., proxymetacaine) into the left nostril.

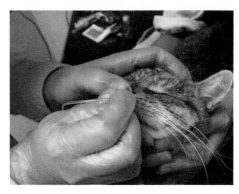

Figure 4.3 Nasoesophagel feeding tube being fed through the nostril of a cat.

6 The tube should pass without resistance and the patient may swallow as the tube passes the oropharynx (Figure 4.4).

7 If resistance is met the tube should be withdrawn and steps 4–6 should be repeated.

8 Once the tube has been passed to the level of the tape marker it should be secured as closely as possible to the nostril using a single suture or tissue glue to attach the tape marker to the skin with a single suture or to the fur with glue.

9 A second tape marker is then placed further along the tube to attach the tube via a suture or glue to the skin or fur on the head between the eyes (care must be taken to avoid the tube touching the whiskers in cats).

10 An Elizabethan collar is then placed to avoid inadvertent removal of the tube by the patient (Figure 4.5).

Confirmation of accurate placement

Several techniques are available to check accurate placement of a nasoesophageal feeding tube and include:

1 Applying suction to the tube using a 5 or 10 mL syringe; if negative pressure is not achieved the tube may be in the airways (or stomach).

2 Injecting 5–10 mL of air to the tube and auscultating the cranial abdomen for borborygmal sounds.

3 Instilling 3–5 mL of sterile saline into the tube and observing for a cough response (this indicates incorrect placement in the airway).

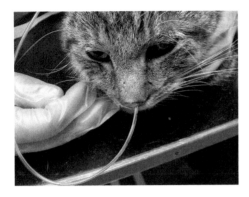

Figure 4.4 The nasoesophageal tube should pass without resistance from the nasal passage into the oropharynx and into the esophagus.

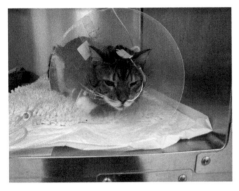

Figure 4.5 A cat is fitted with an Elizabethan collar to prevent inadvertent removal of the tube by the patient.

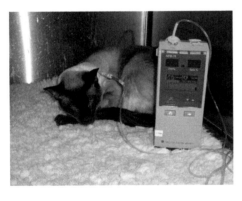

Figure 4.6 Capnography can be used to confirm that the nasoesophageal feeding tube is not in the airway by the lack of a CO_2 tracing being produced.

4 Applying a capnograph to the tube (Figure 4.6). If a CO_2 trace is seen on the monitor, this indicates that the tube is in the airway (Chau et al., 2011).
5 Performing thoracic radiography to check for correct placement of the tube in the distal esophagus and ensuring there is no kinking of the tube.

Monitoring and ongoing care

The tube exit site from external nares should be checked once to twice daily for any discharge or bleeding. Any crusting can be cleaned using moistened cotton wool. The tube should be checked for patency.

Diets and tube feeding

Nasoesophageal feeding tubes are somewhat limited in the choices of diets that can be administered through them as the narrow lumen of these tubes limits anything other than a pure liquid diet. These diets tend to be relatively energy dense (i.e, 1 kcal/ml) and have high concentrations of protein and salt. For these reasons, these diets and thus nasoesophageal feeding tubes may be relatively contraindicated in patients with intolerance to high protein (e.g., renal or hepatic failure) or to high sodium (e.g., cardiac failure). However, some of the diets have a lower protein and sodium content that may be tolerated in this subset of patients. Alternatively the diets can be further diluted with water, however in this case, a relatively large volume may be necessary to meet the energy requirements of the patients.

Feeding via nasoesophageal tubes can be performed either via bolus administration or as a constant rate infusion. For bolus feeding, the daily amount of the diet to be delivered is divided into 3–6 meals to find a balance between practicality and individual meal sizes. In general, a meal size (including tube flush volumes) should not exceed 10–12 mL/kg. Setting up a constant rate infusion using liquid diets is relatively straightforward as these diets can be administered using a syringe driver or fluid pump (Figure 4.7). However, it is vital to ensure that the enteral nutrition bag, syringes and infusion lines are clearly labelled to prevent accidental administration of enteral feed into intravenous catheters (Figure 4.8).

Prior to each bolus feeding, a small volume (e.g., 3–5 mL) of sterile water or saline should be administered via the tube to confirm patency and correct position. If resistance is encountered or if the patient coughs after the flush, the planned feeding should be stopped and measures taken to investigate and correct the problem. This may include thoracic radiography (and or capnography) to confirm correct tube position or steps to unblock the tube (see troubleshooting). The tube should also be flushed with a small volume (5 mL) of water at the end of feeding to prevent blockages. When using a constant rate infusion to feed via a nasoesophageal feeding tube the patient should be hospitalized in an area where it will be monitored constantly, for example, an intensive care unit. This is to prevent inadvertent feeding into the airways if the tube dislodges from the oesophagus to the trachea.

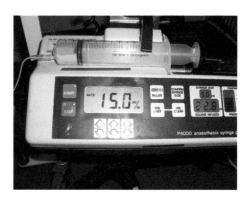

Figure 4.7 Nasoesophageal feedings may be delivered as constant rate infusion via syringe drivers or fluid pumps.

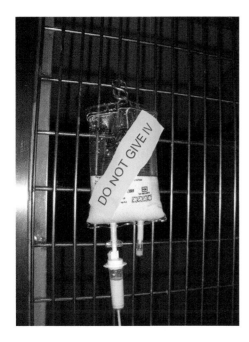

Figure 4.8 A bag of enteral feeding clearly labelled to indicate that it must not be administered intravenously.

Complications and troubleshooting

The complications associated with nasoesophageal feeding tubes are relatively minor and are unlikely to result in death or significant morbidity. In one study, the most common complications seen with the use of nasogastric feeding tubes were vomiting, diarrhea and inadvertent tube removal, which occurred in 37% of patients (Abood and Buffington, 1992). Other minor complications (e.g., irritation of nasal passages, sneezing) can occur during the placement of the tube or as a consequence of the in-dwelling tube. A recent study comparing complications associated with nasoesophageal versus nasogastric feeding tubes found no difference in rates of complications (Yu et al., 2013). To prevent inadvertent use of the nasoesophageal tube for anything other than feeding, the feeding tube should be clearly labelled. The use of special safety enteral feeding syringes[1,2] and tube adaptors also prevents accidental injection of food into intravenous catheters (e.g., jugular catheters) (Guenter et al., 2008).

Tracheal intubation
The most serious complication associated with placement of this type of tube is inadvertent tracheal intubation. This can be avoided by careful technique and confirmation of correct placement within the oesophagus. It is also possible that a previously correctly placed tube can be vomited and then inadvertently passes into the trachea. For this reason, it is important to confirm that the tube is still in the correct place prior to each feeding. If there is any concern that tracheal intubation may have occurred, follow-up thoracic radiography should be performed.

Vomiting

Vomiting may occur with nasoesophageal tubes but this may be less frequently encountered than with esophagostomy feeding tubes. Patients that are experiencing frequent vomiting as a pre-existing condition prior to tube placement may require an alternate feeding technique or have vomiting controlled with anti-emetic therapy before implementation of tube feeding. Despite these concerns, recent studies have not reported an increase in vomiting episodes following implementation of nasoesophageal feeding (Mohr et al., 2003, Campbell et al., 2010, Holahan et al., 2010).

Tube blockage

Nasoesophageal tubes may be particularly prone to blockage due to their narrow lumen diameter. Tube blockages are best prevented by using pure liquid diets and by flushing the tube following each feeding using a small volume of water (i.e. 5 mL). If a blockage does occur, flushing and applying suction using warm water may dislodge the blockage. Alternatively a combination of pancreatic enzymes and sodium bicarbonate in water should be injected into the clogged feeding tube and left for a few minutes before attempting flushing again with water to release the blockage (Parker and Freeman, 2013). Other compounds such as carbonated drinks may also be attempted but this has been shown to be less effective than water in an *in vitro* experiment (Parker and Freeman, 2013).

Rhinitis, epistaxis and dacrocystitis

Local irritation of the nasal cavity and tear ducts may occur with nasoesophageal tubes. These complications are especially likely following lengthy periods of use and if there is pre-existing disease in these areas. Tube removal may be necessary if these signs are particularly severe.

Reflux esophagitis

Regurgitation and reflux esophagitis may occur if the tube is inadvertently placed (across the lower esophageal sphincter) into the stomach. However, this complication is rarely reported and believed to be more common with large bore feeding tubes such as esophageal feeding tubes than with narrower nasoesophageal feeding tubes.

Removal and transition to oral feeding

Food can be offered to the patient throughout the period this feeding tube is in place as its presence is unlikely to cause any hindrance to the patient's appetite or swallowing. In one study into the use of nasogastric feeding tubes, about half of the patients started eating voluntarily while still hospitalized (Abood and Buffington, 1992).

Nasoesophageal feeding tubes enable nutrition to be provided while a patient is stabilized with other treatments. Once the patient has been stabilized (and if it is still inappetent), a longer term feeding tube option (e.g., esophagostomy or gastrostomy feeding tube) can be placed.

KEY POINTS

- Nasoesophageal feeding tubes can be a very useful feeding technique in clinical cases where a relatively short-term nutritional intervention is required.

- This type of feeding tube does not require any specialized equipment or expertise for placement and thus can be a very useful technique in general practice.

- Nasoesophageal feeding tubes are unlikely to be tolerated for extended periods of time and thus are not suitable for long-term or at home feeding.

- Tube choice is dependent on the size of the patient but in general, tube sizes between 3.5 and 5 French are adequate in cats, whereas tubes with sizes > 6 French may be appropriate in dogs.

- Food can be offered to the patient throughout the period the feeding tube is in place as its presence is unlikely to cause any hindrance to the patient's voluntary food intake.

References

Abood, S.K. and Buffington, C.A. (1991) Improved nasogastric intubation technique for administration of nutritional support in dogs. *Journal of the American Veterinary Medical Association*, **199**(5), 577–579.

Abood, S.K. and Buffington, C.A. (1992) Enteral feeding of dogs and cats: 51 cases (1989–1991). *Journal of the American Veterinary Medical Association*, **201**(4), 619–622.

Campbell, J.A., Jutkowitz, L.A., Santoro, K. A. et al. (2010) Continuous versus intermittent delivery of nutrition via nasoenteric feeding tubes in hospitalized canine and feline patients: 91 patients (2002–2007). *Journal of Veterinary Emergency and Critical Care*, **20**(2), 232–236.

Chau, J.P., Lo, S.H., Thompson, D.R. et al (2011) Use of end-total carbon dioxide detection to determine correct placement of nasogastric tube: a meta-analysis. *International Journal of Nursing Studies*, **48**(4), 513–521.

Guenter, P., Hicks, R.W., Simmons, D. et al. (2008) Enteral feeding misconnections: A Consortium Position Statement. *The Joint Commission Journal on Quality and Patient Safety*, **34**(5), 285–292.

Holahan, M., Abood, S., Hauptman, J. et al. (2010) Intermittent and continuous enteral nutrition in critically ill dogs: a prospective randomized trial. *Journal of Veterinary Internal Medicine*, **24**(3), 520–526.

Mohr, A.J., Leisewitz, A. L., Jacobson, L. S. et al. (2003) Effect of early enteral nutrition on intestinal permeability, intestinal protein loss, and outcome in dogs with severe parvoviral enteritis. *Journal of Veterinary Internal Medicine*, **17**(6), 791–798.

Parker, V. J. and Freeman, L. M. (2013) Comparison of various solutions to dissolve critical care diet clots. *Journal of Veterinary Emergency and Critical Care*, **23**(3), 344–347.

Yu, M. K., Freeman, L. M., Heinze, C. R. et al. (2013) Comparison of complications in dogs with nasoesophageal versus nasogastric tubes. *Journal of Veterinary Emergency and Critical Care*, **23**(3) 300–304.

CHAPTER 5

Esophagostomy feeding tubes in dogs and cats

Laura Eirmann

Oradell Animal Hospital; Nestle Purina PetCare, Ringwood, NJ, USA

Introduction

Esophagostomy tube feeding was first described as a means to provide nutritional support for people with cranial esophageal cancer in 1951 (Klopp, 1951). In the mid-1980s Crowe developed a similar technique for veterinary patients (Crowe, 1990). Esophagostomy tube feeding proved to be a safe and effective means of providing enteral nutrition for appropriate patients. This modality of nutritional support entails a relatively easy placement technique that is minimally invasive and well tolerated. Placement of the feeding tube into the midcervical region mitigates complications associated with pharyngostomy tubes, including gagging and partial airway obstruction (Crowe, 1990). Esophagostomy tubes can provide at-home nutritional support for weeks to months for patients unable or unwilling to meet nutritional needs orally. The larger diameter tube compared to nasoesophageal or jejunostomy tubes allows for a wider selection of diet options, including blenderized pet foods formulated for specific medical conditions.

Indications and contraindications for esophagostomy tubes

Enteral feeding is preferred over the parenteral route because it is physiologically sound, less costly, and safer (Prittie and Barton, 2004). Physiological benefits include maintenance of intestinal mucosal integrity and preservation of gastrointestinal immune function. General contraindications for enteral nutrition include uncontrolled vomiting, ileus, gastrointestinal obstruction, severe maldigestion or malabsorption and an inability to protect the airway.

An esophagostomy feeding tube allows delivery of nutrients to patients with inadequate intake who cannot prehend, masticate, or swallow food in a normal or safe manner. It can be used to meet the nutritional needs of anorexic patients, such as cats with hepatic lipidosis. This device is indicated in patients with nasal, oral, or pharyngeal disease since the midcervical placement of the

---

Nutritional Management of Hospitalized Small Animals, First Edition. Edited by Daniel L. Chan.
© 2015 John Wiley & Sons, Ltd. Published 2015 by John Wiley & Sons, Ltd.

Table 5.1 Indications and contraindications for esophagostomy feeding tubes.

Indications	Contraindications
Prolonged inadequate intake	High risk for general anesthesia or coagulopathy
Anticipated need for nutritional support > 7 days	Esophageal disease or marked gastrointestinal dysfunction precluding the enteral feeding route
Nasal, oral or pharyngeal disease or surgery	Inability to protect the airway (poor mentation, poor gag reflex)

Table 5.2 Advantages and disadvantages of esophagostomy feeding tubes.

Advantages	Disadvantages
Relatively easy and fast placement	Requires general anesthesia
Cost effective	Risk of cellulitis or infection at stoma site
Does not require specialized equipment	Esophagus and more distal gastrointestinal tract must be functional
Well tolerated by the patient	Potential to dislodge if patient vomits
Broad options for diet selection when larger feeding tubes are placed	Potential esophageal reflux or irritation if malpositioned
Can be used immediately and removed immediately if necessary	
Appropriate for long-term and at-home use	

tube bypasses these anatomic regions. Patients with oropharyngeal neoplasia, mandibular or maxillary trauma, oronasal fistulas or dysphagia are potential candidates for an esophagostomy feeding tube.

Patients must undergo general anesthesia for placement of the feeding tube, so the anesthetic risk must be considered. Sedation alone for placement of esophagostomy is not recommended as suppression of the gap reflex is not achieved, making placement extremely difficult. Esophagostomy tube placement should be considered contraindicated in patients with coagulopathy as this would lead to an unacceptable risk of bleeding. The esophagus and more distal gastrointestinal tract must be functional for this mode of nutrition to be effective. Patients with megaesophagus, esophagitis, or esophageal strictures are not good candidates for an esophagostomy tube, but may benefit from a more distally placed feeding device such as a gastrostomy tube. Patients at risk of vomiting must be able to protect their airway. A summary of indications and contraindications and a list of advantages and disadvantages are provided in Table 5.1 and Table 5.2.

Esophagostomy tube placement and feeding guidelines

Several techniques are described for placing esophagostomy tubes including percutaneous techniques utilizing curved forceps, needle catheters, or feeding tube applicators (Crowe, 1990; Rawlings, 1993; Crowe and Devey, 1997;

Devitt and Seim 1997, Levine, Smallwood and Buback, 1997; Von Werthern and Wess, 2001). A recent prospective study comparing the forceps technique (discussed in detail in this chapter) versus applicator according to Von Werthern in dogs and cats showed similar rapid placement time but identified some serious complications in some cases (Hohensinn et al., 2012). The technique preferred by the author is demonstrated in Figures 5.1–5.11 and detailed below:

1 The patient is anesthetized, intubated, and placed in right lateral recumbency (Figure 5.1) with the mouth held open by an oral speculum.

2 The surgical field is aseptically prepared from the mandibular ramus to the thoracic inlet and extended to the dorsal and ventral midlines. Placement of the tube on the left side is preferred due to the anatomical location of the esophagus.

3 A feeding tube is premeasured and marked from the midcervical esophagus caudal to the larynx to the 7th to 8th intercostal space so that the aboral (distal) tip will lie in the distal esophagus. Termination in the distal esophagus rather than the stomach decreases the risk of gastroesophageal reflux (Balkany et al., 1997). The feeding tube should be long enough to allow several centimetres to remain exterior to the skin post-placement. The size of the feeding tube depends upon patient size but commonly ranges from 12 to 14 French for cats and up to 20 French for dogs. Red rubber, polyurethane, or silicone tubes may be used (Marks, 2010). Selection of catheter material depends upon clinician preference recognizing differences in stiffness, flexibility and internal diameter (DeLegge and DeLegge, 2005).

4 Depending upon the feeding tube, the distal rounded end may be removed or the exit side hole may be elongated to facilitate passage of the gruel (Figure 5.2).

5 Curved forceps (e.g., Kelly, Carmalt, Mixter, or Schnidt, based on the size of the patient) are placed in the mouth and advanced to the midcervical esophagus distal to the hyoid apparatus. With the patient in lateral recumbency, the curved tip of the forceps is pushed dorsally, tenting the skin, and palpated externally (Figure 5.3). The jugular groove is identified to avoid major vasculature and nerves.

6 A small incision is made on the tented skin over the tip of the forceps through the esophageal wall (Figure 5.4).

7 The forceps tip is exteriorized by blunt dissection and excision of the esophageal mucosa (Figure 5.5).

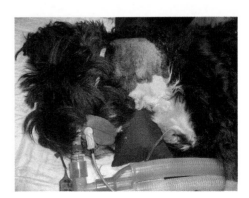

Figure 5.1 Patient is anesthetized and positioned on right lateral recumbency for placement of esophagostomy tube.

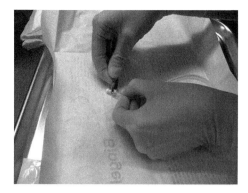

Figure 5.2 The distal exit side hole may be elongated with a blade to facilitate passage of food.

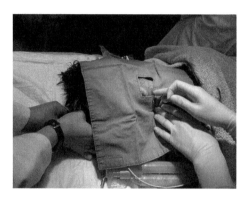

Figure 5.3 A curved Carmalt forceps clamp is placed through the oral cavity and its tip is palpated in the cervical area to identify the site of surgical incision.

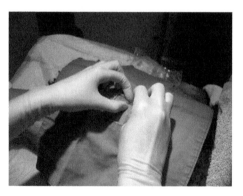

Figure 5.4 A small incision is made over the tips of the forceps through the skin and esophageal wall.

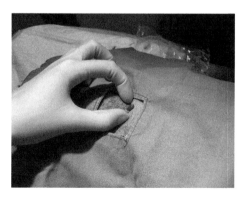

Figure 5.5 The tips of the forceps are exteriorized through the incision.

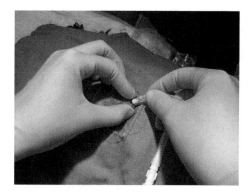

Figure 5.6 The tip of the feeding tube is grasped with the forceps.

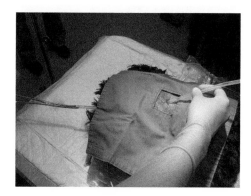

Figure 5.7 The feeding tube is pulled through the oral cavity.

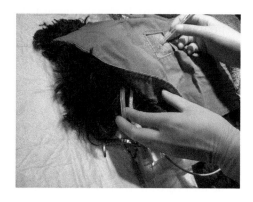

Figure 5.8 The tip of the feeding tube is retroflexed and redirected into the esophagus.

8 The distal end of the feeding tube is grasped with the forceps and pulled through the incision and out of the oral cavity (Figures 5.6 and 5.7). The tongue is retracted to facilitate redirection of the feeding tube.

9 The end of the tube is lubricated, retroflexed, and pushed down the esophagus while the proximal end of the tube is slowly retracted a few centimetres (Figures 5.8 and 5.9).

10 The proximal end of the tube will rotate cranially as the tube straightens to the proper orientation (Figure 5.10). The tube should slide easily back and forth a few millimetres and can be advanced to the premarked site on the tube.

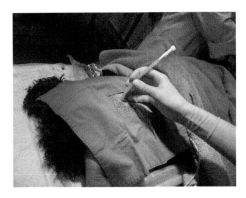

Figure 5.9 While the retroflexed tube is pushed into the oropharynx, gentle traction is applied to the end of the tube until it "flips" into its intended orientation.

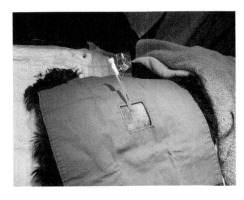

Figure 5.10 The feeding tube is advanced such that the tip lies in the caudal esophagus prior to suturing.

11 The oropharynx is visually inspected to confirm that the tube is no longer present.
12 The incision site is re-scrubbed and the tube is secured with purse-string and Chinese finger-trap sutures using polypropylene suture material (Figure 5.11).
13 Several techniques may be performed to verify correct placement of the feeding tube, including use of capnography (Figure 5.12); however, radiographic confirmation is recommended (Figure 5.13).
14 Antibiotic ointment on a non-adherent pad is placed over the surgical site and a light wrap is applied.
15 The tube is marked at the exit site to monitor for migration. The tube should be flushed with sterile saline to assess for a cough response and to introduce a column of liquid in the tube. The tube remains capped when not in use.
16 To avoid accidental administration of food into an intravenous catheter (termed 'enteral misconnection') all feeding tubes should be clearly labelled (Figure 5.14).

Additional measures to prevent inadvertent feeding into intravenous catheters include the implementation of enteral feeding safety devices.[1,2] This entails capping every feeding tube with special adaptors that are non-luer lock compliant and that can only be connected to special color-coded safety enteral syringes or tubing (Figures 5.15, 5.16, 5.17). These precautionary measures can be cost effective (i.e., are relatively inexpensive) but can be quite effective in preventing

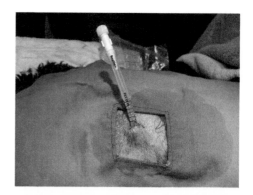

Figure 5.11 The tube is secured with a purse string suture and a 'Chinese Finger Trap' sutures pattern is applied.

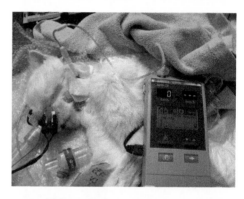

Figure 5.12 Capnography may be attached to the feeding tube to confirm correct placement as the esophagus should produce no discernible carbon dioxide tracing.

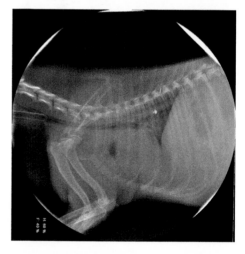

Figure 5.13 Confirmation of appropriate placement of esophageal feeding tube within the distal esophagus is best determined with fluouroscopy or radiography.

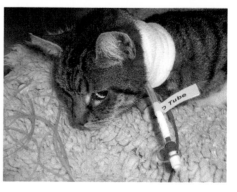

Figure 5.14 Feeding tubes should be clearly labelled to decrease risk of inadvertent feeding into intravenous catheters.

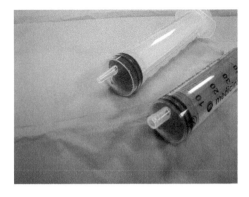

Figure 5.15 A special safety enteral syringe with non-luer tip (on right) is compared with a standard syringe with luer compatible tip.

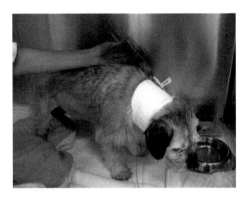

Figure 5.16 The dog in this image is being fed through its esophagostomy tube using a safety enteral feeding system that includes fitting the tube with a non-luer adaptor (purple adaptor) and administering food via special safety enteral syringes.

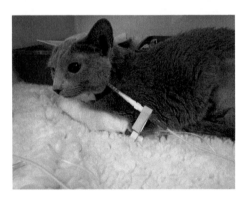

Figure 5.17 A cat receiving esophagostomy enteral feeding via a continuous rate infusion. Note that a special enteral infusion set is connected to a non-luer lock compliant safety feeding adaptor.

serious, if not fatal, medical errors associated with feeding (Guenter et al., 2008). Although these are not yet adopted universally in human medicine, there is growing pressure to make such measures mandatory (Guenter et al., 2008).

The esophagostomy tube can be used as soon as the patient recovers from anesthesia. Diet selection and preparation will be addressed in a later chapter (see Chapter 9). Veterinary liquid diets or properly blenderized pet foods can be utilized. Food may be delivered via multiple bolus feedings or by constant rate infusion. Bolus feeding can be continued at home. The daily caloric requirement is calculated and divided by the number of meals per day (often 4–6 meals per day initially). Based on nutritional assessment, the clinician may initiate feeding at 1/3–1/2 of the calculated energy requirement (typically resting energy requirement) on the first day, not to exceed 5 mL gruel/kg body weight per meal (Delaney, Fascetti and Elliott, 2006). Caloric intake is increased based on patient tolerance over the following days to reach the calculated goal. In most cases, the volume administered per meal can be increased up to 15 mL/kg and the number of meals per day can be decreased to 3 to 4 to accommodate an owner's schedule. Prior to feeding, the position of the tube should be inspected for migration and the tube should be flushed with warm water. Coughing may indicate tube migration. The patient should not be fed until the proper position of the tube has been verified. The patient should be comfortably positioned in an upright or sternal position. The gruel should be warmed to near body temperature and administered over 10–15 minutes, followed with a warm water flush (Vannatta and Bartges, 2004). Feeding should be discontinued if there is nausea, vomiting, coughing or discomfort and the patient and tube should be reassessed.

Monitoring

The stoma site should be examined daily for the first week for evidence of infection or food leakage and the site should be cleaned with an antiseptic solution (Marks, 2010). Daily nutritional assessment includes body weight, physical exam, review of previous 24 hour caloric intake and diagnostics based on the underlying disease. Oral food can be offered when deemed appropriate and voluntary intake recorded. Tube feeding can be reduced or discontinued based on the amount of voluntary intake. Patients with chronic disease may need a feeding tube indefinitely. The tube should not be removed until the patient's body weight is stable and the voluntary intake has been consistently sufficient for at least 1–2 weeks. The tube should be flushed with water twice daily if it is not being utilized. The tube is removed by cutting the anchoring suture, occluding the tube, and pulling gently. The ostomy site should be kept clean and a light dressing may be applied for the first 24 hours or until sealed. The wound will heal by second intention and should not be sutured closed.

Complications

Complications associated with esophagostomy feeding tubes are relatively uncommon and typically minor to moderate (Crowe and Devey, 1997; Levine et al., 1997). There was no difference in complication rate or severity in one retrospective study comparing esophagostomy tubes to percutaneous endoscopic gastrostomy tubes (Ireland et al., 2003). Serious complications, such as inadvertent placement in the airway or mediastinum, or damage to the major vessels and nerves can be avoid by proper placement technique and verifying the position of the tube radiographically. Midcervical placement minimizes the risk of gagging and partial airway obstruction (Crowe, 1990). Ensuring the tube terminates in the mid to distal esophagus rather than the stomach decreases the risk of gastroesophageal reflux with secondary esophagitis or stricture (Balkany et al., 1997). Proper tube size and material decrease the risk of esophageal irritation. Proper patient evaluation to ensure the pet can protect his airway in the event of vomiting is critical to lessen the risk of pulmonary aspiration. If the patient vomits, tube placement should be verified to ensure it has not been displaced.

Complications related to the stoma site or mechanical issues with the tube are possible. Peristomal cellulitis, infection or abscess may occur (Crowe and Devey, 1997: Devitt and Seim, 1997; Levine et al., 1997; Ireland et al., 2003). Peristomal inflammation is a more common complication (Levine et al., 1997). It can be managed in mild cases with through cleaning and topical antibiotics (Levine et al., 1997) while more severe cellulitis or abscessation may require systemic antibiotics and tube removal (Michel, 2004). These risks can be minimized by ensuring the tube is secured properly and the stoma site is kept clean and protected (Michel, 2004). Mechanical issues with the tube include premature removal, kinking or clogging. Risk of premature removal can be minimized by using an appropriate tube size for patient comfort. The tube should be securely sutured and wraps should be comfortable. An Elizabethan collar may be needed in some cases. Kinking can occur during tube placement or after vomiting and can be detected radiographically. Completely flushing the tube with water after every use decreases the risk of tube obstruction. The gruel should be a proper consistency and administration of medications through the tube should be avoided or done with caution (Michel, 2004). Tube obstructions may dislodge with warm water by applying pressure and suction. Other methods include infusing a carbonated beverage or a solution of pancreatic enzyme and sodium bicarbonate (Ireland et al., 2003; Michel, 2004; Parker and Freeman, 2013).

As with any mode of enteral support, gastrointestinal and metabolic complications can occur. Nutritional assessment, monitoring, and treatment modifications are indicated for every patient. Vomiting may occur if the gruel is not warmed to a proper temperature or delivered too quickly. Decreasing the bolus volume and increasing feeding frequency may help patients with vomiting or diarrhea. Antiemetics or motility modifiers may also be indicated. The nutrient composition of the diet or some medications may contribute to adverse gastrointestinal signs and may need to be modified.

Summary

Esophagostomy tube feeding is a safe and well-tolerated technique and offers an effective means of enteral nutritional support in animals. Appropriate patient selection and adherence to proper placement and feeding techniques are imperative. As with any mode of nutritional support, diligent patient monitoring and client education are required. Several studies have documented owner satisfaction with this mode of nutritional support (Devitt and Seim, 1997; Ireland et al., 2003).

KEY POINTS

- Esophagostomy feeding tubes are a safe and effective means of providing enteral nutritional support for appropriately selected veterinary patients.

- Candidates for esophagostomy feeding tubes must have a functional gastrointestinal tract distal to the oropharynx, be able to undergo short duration general anesthesia, and not have a coagulopathy that would place them at risk of hemorrhage.

- Proper placement technique, tube management, and feeding protocols minimize complication risks.

- Esophagostomy feeding tubes can be managed by clients long-term with a variety of diets.

- Potential complications include improper placement or displacement of the tube, mechanical or infectious complications, and gastrointestinal complications.

- Nutritional assessment and monitoring is critical for successful patient outcome.

Notes

1 Safety syringes. Medicina. Blackrod, Bolton, UK.
2 BD Enteral syringe, UniVia. BD, Franklin Lakes, NJ, USA.

References

Balkany, T.J., Baker, B.B., Bloustein, P.A. et al. (1997) Cervical esophagostomy in dogs: endoscopic, radiographic, and histopathologic evaluation of esophagitis induced by feeding tubes. *Annals of Otology, Rhinology and Laryngology*, **86**, 588–593.

Crowe, D.T. (1990) Nutritional support for the hospitalized patient: An introduction to tube feeding. *Compendium for Continuing Education for the Practicing Veterinarian*, **12**(12), 1711–1721.

Crowe, D.T. and Devey J.J. (1997) Esophagostomy tubes for feeding and decompression: clinical experience in 29 small animal patients. *Journal of the American Animal Hospital Association*, **33**, 393–403.

Delaney, S.J., Fascetti, A.J. and Elliott, D.A. (2006) Critical care nutrition of dogs, in *Encyclopedia of Canine Clinical Nutrition* (eds P. Pibot, V. Biourge and D Elliott) Aniwa SAS, Aimrgues, France, pp. 426–450.

DeLegge, R.L. and DeLegge, M.H. (2005) Percutaneous endoscopic gastrostomy evaluation of device material: are we "failsafe"? *Nutrition in Clinical Practice*, **20**, 613–617.

Devitt, C.M. and Seim, H.B. (1997) Clinical evaluation of tube esophagostomy in small animals. *Journal of the American Animal Hospital Association*, **33**, 55–60.

Guenter, P., Hicks, R.W., Simmons, D. et al. (2008) Enteral feeding misconnections: A Consortium Position Statement. *The Joint Commission Journal on Quality and Patient Safety*, **34**(5), 285–292.

Hohensinn, N., Doerfelt, R., Doerner, J. et al. (2012) Comparison of two techniques for oesophageal feeding tube placement (Abstract). *Journal of Veterinary Emergency and Critical Care*, **22**(S2), S21.

Ireland, L.M., Hohenhaus, A.E., Broussard, J.D. et al. (2003) A comparison of owner management and complications in 67 cats with esophagostomy and percutaneous endoscopic gastrostomy feeding tubes. *Journal of the American Animal Hospital Association*, **39**, 241–246.

Klopp, C.T. (1951) Cervical esophagostomy. *Journal of Thoracic Surgery*, **21**, 490–491.

Levine, P.B., Smallwood, L.J. and Buback, J.L. (1997) Esophagostomy tubes as a method of nutritional management in cats: a retrospective study. *Journal of the American Animal Hospital Association*, **33**, 405–410.

Marks, S.L. (2010) Nasoesophageal, esophagostomy, gastrostomy, and jejunal tube placement techniques, in *Textbook of Veterinary Internal Medicine*, 7th edn (eds S.J. Ettinger and E.C. Feldman) Saunders Elsevier, St. Louis. pp. 333–340.

Michel, K.E. (2004) Preventing and managing complications of enteral nutritional support. *Clinical Techniques in Small Animal Practice*, **19**(1), 49–53.

Parker, V.J. and Freeman, L.M. (2013) Comparison of various solutions to dissolve critical care diets. *Journal of Veterinary Emergency and Critical Care*, **23**(3), 344–347.

Prittie, J. and Barton, L. (2004) Route of nutrient delivery. *Clinical Techniques in Small Animal Practice*, **1**(1), 6–8.

Rawlings, C.A. (1993) Percutaneous placement of a midcervical esophagostomy tube: new technique and representative cases. *Journal of the American Animal Hospital Association*, **29**, 526–530.

Vannatta, M. and Bartges, J. (2004) Esophagostomy feeding tubes. *Veterinary Medicine*, **99**, 596–600.

Von Werthern, C.J. and Wess, G. (2001) A new technique for insertion of esophagostomy tubes in cats. *Journal of the American Animal Hospital Association*, **37**, 140–144.

CHAPTER 6

Gastrostomy feeding tubes in dogs and cats

Isuru Gajanayake[1] and Daniel L. Chan[2]

[1] Willows Veterinary Centre and Referral Service, Shirley, Solihull, West Midlands, UK
[2] Department of Veterinary Clinical Sciences and Services, The Royal Veterinary College, University of London, UK

Introduction

The advent of gastrostomy tubes (G-tubes) in small animal medicine has dramatically facilitated feeding of animals with a variety of diseases and conditions. Gastrostomy tubes include several different types of tubes that vary in their composition and technique of placement, but they all allow delivery of nutrients distal to the esophagus, enabling enteral feeding in patients with oral, pharyngeal or esophageal disease. Gastrostomy tubes are generally well tolerated (Seaman and Legendre, 1998; Yoshimoto et al., 2006), can be placed with less invasive techniques (i.e., percutaneously placed with endoscopy), and are highly effective as a means of providing nutritional support (Smith et al., 1998; McCrakin et al., 1993). They also permit bolus meal feeding, and can be used for long-term at-home feeding.

Gastrostomy tubes can be placed percutaneously in one of two ways: blindly using a special tube placing device (e.g., the Eld device)[1] or with the aid of an endoscope (i.e., percutaneous endoscopic-guided gastrostomy (PEG) tube). Gastrostomy tubes can also be placed surgically and this is an especially useful technique when abdominal surgery is already being performed for other reasons (e.g., intestinal surgery, biopsy). Gastrostomy tubes can also be used as a conduit to the jejunum, allowing the upper gastrointestinal tract to be completely bypassed without the need for a surgical jejunostomy (Cavanaugh et al., 2008; Jergens et al., 2007). Additionally, G-tubes can also be replaced with low-profile gastrostomy feeding tubes (Figure 6.1) suitable for long-term use (Bright, DeNovo and Jones, 1995).

Nutritional Management of Hospitalized Small Animals, First Edition. Edited by Daniel L. Chan.
© 2015 John Wiley & Sons, Ltd. Published 2015 by John Wiley & Sons, Ltd.

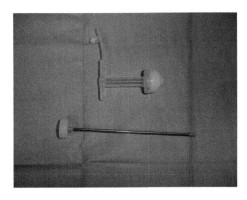

Figure 6.1 Picture of a low profile gastrostomy tube and introducer tool which is used to elongate the tube and facilitate its placement into an existing and mature stoma site. This is a more cosmetic and practical approach for animals with very long term need for assisted feeding.

Table 6.1 Advantages and disadvantages of gastrostomy feeding tubes.

Advantages	Disadvantages
Relatively easy and fast placement	Requires general anesthesia
Ready-to-use kits readily available	Risk of cellulitis or infection at stoma site
Well tolerated by the patient	Risk for peritonitis secondary to leakage
Broad options for diet selection – can liquidize pet foods	Requires specialized equipment
Appropriate for long-term and at-home use	Must wait 14 days before safe removal
Allows for placement of jejunal tubes through gastrostomy tubes	Endoscopic placement may affect gastric motility for up to 72 hours
Gastrostomy tubes can be replaced with low-profile tubes for prolonged use	

Indications and contraindications for gastrostomy tubes

Gastrostomy feeding tubes have three main advantages: (i) they by-pass the pharynx and esophagus, (ii) they generally have the widest bore and so can accommodate almost any diet and (iii) they can be used for long-term feeding (Table 6.1). Bypassing the pharynx and esophagus is important when there is disease in these areas (especially in esophageal disease such as megaesophagus or esophagitis). The use of wide-bore feeding tubes such as G-tubes is useful in patients with specific nutritional requirements (e.g., pancreatitis, adverse food reactions) that require diets not normally available as liquid diets, as almost any therapeutic diet can be modified to enable feeding through G-tubes. Finally, in some patients that require very long-term assisted feeding (e.g., neoplasia, kidney failure, megaesophagus) G-tubes have been used effectively.

Despite several advantages, G-tubes may not be a viable option when there are contraindications for enteral feeding (e.g., severe vomiting, ileus), for anesthetizing the patient, due to cardiovascular instability or for performing surgery (e.g., coagulopathy, compromised wound healing due to severe hypoproteinemia)

Table 6.2 Indications and contraindications for gastrostomy feeding tubes.

Indications	Contraindications
Prolonged inadequate food intake	High risk for general anesthesia or coagulopathy
Anticipated need for nutritional support > 7 days	Gastrointestinal dysfunction precluding the enteral feeding route
Nasal, oral, pharyngeal, esophageal disease or surgery	

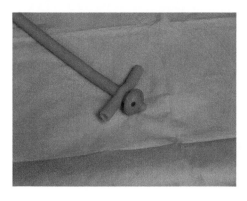

Figure 6.2 This pezzer catheter has been modified to be used as a gastrostomy tube.

(Table 6.2). This mode of nutritional support may also be ineffective when there is severe gastric pathology present (e.g., gastric lymphoma).

Gastrostomy tube placement

Surgical placement of a gastrostomy tube can be performed at the time of abdominal surgery for another reason (e.g., mass excision or biopsy collection). With surgical placement, the tube is secured with sutures to the abdominal wall and this site is sealed with omentum to minimize the risk of leakage of luminal contents. For this technique, balloon-tipped Foley catheters designed for use in the urinary bladder should be avoided owing to the possibility of balloon rupture and displacement of the catheter, thereby increasing the risk of peritoneal cavity contamination and septic peritonitis.

Techniques for blind placement of gastrostomy tubes have been described (Glaus et al., 1998; Fulton and Dennis, 1992) but the risk of complications such as laceration and impalement of the spleen would be greater than with endoscopic placement (Marks, 2010).

Requirements for PEG feeding tube placement

Although a pezzer catheter tube can be modified (Figure 6.2) for use as a gastrostomy catheter and placed via endoscopy, commercial PEG tube kits are available that contain the appropriate tube and necessary equipment for placement (e.g,. large bore needle, suture reel and tube attachments (Figure 6.3). One end

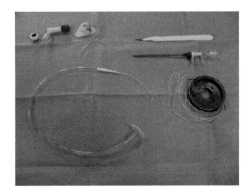

Figure 6.3 Commercially available kit for percutaneous endoscopically guided gastrostomy tubes containing all necessary components.

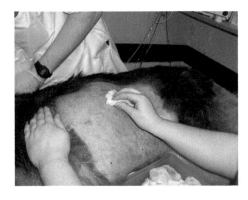

Figure 6.4 For placement of percutaneous endoscopically guided gastrostomy tube, patient should be anesthetized, placed in right lateral recumbency and a wide skin clip and aseptic preparation is required.

of the tube contains a mushroom tip (i.e., the end that ends up inside the stomach) and the other end tapers to a point with a swaged on loop of suture (i.e., the end of the tube that ends up outside the stomach). Detailed instructions are usually provided in these commercial kits to demonstrate accurate placement of the tube. Tube sizes vary depending on the available kits but in general a 15 French tube is suitable for cats and small dogs and a 20–24 French tube for medium-sized dogs. PEG tube placement also requires flexible video endoscopy and competency in its use (Armstrong and Hardie, 1990).

Technique for PEG tube placement

A step-by-step description of the PEG tube technique is described below:

1 The patient is anesthetized and placed in right lateral recumbency.
2 The skin on the left flank is clipped and surgically prepared encompassing an area extending from the costal arch to the mid-abdomen in a cranial to caudal direction, and from the transverse processes of the lumbar vertebrae to the level of the ventral end of the last rib in a dorso-ventral direction (Figure 6.4).
3 The endoscope is passed into the stomach and the stomach is distended with air (Figure 6.5).
4 The endoscopist finds an appropriate place for the feeding tube placement in the stomach in an area of the gastric body (e.g., away from the pylorus) – this position on the external body wall can be identified by trans-illuminating the area with the endoscope.

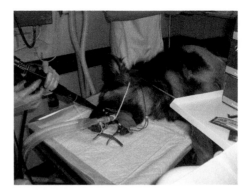

Figure 6.5 The endoscope is passed down the esophagus and into the stomach, which should be insufflated with air to enable visualization and allow percutaneous placement of gastrostomy tube.

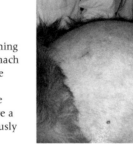

Figure 6.6 To ensure that there is nothing between the abdominal wall and stomach wall, an assistant should press into the body wall with a finger and the endoscopist should confirm seeing the indentation of the stomach wall before a trocar catheter is inserted percutaneously into the stomach.

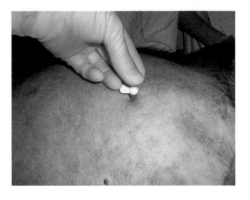

Figure 6.7 A wide bore trocar catheter is inserted percutaneously into the insufflated stomach. The catheter should be visualized inside the stomach via endoscopy.

5 This position is then confirmed by an assistant pushing into the abdominal wall with a finger, whilst the endoscopist observes the indentation on the internal surface of the stomach via the endoscope. This procedure also confirms that there are no organs between the gastric and abdominal walls (Figure 6.6).

6 A small stab incision is made at this site with a scalpel blade.

7 A large bore needle is then passed through this stab incision into the inflated stomach (Figure 6.7) (the entry of the needle into the stomach can be visualized endoscopically).

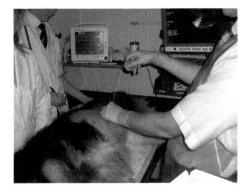

Figure 6.8 A suture with a loop at the end is inserted into the stomach via the trocar and visualized via the endoscope.

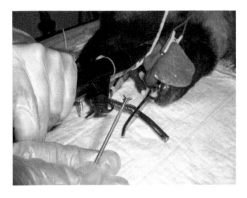

Figure 6.9 Endoscopic forceps are used to grab the suture from the stomach.

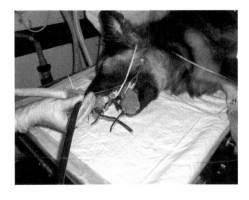

Figure 6.10 The suture obtained with endoscopic forceps should be gently pulled from the stomach through the mouth with the endoscope.

8 The long suture reel is then fed through this needle into the stomach by the assistant, without releasing the external end (Figure 6.8).

9 The suture inside the stomach is grabbed with endoscopic forceps (Figure 6.9) and the suture is pulled out of the stomach while gently retracting the endoscope out of the stomach and mouth (Figure 6.10). This leaves a suture line running down the mouth and esophagus into the stomach and out through the gastric and abdominal wall to the assistant.

10 The mouth end of the suture is then looped and knotted to the swaged-on suture at the end of the feeding tube (Figure 6.11).

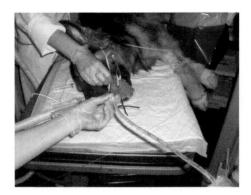

Figure 6.11 The gastrostomy catheter is secured to the suture before it is pulled into the stomach via the suture.

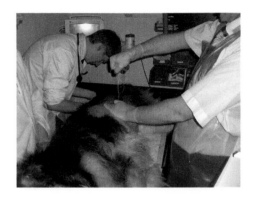

Figure 6.12 Gentle and firm traction is applied to the suture to pull the gastrostomy catheter into the stomach and out through body wall.

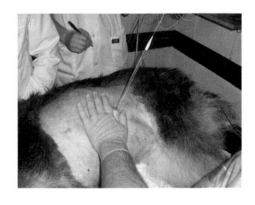

Figure 6.13 The suture attached to the gastrostomy catheter is pulled until the mushroom tip is against the stomach wall. This can be confirmed endoscopically.

11 The feeding tube is lubricated with gel to facilitate passage within the esophagus and stomach.
12 The assistant holding the suture line at the abdominal wall then gently pulls on this, thereby pulling the feeding tube into the esophagus and stomach (Figure 6.12).
13 With further pressure the tube will be pulled out of the abdominal wall, but it may be necessary to widen the skin incision slightly to enable easy passage of the tube (Figure 6.13).

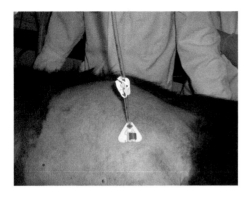

Figure 6.14 Once correct placement is confirmed, the catheter is secured to the external body wall to prevent movement.

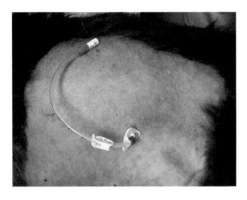

Figure 6.15 This picture shows the gastrostomy tube anchored to the body wall with its clamps and adaptors.

14 Once the mushroom end of the tube feels firmly against the abdominal wall, the internal position of the tube can be checked with endoscopy to ensure the mushroom tip is against the gastric wall.

15 The tube can then be secured to the abdominal wall using the flanges provided with the kit – it may also be necessary to place an additional Chinese finger trap suture to prevent tube migration (Figure 6.14).

16 Once the tube is secured, the endoscope can be removed and the external end of the feeding tube is cut to a suitable length to enable placement of the feeding adaptors (Figure 6.15).

17 Finally a sterile dressing is applied at the tube stoma site and the remainder of the tube is secured with a light body wrap or stockinet so that the patient cannot reach and pull out the tube (an Elizabethan collar may also be necessary for this purpose).

Feeding via gastrostomy tubes

Gastrostomy feeding tubes allow the use of liquid, semi-solid and gruel-type diets. Because of their wider bore, there is less risk of these tubes becoming blocked with food as long as proper precautions are taken (e.g., flushing the tube with water before and after each feed). Traditionally, there was a recommendation that feeding through gastrostomy tubes placed endoscopically should be withheld for the first 24 hours to allow the formation of a fibrin seal at the stoma site. However, more recent recommendations regarding the use of percutaneously placed gastrostomy tubes downplay the importance of delaying feeding. In people, PEG tubes can be placed on an outpatient basis and feeding can start on the same day of placement (Stein et al., 2002).

There is also some controversy regarding the effects of percutaneous placement of gastrostomy tubes on gastric motility. Smith and others (1998) found that placement of PEG tubes in healthy cats did not delay gastric emptying (as assessed by nuclear scintigraphy of radiolabelled food). However, a subsequent study documented delayed gastric emptying for up to 5 days after tube placement (Foster, Hoskinson and Moore, 1999). For this reason, patients should not be fed the full-prescribed amount of food until 72 hours following placement. Once placed, gastrostomy tubes should be left in place for at least 10–14 days prior to removal. In some instances, such as when delayed wound healing is likely to be present due to hypoalbuminemia or immune-compromise, the tube will need to be left in for a longer period.

Monitoring of gastrostomy tubes, transition to oral feeding and tube removal

The stoma site should be examined once daily for the first week, for evidence of infection or food leakage and following examination the site should be cleaned with an antiseptic solution (Marks, 2010). The patient should also be assessed each day to monitor vital parameters (especially body temperature), body weight, caloric intake and tolerance of feeding. Oral food can be offered when deemed appropriate and the amount of food eaten should be recorded. Tube feedings can then be reduced or discontinued on the basis of the amount of voluntary intake. Patients with chronic disease may need a feeding tube in place indefinitely. The tube should not be removed until the patient's body weight is stable and the voluntary intake has been consistently sufficient for at least 1–2 weeks. The tube should be flushed with water twice daily if it is not being used for feeding.

Tube removal
When the animal is deemed to be eating an appropriate amount of food voluntarily (e.g., 75% resting energy requirements (RER), the G-tube can be removed. In medium- to large-sized dogs, the tube can be cut and the mushroom tip left to pass in the faeces. To do this, the anchoring attachments are removed and the tube is cut close to the skin and pushed in (Figure 6.16). However, in smaller dogs and cats there is a risk that the mushroom tip will lead to an intestinal obstruction. As such, endoscopic removal of the mushroom tip is necessary (Figure 6.17). Following removal, the tube stoma site is kept clean with a light dressing for the first 24 hours or until it seals. The wound is left to heal by second intention.

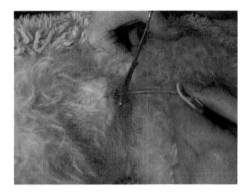

Figure 6.16 This picture depicts a gastrostomy tube being removed. In larger dogs, the catheter is simply cut at the level of the skin and the remaining portion is pushed into the stomach.

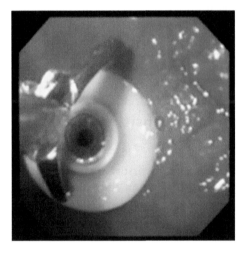

Figure 6.17 In smaller patients, the internal disk of the catheter should be retrieved endoscopically and the tube is not cut until the tip is secured.

Complications

Major complications associated with G-tubes include abdominal visceral injury during percutaneous placement, or peritonitis if stomach contents leak into the abdominal cavity secondary to tube dislodgement or dehiscence of the stoma (Armstrong and Hardie 1990; Fulton and Dennis, 1992; Glaus et al., 1998). As with any surgically placed feeding device, cellulitis or infection at the stoma site is also possible. Improperly placed G-tubes may cause pyloric outflow obstruction. Pressure necrosis of the gastric wall may also occur if the tube is secured too tightly, and this can ultimately lead to dislodgement of the tube (Elliott, Riel and Rodgers, 2000).

Many complications associated with gastrostomy feeding tubes can be easily prevented by careful patient evaluation, patient selection, appropriate feeding tube selection, adhering to good feeding protocols and close patient monitoring. Most enteral feeding complications are minor in nature but aspiration, tube dislodgement and certain metabolic derangements can be life threatening. Intolerance to enteral feeding may manifest as vomiting, diarrhea, abdominal pain and ileus. Signs of gastrointestinal intolerance commonly lead to failure to reach target provision of nutritional support as feedings may be reduced or suspended. Intolerance to enteral feeding may also arise when patients may have impaired gastrointestinal motility or perfusion. Ileus may be minimized by warming the food (to approximate body temperature) prior to feeding. Use of prokinetic therapy may also help to address ileus (see Chapter 17).

Anticipating specific intolerances during the nutritional assessment and setting initially conservative caloric goals (i.e., not exceeding the patient's RER), may minimize risk for metabolic complications. Refeeding syndrome (Chapter 16) is a life-threatening metabolic complication that may occur in certain patients after prolonged anorexia or with certain catabolic states. Briefly, this syndrome is thought to result from rapid shifts of key intracellular electrolytes (e.g., potassium, phosphorus and magnesium) from the intravascular to intracellular space, a process that is triggered by reintroduction of feeding.

Aspiration is a potentially life-threatening complication that could be minimized by careful patient selection and monitoring. The development of vomiting, regurgitation, pyrexia, tachypnea or dyspnea should prompt patient evaluation. Infections may occur at the stoma site, along fascial planes or within the peritoneum. In one study, stoma site complications were noted in 46% of patients, but all dogs in this study had chronic kidney disease which may have resulted in compromised immunity and healing (Elliot et al., 2000). Infectious complications can be minimized with proper tube placement technique and careful monitoring of the tube site (e.g., daily bandage and stoma checks). Systemic prophylactic antimicrobials are not recommended but may become indicated if the stoma site becomes infected.

Mechanical complications include obstructed tubes or tube migration. If the latter complication is suspected, a contrast radiographic study can be performed to check for correct tube positioning. To perform this, a small amount of iodinated radiographic contrast medium is instilled into the tube and if the tube is correctly positioned in the stomach the contrast will be visible within the gastric rugal folds (Figure 6.18). Tube blockages can be prevented by proper tube management, such as flushing the tube with warm water before and after feeding. Using feeding tubes for administration of medications (especially sucralfate or aluminum hydroxide) should also be avoided as they can obstruct tubes. Proper preparation of the food (e.g., using a blender) before tube feeding can also

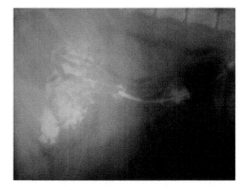

Figure 6.18 In cases requiring checking whether there is any leakage of contents from the stoma in the stomach, iodinated contrast media can be injected through the gastrostomy tube and the abdomen is immediately radiographed.

reduce the risk of tube obstruction. Liquidized diets should have a smooth consistency and be easily syringed without much resistance. Tubes that become obstructed can sometimes be unobstructed by forcibly flushing with warm water. Use of carbonated soft drinks, solutions containing pancreatic enzymes and bicarbonate have been reported as ways to unobstruct feeding tubes (Ireland et al., 2003; Michel, 2004; Parker and Freeman, 2013).

Summary

Gastrostomy tube feeding is one of the most effective means of providing enteral nutritional support to small animals. There are various options in regards to tube types and placement techniques and this enables the clinician to choose the most appropriate type of tube to be used on a particular patient. Appropriate patient selection and adherence to proper placement and feeding techniques are imperative. As with any mode of nutritional support, diligent patient monitoring and client education are required.

KEY POINTS

- Gastrostomy feeding tubes are one of the most effective means of providing enteral nutritional support for appropriately selected veterinary patients.
- Candidates for gastrostomy feeding tubes must have a functional gastrointestinal tract distal to the stomach, be able to undergo short duration general anesthesia, and not have a coagulopathy that would place them at risk of hemorrhage.
- Proper placement technique, tube management, and feeding protocols minimize complication risks.
- Placement techniques include percutaneous techniques (e.g., endoscope guided or blind) and surgical techniques.
- Gastrostomy tubes may also be replaced with low-profile gastrostomy ports for long-term usage.
- Gastrostomy feeding tubes can be managed by clients long-term with a variety of diets.
- Potential complications include improper placement or displacement of the tube, mechanical or infectious complications and gastrointestinal complications.
- Nutritional assessment and monitoring is critical for successful patient outcome.

Note

1 ELD gastrostomy tube applicator. Jorgensen Labs Inc., Loveland, CO.

References

Armstrong, P.J. and Hardie, E.M., (1990) Percutaneous endoscopic gastrostomy. A retrospective study of 54 clinical cases in dogs and cats. *Journal of Veterinary Internal Medicine*, **4**, 202–206.

Bright, R.M., DeNovo, R.C. and Jones, J.B. (1995) Use of a low-profile gastrostomy device for administrating nutrients in two dogs. *Journal of the American Veterinary Medical Association*, **207**(9), 1184–1186.

Cavanaugh, R.P., Kovak, J.R., Fischetti, A.J. et al. (2008) Evaluation of surgically placed gastro-jejunostomy feeding tubes in critically ill dogs. *Journal of the American Veterinary Medical Association*, **232**(3), 380–388.

DeLegge, R.L. and DeLegge, M.H. (2005) Percutaneous endoscopic gastrostomy evaluation of device material: are we "failsafe"? *Nutrition in Clinical Practice*, **20**, 613–617.

Elliot, D.A., Riel, D.L. and Rodgers, Q.R. (2000) Complications and outcomes associated with the use of gastrostomy tubes for nutritional treatment of dogs with renal failure. *Journal of the American Veterinary Medical Association*, **217**, 1337–1342.

Foster, L.A., Hoskinson, J.J. and Moore, T.L. (1999) Effect of implanting a gastrostomy tube on gastric emptying in cats. (Abstract) Proceedings of the Purina Forum, St. Louis, MO.

Fulton R.B. and Dennis, J.S. (1992) Blind percutaneous placement of a gastrostomy tube for nutritional support in dogs and cats. *Journal of the American Veterinary Medical Association*, **201**, 697–700.

Glaus, T.M., Cornelius , L.M., Bartges, J.W. et al. (1998) Complications with non-endoscopic percutaneous gastrostomy in 31 cats and 10 dogs: a retrospective study. *Journal of Small Animal Practice*, **39**, 218–222.

Ireland, L.M., Hohenhaus, A.E., Broussard, J.D. et al. (2003) A comparison of owner manage-ment and complications in 67 cats with esophagostomy and percutaneous endoscopic gas-trostomy feeding tubes. *Journal of the American Animal Hospital Association*, **39**, 241–246.

Jergens, A.E., Morrison, J.A., Miles, K.G. et al. (2007) Percutaneous endoscopic gastrojejunos-tomy tube placement in healthy dogs and cats. *Journal of Veterinary Internal Medicine*, **21**, 18–24.

McCrakin, M.A., DeNovo, R.C., Bright, R.M. et al. (1993) Endoscopic placement of a percuta-neous gastroduodenostomy feeding tube in dogs. *Journal of the American Veterinary Medical Association*, **203**, 792–797.

Marks, S.L. (2010) Nasoesophageal, esophagostomy, gastrostomy, and jejunal tube placement techniques. in *Textbook of Veterinary Internal Medicine*. 7th edn (eds S.J. Ettinger and E.C. Feldman) Saunders Elsevier, St. Louis. pp. 333–340.

Michel, K.E. (2004) Preventing and managing complications of enteral nutritional support. *Clinical Techniques in Small Animal Practice*, **19**(1), 49–53.

Parker, V. J. and Freeman, L. M. (2013) Comparison of various solutions to dissolve critical care diet clots. *Journal of Veterinary Emergency and Critical Care*, **23** (3), 344–347.

Seaman, R. and Legendre, A.M. (1998) Owner experience with home use of gastrostomy tubes in their dogs or cat. *Journal of the American Veterinary Medical Association*, **212**,1576–1578.

Smith, S.A., Ludlow, C.L., Hoskinson, J.J. et al. (1998) Effect of percutaneous endoscopic gas-trostomy on gastric emptying in clinically normal cats. *American Journal of Veterinary Research*, **59**(11), 1414–1416.

Stein, J., Schulte-Bockholt, A., Sabin, M. et al. (2002) A randomized trial of immediate vs. next-day feeding after percutaneous endoscopic gastrostomy in intensive care patients. *Intensive Care Medicine*, **28**, 1656–1660.

Yoshimoto, S.K., Marks, S.L., Struble, A.L. et al. (2006) Owner experience and complications with home use of a replacement low profile gastrostomy device for long-term enteral feeding in dogs. *Canadian Veterinary Journal*, **47**, 144–150.

CHAPTER 7

Jejunostomy feeding tubes in dogs and cats

F. A. (Tony) Mann[1] and Robert C. Backus[2]

[1] *Veterinary Medical Teaching Hospital, College of Veterinary Medicine, University of Missouri, Columbia, MO, USA*
[2] *Department of Veterinary Medicine and Surgery, College of Veterinary Medicine, University of Missouri, USA*

Introduction

Optimal wound healing requires ample nutrition and animals undergoing abdominal surgery often have multiple factors contributing to nutritional compromise. The underlying disease or trauma may have led to anorexia or increased metabolic demands. Vomiting and diarrhoea may also have been components of the underlying disease, contributing to a malnourished state. Abdominal surgery itself causes tissue trauma and the manipulation of organs may contribute to postoperative nausea and vomiting. Unquestionably, nutritional support will improve clinical outcomes in postoperative abdominal surgery patients, but achieving this can be challenging, especially when vomiting is a clinical sign. Parenteral nutritional support may be used, but enteral feeding is preferred because it is more physiologically sound, associated with fewer infectious and metabolic complications, and is generally less expensive. (Hegazi et al., 2011).

Indications for a jejunostomy feeding tube

When vomiting is a persistent clinical sign, the most effective feeding tube may be one that delivers nutrients distal to the stomach. Nasojejunal feeding tubes is one such example in patients not undergoing abdominal surgery (Wohl, 2006; Beal and Brown, 2011) but use of this technique is currently limited. If the abdominal cavity is exposed because of the necessity for celiotomy, then surgical jejunostomy tube placement should be considered. Although performing an abdominal surgery for the mere placement of a feeding tube would be considered rather invasive, if performed as part of an already planned abdominal surgery, jejunostomy tube placement can be quickly and effectively accomplished, adding less than 10 minutes to the surgical duration. At the authors' institution the indication for jejunostomy tube placement includes any abdominal surgery performed in a patient that has vomiting as a clinical sign of illness or may have

---

Nutritional Management of Hospitalized Small Animals, First Edition. Edited by Daniel L. Chan.

vomiting as a consequence of the surgical manipulations. Because of the latter indication, most patients undergoing abdominal surgery at the authors' institution receive a jejunostomy tube. This pre-emptive approach may result in tubes placed in some animals that do not necessarily need the tube but, using the interlocking box jejunopexy technique described in this chapter, the tube can be removed as soon after surgery as desired. Removing an unnecessary jejunostomy tube is simple; whereas, trying to later provide nutritional support in a postoperative vomiting patient can be quite difficult and may be limited to parenteral nutrition administration. In the authors' experience, though, very few jejunostomy tubes go unused, because many abdominal surgery patients will be on pain medication and sedatives that alter mentation and contribute to nausea and anorexia in the early postoperative period. Jejunostomy feedings permit early institution of enteral support, even in neurologically obtunded patients.

Jejunostomy feeding tube placement technique

1 A small diameter (5, 8 or 10 French) tube is chosen for jejunostomy. Most commonly, 8 French is used. Multiple tube biomaterial choices are available. Some common choices are red rubber,[1] polyurethane,[2] polyvinyl chloride,[3] and silicone[4] tubes. Silicone (Figure 7.1) is preferred because of minimal tissue reactivity compared to other tube biomaterials (Apalakis, 1976). If not damaged, silicone tubes can be cleaned, steam sterilized and used again.
2 Upon completion of the surgical procedures for which the celiotomy was performed, the surgeon should identify the site in the abdominal wall where the tube will exit. The exit stoma for the tube should be located in the right lateral

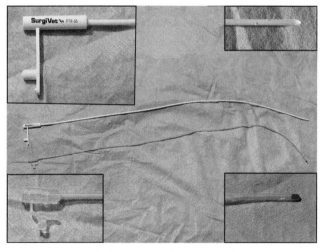

Figure 7.1 Silicone nasogastric tube for use as a jejunostomy tube. Manufacture of the white tube was discontinued in 2009 but is used in this chapter for ease of viewing in the illustrations. The clear tube substitute is less stiff, more stretchable, and a little more collapsible than the white tube. (Mann et al., 2011. Reproduced with permission from Wiley & Sons.).

abdominal wall in the mid-abdomen caudal to where a gastropexy would typically be performed (Figure 7.2). Whereas a left abdominal wall stoma would be acceptable, the authors find the right abdominal wall more practical for a right-handed surgeon and more anatomically appropriate for the segment of small intestine that will accommodate the tube.

3 The loop of intestine into which the jejunostomy tube will be introduced should be isolated and a stay suture should be placed to maintain orientation (Figure 7.3). The tube should enter the jejunum as cranially as is practical. It

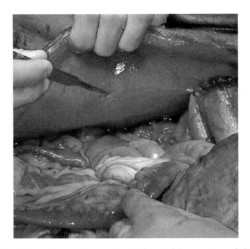

Figure 7.2 Location for jejunostomy tube entry in the middle portion of the right abdominal wall. (Cranial is to the right; view is from the perspective of an assistant to a right-handed surgeon.) Note the location of the incisional gastropexy cranial to the proposed jejunostomy tube entry site. The number 11 scalpel blade points to the proposed tube exit site. (Mann et al., 2011. Reproduced with permission from Wiley & Sons.).

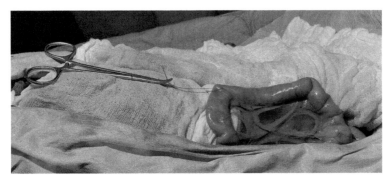

Figure 7.3 A 3-0 poliglecaprone 25 stay suture placed just cranial to the proposed jejunostomy site. (Cranial is to the left; view is from a right-handed surgeon's perspective.) A full-thickness bite of intestine is made, the stay suture is tagged with mosquito hemostatic forceps, and the jejunal loop is moved to the animal's left. The stay suture maintains orientation while the tube is introduced into the abdomen. (Mann et al., 2011. Reproduced with permission from Wiley & Sons.)

is acceptable for the tube to span an enterotomy or anastomosis site, but having the tip of the tube come to rest at such sites should be avoided.

4 The tube is introduced into the abdomen before placing it in the jejunum (Figure 7.4). From within the abdomen, a tiny stab incision is made with a number 11 scalpel blade in the transversus abdominis muscle in the mid-abdomen just caudal to the typical gastropexy location and approximately 4 cm from the midline incision.

5 A mosquito hemostatic forceps is introduced into the stab incision and force applied in a craniolateral direction until the tip can be palpated just lateral to the nipples of the mammary chain.

6 A tiny stab incision is made in the skin over the tip of the forceps, taking care to not make the incision any larger than necessary to permit exposure of the forceps' tip.

7 Then, the tip of the jenunostomy tube is grasped with the forceps and the tube is pulled into the abdomen.

8 After it is in the abdomen, the tube is placed into the jejunum (Figure 7.5).

9 A purse-string suture (or horizontal mattress suture, as preferred by the principal author) is placed in the antimesenteric border of the previously isolated cranial segment of jejunum using 3-0 absorbable monofilament suture material (such as poliglecaprone 25 or glycomer 631).

10 A tiny stab incision just large enough to accommodate the tube is made with a number 11 blade in the centre of the horizontal mattress suture, and the jejunostomy tube is introduced into the stab and advanced caudally for a

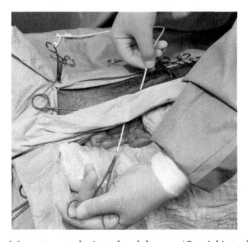

Figure 7.4 Pulling the jejunostomy tube into the abdomen. (Cranial is to the right; view is from an assistant surgeon's perspective, assuming that the surgeon is right-handed.) After a tiny puncture is made in the transversus abdominis muscle with a number 11 scalpel blade, a mosquito hemostatic forceps is introduced into the tiny puncture and advanced in a craniolateral direction until the tip can be felt under the skin just lateral to the nipple line. A number 11 scalpel blade is used to make a tiny incision over the forceps' tips just large enough to permit the tips to exit the skin immediately lateral to the nipple line. Then, the forceps' tips are opened to grab the tip of the tube and pull the tube into the abdominal cavity. (Mann et al., 2011. Reproduced with permission from Wiley & Sons.).

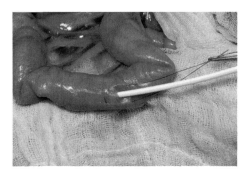

Figure 7.5 Placing the jejunostomy tube into the intestine. (Cranial is to the right; view is from an assistant surgeon's perspective, assuming that the surgeon is right handed.) The tube is positioned in the cranial aspect of the field while the purse-string suture (actually a horizontal mattress suture) is placed using full-thickness bites. The properly executed mattress suture resembles a "smiley face". A number 11 blade is used to make a hole in the centre of the mattress suture (a "nose" in the "smiley face"). The blade is held upside down with the sharp edge toward the "eyes" of the "smiley face" to avoid cutting the suture as could occur if the blade penetrated too close to the "mouth" of the "smiley face". Note that the cranial stay suture has been removed and the tube is threaded into the hole made in the intestine. The hole in the intestine should be just large enough to accommodate the tube. The tube is threaded caudally in the jejunum while gentle counter tension is applied to the tagged ends of the mattress suture. Saline is periodically injected via the tube into the intestine to provide mild distention and lubrication for ease of tube passage. The tube is advanced for a generous distance (the amount of intestine supplied by about three vascular arcades). Then, the horizontal mattress suture is tied to prevent leakage around the tube during remaining manipulations. The tube can still slide through the hole in the intestine so care must be taken to make sure the tube does not back out during the remainder of the procedure. The strands of the tied mattress suture are cut and the jejunum is aligned with the body wall in preparation for jejunopexy. (Mann et al., 2011. Reproduced with permission from Wiley & Sons.).

generous distance (one long intestinal loop, the length supplied by at least three vascular arcades).

11 The mattress suture is tied and the jejunum is secured to the body wall using 3-0 monofilament suture (e.g., poliglecaprone 25 or glycomer 631) in an interlocking box pattern (Figure 7.6).

12 The interlocking box pattern is chosen instead of simple interrupted sutures that tack the jejunum to the body wall because the interlocking boxes keep fluid that might leak around the tube in the intestine. Fluid could potentially leak around the tube into the subcutaneous tissues, but intestinal fluid should not be able to leak into the abdominal cavity. There is no need to wait for adhesions to seal the area around the tube for safe tube removal as is the case with simple tacking sutures. With the interlocking box technique the tube may be safely removed at any time (Daye, Huber and Henderson, 1999), and there should be little concern for peritonitis if the tube is prematurely removed by the patient. Prior to the development of the interlocking box suture pattern, jejunostomy tubes were left in place for 5 to 7 days to wait for the adhesive seal, regardless of whether or not the feeding tube was being used.

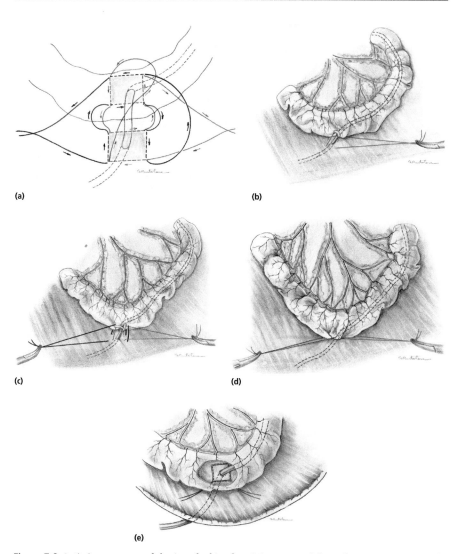

(a)

(b)

(c)

(d)

(e)

Figure 7.6 Artistic summary of the interlocking box jejunopexy. (These drawings are oriented from the perspective of a right-handed surgeon, with cranial to the left and caudal to the right.) **a**) The red (caudal) suture represents the first box with suture passes in the following order: (1) caudal to cranial in the body wall superficial to the tube, (2) superficial to deep in the intestine cranial to the tube, (3) cranial to caudal in the body wall deep to the tube, and (4) deep to superficial in the intestine caudal to the tube. The black (cranial) suture represents the second box with suture passes in the following order: (1) superficial to deep in the body wall cranial to the tube, (2) cranial to caudal in the intestine deep to the tube, (3) deep to superficial in the body wall caudal to the tube, and (4) caudal to cranial in the intestine superficial to the tube. **b**) The first box is completed and the (red) suture strands tagged with the forceps in the caudal aspect of the surgical field. **c**) Both boxes are completed with the black suture strands tagged with forceps in the cranial aspect of the surgical field. **d**) When the strands of both boxes are pulled the tube is no longer visible. **e**) The holes in the body wall and jejunum are juxtaposed and sandwiched between the jejunum and body wall within the interlocking boxes. Therefore, any fluid around the tube will stay in the intestine or could potentially leak into the subcutaneous tissues, but intestinal fluid should not be able to leak into the abdominal cavity. The suture strands are retained in this drawing for orientation purposes, but would be knotted and cut at this point. (Mann et al., 2011. Reproduced with permission from Wiley & Sons.).

13 The feeding tube is placed into the intestine as described above before the interlocking box sutures are placed. Then, the box sutures are placed in the following order (Figure 7.6).

14 The first box is started by passing caudocranially in the abdominal wall ventral (superficial) to the jejunostomy site.

15 The suture is then passed transversely across the jejunum (full-thickness bite) ventrodorsally just cranial to the jejunostomy.

16 The third pass is from cranial to caudal in the abdominal wall dorsal (deep) to the jejunostomy, and the final pass is from dorsal to ventral transversely in the intestine caudal to the jejunostomy. The suture strands are left long and tagged with hemostats.

17 The second box is started by passing ventrodorsally in the abdominal wall cranial to the jejunostomy.

18 The second suture is passed craniocaudally in the intestine dorsal (deep) to the jejunostomy.

19 The third suture is passed dorsoventrally in the body wall caudal to the jejunostomy, and the final pass is from caudal to cranial in the intestine ventral (superficial) to the jejunostomy. All suture passages in the jejunum are full-thickness bites.

20 The cranial suture strands are pulled together as are the previously placed caudal strands.

21 The caudal strands are tied to secure the first box and the cranial strands are tied to secure the second box.

22 Externally, the jejunostomy tube is anchored to skin and underlying fascia with four interrupted friction sutures placed 1 cm apart (Song, Mann and Wagner-Mann; Figure 7.7). Size 2-0 nylon or polypropylene is preferred for anchoring 8 French and 10 French tubes; size 3-0 is used for 5 French tubes.

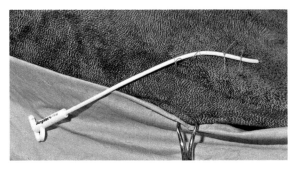

Figure 7.7 Anchoring the jejunostomy tube to the skin and underlying fascia with four friction sutures on the right side of the abdomen. (Cranial is to the left.) The first friction suture is placed as soon as the interlocking box jejunopexy is complete so that inadvertent tube withdrawal does not occur during remaining surgical manipulations. The first friction suture is placed immediately cranial and slightly lateral to the tube exit site, ensuring that the friction suture penetrates underlying fascia without entering the abdomen. Saline is injected into the tube after each friction suture is placed to make sure that the lumen of the tube is not obstructed by the suture. Three additional friction sutures are placed after the abdominal incision is closed. (Mann et al., 2011. Reproduced with permission from Wiley & Sons.)

23 Inject a small amount (0.5 to 1.0 mL) of saline into the tube after each friction suture is placed to ensure that the friction suture has not occluded the tube lumen.

Administration of liquid diets

The small diameter of jejunostomy tubes dictates the use of liquid diets. Of the many liquid diets available on the market, the authors have most experience with Canine/Feline CliniCare[5] (Abbott Laboratories, North Chicago, IL) and Formula V EnteralCare™ HPL[6] (PetAg, Hampshire, IL). These diets are alike in their formulations, being isotonic and containing polymeric ingredients that are principally mixtures of intact and hydrolyzed milk protein fractions and maltodextrins. Manufacturers of both diets claim that the nutrient profiles of their products meet established adult maintenance requirements of dogs and cats. However, compared to most commercially available maintenance diets for dogs, these two diets are much higher in protein (30% of metabolizable energy) and fat (40 to 45% of metabolizable energy) and lower in fibre (< 1% crude fibre as dry weight). The CliniCare product uniquely contains a marine fish oil, which through activity of long-chain n-3 fatty acids might modulate the systemic inflammatory response (Weimann et al., 1998). The EnteralCare HPL ("high protein-level") has been discontinued and substituted with a lower protein formulation called EnteralCare MPL[7] ("moderate protein-level").

These liquid diets have been administered via constant rate infusion using a specifically designed liquid diet feeding pump[8] and feeding administration set,[9] but intravenous fluid pumps, fluid bags and administration sets may be adapted for enteral feeding. In the latter case, particular attention must be paid to avoid inadvertent connection of an enteral feeding line to an intravenous catheter. The use of enteral safety devices with non-luer connections may prevent these inadvertent connections (see Chapter 5). The amounts and concentrations of enteral diet infused have varied but administration is typically begun within 24 hours of surgery (often within a couple hours of anaesthetic recovery) at a slow (5 mL per hour) rate with a ramping rate at the clinician's discretion to eventually meet resting energy requirement (RER). Rarely is the RER target met before the animal begins oral intake, demonstrating that the jejunostomy tube does not impair appetite, which is important because interest in food is a clinical indicator of recovery. For animals in which RER is not met, a benefit beyond supplying substrate for protein and energy needs may be gained from effects on the gut mucosal barrier and immune function (Hermsen, Sano and Kudsk, 2009), stimulation of intestinal blood flow (de Aguilar-Nascimento, 2005), and prevention of gut atrophy (Hartl and Alpers, 2011).

For those animals that do not eat enough or at all, jejunostomy feeding may be continued for as long as the animal is hospitalized. No maximum duration for leaving jejunostomy tubes in place has been reported. In the authors' experience, the median duration has been 2 to 3 days, with usages as long as 12 to 13 days. Jejunostomy tubes are not left in animals upon hospital dismissal because it is the rare pet owner who can maintain constant rate infusion. Bolus infusion into the jejunum is discouraged to avoid intestinal distention that may cause abdominal discomfort and to avoid lack of absorption and resultant diarrhea.

Passage of feces is absent in many animals undergoing jejunal feeding; whereas, in other animals, feces are not liquid but soft and variably formed. Soft feces may reflect the lack of fiber in the diets. To the authors' knowledge, fecal scores in normal healthy dogs given liquid diets have not been reported.

Complications of jejunostomy tubes

Complications of jejunostomy tubes include local cellulitis, inadvertent complete or partial removal of the tube, tube occlusion, stomal infection, and peritonitis (Swann, Sweet and Mitchell, 1997; Crowe and Devey, 1997; Yagil-Kelmer, Wagner-Mann and Mann, 2006). Self-limiting local cellulitis is the most common complication. Premature tube removal is typically inconsequential with the interlocking box jejunopexy technique, other than the loss of a feeding route. Incompletely removed tubes rarely require intervention other than monitoring for the retained portion in the intestine to be eliminated in the feces. Tube occlusion is usually the result of not flushing the tube when liquid diet administration is interrupted. Instilling carbonated beverage into the tube may solve this complication in most situations. Peritonitis is rare with the technique described here and often cannot be specifically attributed to the jejunostomy.

Removal of jejunostomy tubes

When removing a jejunostomy tube, inject the tube with approximately 5 mL of water or saline to ensure that residual food is flushed into the intestinal lumen and not dragged through the subcutaneous tissues of the abdominal wall. Cut the friction sutures and gently extract the tube. Although jejunostomy tube removal is well tolerated by dogs and cats, infiltration with local anesthetic around the exit stoma skin and body wall will lessen tube removal discomfort. Periodically cleanse the stoma as needed to remove secretions. Secretions from the stoma are usually mild and typically resolve in 3 to 5 days.

Summary

Jejunostomy tubes are placed during celiotomy with a pre-emptive approach to ensure a reliable method of feeding should postoperative vomiting ensue. The interlocking box jejunopexy technique permits early jejunostomy tube removal from patients with early adequate caloric intake and allays concerns about abdominal sepsis in animals that prematurely remove their tubes. Serious complications with jejunostomy tube placement technique described here are rare and others are self-limiting or easily managed.

KEY POINTS

- When vomiting is a persistent clinical sign, the most effective feeding tube may be one that delivers nutrients distal to the stomach.

- If the animal requires a celiotomy and nutritional support, then a surgical jejunostomy tube placement should be considered.

- Jejunostomy tube placement can be performed quickly and effectively accomplished, adding less than 10 minutes to the surgery time.

- Using a pre-emptive approach of jejunostomy tube placement may result in tubes placed in some animals that do not necessarily need the tube, but using the interlocking box jejunopexy technique, the tube can be removed as soon after surgery as desired.

- The small diameter of jejunostomy tubes dictates the use of liquid diets.

- Serious complications associated with the jejunostomy tube placement technique described in this chapter are rare and others are self-limiting or easily managed.

Notes

1 SOVEREIGN Feeding Tube and Urethral Catheter, Covidien Animal Health & Dental Division, Mansfield, MA.
2 Argyle Indwell Polyurethane Feeding Tube, Covidien Animal Health & Dental Division, Mansfield, MA.
3 Argyle Polyvinyl Chloride Feeding Tube with Sentinel Line, Covidien Animal Health & Dental Division, Mansfield, MA.
4 Nasal Oxygen/Feeding Tube-Silicone, Smiths Medical, Waukesha, WI.
5 Canine/Feline CliniCare, 2009 formulation: 340 mOsm/kg, 1 kcal/mL, 8.2 g/100 kcal crude protein, 5.2 g/100 kcal crude fat, 0.1 g/100 kcal crude fiber, 56 mg/100 kcal eicosapentaenoic acid, 36 mg/100 kcal docosapentaenoic acid, Abbott Laboratories, North Chicago, IL.
6 Formula V EnteralCare™ HPL: 312 mOsm/kg, 1.2 kcal/mL, 8.5 g/100 kcal crude protein, 4.8 g/100 kcal crude fat, 0.2 g/100 kcal crude fiber, 1.3 mg/100 kcal docosapentaenoic acid (typical analysis, dated April 26, 2007), provided from PetAg, Inc., Hampshire, Il, September 10, 2010, after request by author, RCB.
7 Formula V EnteralCare™ MPL: 258 mOsm/kg, 1.2 kcal/mL, 7.5 g/100 kcal crude protein, 6.6 g/100 kcal crude fat, 0.2 g/100 kcal crude fiber, http://www.petag.com/wp-content/uploads/2011/03/Item%2099430%20-%20EnteralCareMLP%20PDS.pdf (accessed June 25, 2011).
8 Kangaroo 224 Feeding Pump, Sherwood Medical, St. Louis, MO.
9 Kangaroo Pump Set, Sherwood Medical, St. Louis, MO.

References

Apalakis, A. (1976) An experimental evaluation of the types of material used for bile duct drainage tubes. *British Journal of Surgery*, **63**, 440–445.

Beal, M.W. and Brown, A.J. (2011) Clinical experience using a novel fluoroscopic technique for wire-guided nasojenual tube placement in the dog: 26 cases (2006–2010). *Journal of Veterinary Emergency and Critical Care*, **21**,151–157.

Crowe, D.T. and Devey, J.J. (1997) Clinical experience with jejunostomy feeding tubes in 47 small animal patients. *Journal of Veterinary Emergency Critical Care*, **7**, 7–19.

Daye, R.M., Huber, M.L. and Henderson, R.A. (1999) Interlocking box jejunostomy: a new technique for enteral feeding. *Journal of the American Animal Hospital Association*, **35**, 129–134.

de Aguilar-Nascimento, J.E. (2005) The role of macronutrients in gastrointestinal blood flow. *Current Opinion Clinical Nutrition Metabolic Care*, **8**, 552–556.

Hartl, W.H. and Alpers, D.H. (2011) The trophic effects of substrate, insulin, and the route of administration on protein synthesis and the preservation of small bowel mucosal mass in large mammals. *Clinical Nutrition*, **30**, 20–27.

Hegazi, R., Raina, A., Graham, T. et al. (2011) Early jejunal feeding initiation and clinical outcomes in patients with severe acute pancreatitis. *Journal of Parenteral and Enteral Nutrition*, **35**, 91–96.

Hermsen, J.L., Sano, Y. and Kudsk, K.A. (2009) Food fight! Parenteral nutrition, enteral stimulation and gut-derived mucosal immunity. *Langenbecks Archives of Surgery*, **394**, 17–30.

Mann F.A., Constantinescu G.M. and Yoon H. (2011) *Fundamentals of Small Animal Surgery*, Wiley-Blackwell, Ames, Iowa.

Song, E.K., Mann, F.A. and Wagner-Mann, C.C. (2008) Comparison of different tube materials and use of Chinese finger trap or four friction suture technique for securing gastrostomy, jejunostomy, and thoracostomy tubes in dogs. *Veterinary Surgery*, **37**, 212–221.

Swann, H.M., Sweet, D.C. and Michel, K. (1997) Complications associated with use of jejunostomy tubes in dogs and cats: 40 cases (1989–1994). *Journal of the American Veterinary Medical Association*, **210**, 1764–1767.

Weimann, A., Bastian, L., Bischoff, W.E. et al. (1998) Influence of arginine, omega-3 fatty acids and nucleotide-supplemented enteral support on systemic inflammatory response syndrome and multiple organ failure in patients after severe trauma. *Nutrition*, **14**, 165–172.

Wohl, J.S. (2006) Nasojejunal feeding tube placement using fluoroscopic guidance: technique and clinical experience in dogs. *Journal of Veterinary Emergency Critical Care*, **16**(S1), S27–S33.

Yagil-Kelmer, E., Wagner-Mann, C. and Mann, F.A. (2006) Postoperative complications associated with jejunostomy tube placement using the interlocking box technique compared with other jejunopexy methods in dogs and cats: 76 cases (1999–2003). *Journal of Veterinary Emergency Critical Care*, **16**(S1), S14–S20.

CHAPTER 8

Minimally invasive placement of postpyloric feeding tubes

Matthew W. Beal

Emergency and Critical Care Medicine, Director of Interventional Radiology Services, College of Veterinary Medicine, Michigan State University, USA

Introduction

The importance of nutritional support in hospitalized small animal patients is widely accepted (Remillard et al., 2001; Chan, 2004; Michel and Higgens, 2006; Chan and Freeman, 2006; Holahan et al., 2010). In people, significant debate still exists as to whether enteral nutritional support (EN) is superior to parenteral nutritional support (PN) (Heyland et al., 2003; Gramlich et al., 2004; Peter, Moran and Phillips-Hughes, 2005; Altintas et al., 2011). Proponents of EN cite advantages including significantly shorter lengths-of-stay (Peter et al., 2005) and significantly fewer infectious complications (Heyland et al., 2003; Gramlich et al., 2004; Peter et al., 2005), especially catheter-related bloodstream infections, and shorter duration of ventilatory support (Altintas et al., 2011) when compared to people fed parenterally. EN may also promote gastrointestinal mucosal health by reducing mucosal atrophy, intestinal permeability and gut bacterial translocation. In addition, EN may be significantly less expensive than PN support (Gramlich et al., 2004). However, the proposed advantages of EN are not uniformly accepted in people and some potential advantages of PN include a decrease in the time to achieving feeding goals and ease of administration (Altintas et al., 2011). Specific benefits imparted by EN (over PN) on hospitalized small animal patients are unknown. However, because of the evidence to support their use in human medicine, EN methods are widely utilized in veterinary medicine (Waddell and Michel, 1998; Heuter, 2004; Hewitt et al., 2004; Han, 2004; Salinardi et al., 2006; Wohl, 2006; Jergens et al., 2007; Campbell et al., 2010; Holahan et al., 2010). Establishing esophageal or gastric feeding tube access for EN is quick and easy to perform (see Chapters 4–6), but sometimes, these methods are either contraindicated or feeding is poorly tolerated, as evidenced by nausea and vomiting (Abood and Buffington, 1992; Holahan et al., 2010). Postpyloric feedings mitigate this problem by bypassing the esophagus and stomach allowing the provision of EN. Surgical jejunostomy techniques are well established (see Chapter 7), however, the methods are invasive and complications occur in approximately 17.5–40% of clinical patients (Crowe and Devey

Nutritional Management of Hospitalized Small Animals, First Edition. Edited by Daniel L. Chan.
© 2015 John Wiley & Sons, Ltd. Published 2015 by John Wiley & Sons, Ltd.

1997; Swann, Sweet and Michel, 1997; Hewitt et al., 2004; Yagil-Kelmer et al., 2006). These complications include, but are not limited to, septic peritonitis, ostomy site infection or inflammation, tube dislodgement, or tube occlusion. Minimally invasive techniques for achieving jejunal access utilizing the nasoje-junal (NJ), gastrojejunal (GJ), and esophagojejunal (EJ) routes with either fluor-oscopic or endoscopic assistance offer an alternative to surgical jejunostomy / gastrojejunostomy (Jennings et al., 2001; Heuter, 2004, Wohl, 2006; Jergens et al., 2007; Papa et al., 2009; Beal, Jutkowitz and Brown, 2007; Beal et al., 2009; Beal and Brown, 2011; Campbell and Daley, 2011).

Indications and patient selection

The small animal patients that will benefit from minimally invasive postpy-loric feeding tubes are those with contraindications to or intolerance of esoph-ageal or gastric feeding. This includes animals with protracted vomiting or regurgitation, those at a high risk of aspiration due to their underlying dis-ease, those with altered levels of consciousness and those with gastric motility disorders. Clinical studies describing NJ and GJ techniques most often included patients with pancreatitis as well as those with protracted vomiting due to peritonitis, parvoviral enteritis, acute renal failure and cholangiohepatitis/cholecystitis, and those with altered levels of consciousness due to post-arrest status, prolonged seizures, the need for ventilatory support and intracranial neoplasia (Jennings et al., 2001; Wohl, 2006; Beal and Brown, 2011; Campbell and Daley, 2011).

General anesthesia is recommended for the placement of GJ, NJ, and EJ tubes although there is one study in which NJ tubes were placed with seda-tion and utilization of local anesthesia techniques (Wohl, 2006). NJ tube placement can be very stimulating even in the face of (intranasal) local anes-thetic infusion due to pain associated with passage of different devices through the nose and the gag reflex that may be associated with pharyngeal stimulation. The patient population undergoing NJ placement often has a history of vomiting or regurgitation and a resulting risk of aspiration pneu-monia. When used in conjunction with intranasal infusion of local anes-thetic agents, general anesthesia will allow endotracheal intubation and protection of the airway while eliminating pain and pharyngeal stimulation. GJ and EJ techniques will require general anesthesia in large part because they are more invasive than NJ techniques. Assessment of primary and secondary hemostasis (platelet count, prothrombin time (PT), activated partial thromboplastin time (aPTT)) is recommended prior to NJ, GJ, or EJ tube placement due to the risk of epistaxis, cervical hemorrhage, peritoneal or gastrointestinal hemorrhage. Animals with evidence of spontaneous bleeding coupled with a hemostatic abnormality, or those with thrombocyto-penia (<35 000/μL) or significant prolongations in PT or aPTT should have their hemostatic abnormalities resolved prior to elective NJ, GJ, or EJ tube placement.

Nasojejunal tube placement

Technique description

Nasojejunal tube placement has been described using various fluoroscopic and endoscopic techniques (Jennings et al., 2001; Wohl, 2006; Papa et al., 2009; Beal et al., 2007; Beal et al., 2009; Beal and Brown, 2011; Campbell and Daley, 2011). Regardless of technique, utilization of local or regional anesthesia of the nose/face, in addition to general anesthesia, will facilitate patient tolerance of the placement procedure.

The original fluoroscopic NJ technique (FNJ) described by Wohl (2006) utilizes fluoroscopic imaging and a weighted feeding tube[1, 2] coupled with positional variation to facilitate passage of the tube across the pylorus, through the duodenum and into the jejunum. The patient is initially positioned in sternal recumbency while the tube is advanced from the nares into the esophagus. The patient is then placed in right lateral recumbency as the tube is advanced into the stomach. Then, the patient is returned to sternal recumbency or placed in left lateral recumbency as the tube is advanced into the body of the stomach. Positioning of the tube can be confirmed by returning the patient to sternal recumbency. The patient is then placed in left lateral recumbency and air can be infused via the tube to help illustrate the pyloric antrum (if not already air filled) and identify the pylorus itself. The tube is then pushed through the pylorus, down the descending duodenum, up the ascending duodenum and into the jejunum. The overall success of transpyloric passage of the tube using this technique was approximately 74% (Wohl, 2006). Amongst dogs in which transpyloric passage was achieved, success at achieving jejunal access was 74% (overall ability to achieve jejunal access was approximately 56%) (Wohl, 2006).

A technique for fluoroscopic, wire-guided NJ (FWNJ) has been previously described by the author in a series of 26 dogs with critical illness (Beal and Brown, 2011). This procedure is best performed with the patient positioned in left lateral recumbency.

1 Once the patient is in a favorable plane of anesthesia and local anesthetic has been infused into the nares, a well-lubricated 8 Fr red rubber feeding tube[3] with the tip removed to create an end-hole is passed ventrally and medially through the ventral nasal meatus and into the proximal esophagus. Intermittent fluoroscopy confirms tube location.

2 Through this catheter, a moistened 260 cm, 0.035 in (0.89 mm) straight-tip, standard stiffness, hydrophilic guide wire (HGW)[4] is advanced down the esophagus and into the stomach (Figure 8.1).

3 The red rubber feeding tube is removed and a 4 Fr or 5 Fr 100 cm Berenstein (angled) catheter[5] is advanced over the HGW and into the stomach. The left lateral positioning facilitates the accumulation of air in the pylorus and illustrates its location (Figure 8.2). If the pylorus is not easily visualized, 5–20 mL of room air is infused into the stomach via the Berenstein catheter.

4 The Berenstein catheter is used to direct the HGW towards and eventually across the pylorus (Figure 8.3). The HGW should always lead the Berenstein

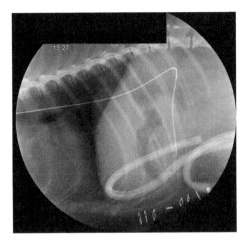

Figure 8.1 A 0.035 in (0.89 mm) straight-tip, standard stiffness, hydrophilic guide wire (HGW)[4] is advanced down the esophagus and into the stomach.

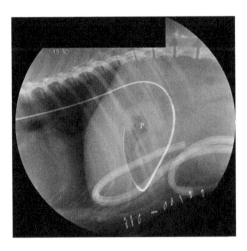

Figure 8.2 A 4–5 Fr 100 cm Berenstein (angled) catheter[5] is advanced over the HGW and into the stomach. The left lateral positioning facilitates the accumulation of air in the pylorus (P).

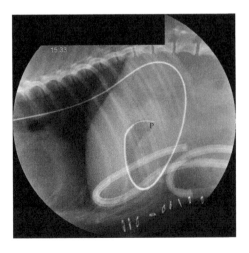

Figure 8.3 The Berenstein catheter is used to direct the HGW towards and eventually across the pylorus (P).

catheter to prevent trauma to the wall of the gastrointestinal tract. The Berenstein is advanced over the HGW and into the duodenum and the HGW is then advanced well into the jejunum. Due to the number of "turns" in the path to the jejunum (esophagus to pylorus, pylorus into descending duodenum, descending to ascending duodenum), advancement of the HGW can sometimes be challenging. Switching to a 0.035 in (0.89 mm) 260 cm straight-tip, stiff, hydrophilic guide wire[6] will sometimes improve the "pushability" of the wire and advancement of the Berenstein catheter over it (and often the feeding tube as well).

5 Once the HGW is advanced into the jejunum, the Berenstein catheter is removed over the HGW and a well lubricated, end-hole-modified (bolus tip removed, tip thermally smoothed, and side holes created), 8 Fr 140 cm (55 in) feeding tube[7] is advanced over the HGW and into the jejunum (Figure 8.4).

6 The HGW is then removed.

Using this technique, ability to achieve transpyloric passage was 92% and ability to achieve jejunal access was 78% (Beal and Brown, 2011). In the remaining dogs, the tube terminated at the caudal flexure of the duodenum or in the ascending duodenum. In this series, the ability to achieve jejunal access in the second half of the study period was 100%. This improvement was attributed to improved technical capability of the operator. Median procedural time was 35±20 minutes (Beal and Brown, 2011).

Endoscopic techniques for NJ tube placement (EndoNJ) have also been described (Papa et al., 2009; Campbell and Daley, 2011). In 2009, Papa et al. described a technique in three normal dogs in which dogs were positioned in left lateral recumbency and a flexible endoscope (9 mm diameter, 130 cm long, 2.8 mm diameter working channel) was inserted orally and advanced into the duodenum. Next, a 450 cm 0.035 in (0.89 mm) guide wire[8] is advanced down the working channel and into the jejunum and an 8 Fr, 250 cm long PVC[9] feeding tube is advanced over the guide wire, also down the working channel of the endoscope and into the jejunum. The endoscope is removed over the feeding

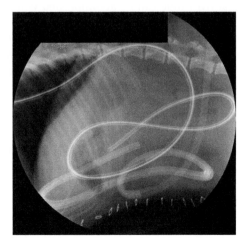

Figure 8.4 Once the HGW is advanced into the jejunum, the Berenstein catheter is removed over the HGW and a well lubricated, end-hole-modified (bolus tip removed, tip thermally smoothed, and side holes created), 8 Fr 137.5 cm (54 in) feeding tube[7] is advanced over the HGW and into the jejunum.

tube and guide wire. To achieve nasal passage of the tube, a lubricated catheter[3] was passed down the nose and exteriorized via the mouth, attached to the feeding tube, and withdrawn, pulling the feeding tube out of the nose. The median procedural time in the study demonstrating this technique was 30 min (range 15–45 min). This technique was associated with achieving jejunal access in all dogs (Papa et al., 2009).

A second EndoNJ technique utilized in 5 clinical cases (dogs) was described by Campbell and Daley (2011). In this technique, the patient is positioned in left lateral recumbency and an 8–9 Fr feeding tube is advanced into the stomach via the nose. A fiberoptic endoscope (9.3 mm diameter, 2.3 mm working channel, 103 cm length) is then advanced via the mouth into the stomach. Under endoscopic visualization, the feeding tube is advanced into the pyloric antrum. Next, a 170 cm, 2.4 mm diameter grasping forceps[10, 11] is advanced via the working channel to grasp the feeding tube approximately 1 cm from its distal tip. The endoscope, forceps, and feeding tube are then positioned just over the pylorus. The grasping forceps and feeding tube are then advanced into the pylorus. The grasping forceps are released and withdrawn and the scope is backed up 3–5 cm. The shaft of the feeding tube is then re-grasped and advanced into the pylorus. This process was repeated until the desired length of feeding tube was advanced beyond the pylorus to achieve jejunal access. In the case series describing this method, median procedural duration was 35 min (range 30–45 min) and jejunal access was achieved in all dogs (Campbell and Daley, 2011). The authors found this EndoNJ technique technically challenging due to difficulty grasping the tube with the grasping forceps.

Regardless of placement technique, securing the NJ tube is of critical importance to prevent external migration or premature removal of the tube by the patient. Folding the tube under the alar fold and securing it at this location utilizing 2-0 or 3-0 nylon[12] in a finger trap pattern and at additional locations along the side of the face is generally effective. Tube security is enhanced when an Elizabethan collar is also utilized.

Removal of the NJ tube or conversion to a nasogastric (NG) or nasoesophageal (NE) tube can be accomplished when the patient no longer demonstrates intolerance of, or contraindications to, gastric feeding. Conversion to a NG or NE can be accomplished with the instillation of 0.2–0.3 mg/kg of lidocaine[13] intranasally q 5 min for 3 doses, removal of the finger trap that secured the tube adjacent to the nose and backing the tube out until it is positioned within the stomach or esophagus as desired. The tube is then resutured adjacent to the alar fold as previously described.

Monitoring

When utilizing the FNJ and FWNJ techniques, the exact location of the tube is always known. EndoNJ techniques will require post-procedural radiography to confirm tube placement. The author routinely infuses 2–3 mL of a sterile, iodine-based contrast agent[14] into the NJ to confirm intraluminal placement during final imaging. Additional monitoring of tube location is probably unnecessary unless the patient exteriorizes a portion of the tube from the nose (suggesting migration) or demonstrates signs suggestive of intolerance of feeding, such as vomiting of the enteral diet (suggesting orad migration), abdominal pain or other clinical signs that could be referable to the procedure.

Complications

Procedural complications associated with NJ tube placement are generally minor. Reported procedural complications include mild epistaxis and inability to achieve transpyloric or jejunal access (Wohl, 2006; Beal and Brown, 2011). There has been the suggestion that the use of IV metoclopramide[15] to increase antral contractions may facilitate passage of NJ tubes (Wohl, 2006).

In the hours to days after the placement procedure, orad migration of the tube is the most common complication (Wohl, 2006; Beal and Brown, 2011). Based on the available literature, it appears that inability to position the tube within the jejunum (duodenal positioning) is one of the greatest risk factors for orad migration (Wohl, 2006; Beal and Brown, 2011). In the study by Wohl (2006), insertion of the tube past the duodenojejunal flexure was associated with a lower incidence of oral migration than that seen in tubes that rested duodenally in which 86% migrated orally. Sneezing and vomiting may be risk factors for oral migration and should be pharmacologically managed for this reason and for patient comfort. Instillation of 0.2–0.3 mg/kg of lidocaine[13] intranasally and resuturing the finger trap suture in a slightly different location may help alleviate sneezing. Vomiting and diarrhoea may occur after NJ tube placement, however, many patients have one or both of these signs prior to placement of the NJ. In one study, the incidence of vomiting and diarrhea was the same post-procedure as it was before the procedure (Beal and Brown, 2011). Additional minor complications in the post-procedural period include mild nasal discharge and facial irritation as well as kinking of the tube as it makes the turn from the nares under the alar fold (Wohl, 2006; Beal and Brown, 2011; Campbell and Daley, 2011).

Gastrojejunal tube placement

Minimally invasive placement of GJ tubes offers additional options for postpyloric feeding for animals that are intolerant of, or have contraindications to esophageal or gastric feeding. Advantages of many GJ systems include the ability to feed enterally while providing gastric decompression, the ability to easily transition from postpyloric feeding to gastric feeding (of a non-liquid diet), and the ability to achieve more aboral placement within the jejunum compared to nasojejunal techniques in dogs (author experience). Disadvantages of GJ tubes in comparison to NJ tubes include the necessity for the tube to remain in place until a healthy ostomy develops, risk of septic peritonitis due to tube dislodgement, a high incidence of minor ostomy complications and a degree of increased technical complexity (Jennings et al., 2001; Jergens et al., 2007; Beal et al., 2009). In addition to a surgical technique (Cavanaugh et al., 2008), many minimally invasive techniques have been described for GJ tube placement including a percutaneous endoscopic gastrojejunal tube (PEGJ)

(Jennings et al., 2001; Heuter, 2004; Jergens et al., 2007) and a percutaneous radiologic gastrojejunal tube placement (PRGJ) (Beal et al., 2009).

Technique description

Numerous PEGJ techniques have been described (Jennings et al., 2001; Heuter, 2004; Jergens et al., 2007), however, the technique described by Jergens et al. (2007) is the most objectively evaluated technique in normal dogs and cats. Commercially available PEGJ kits[16] are recommended because they allow precise interdigitation between the gastric segment of the tube and the jejunal segment, thus minimizing leakage and other complications. An endoscope suitable for upper gastrointestinal endoscopy is required for this method.

1 The technique described by Jergens et al. (2007) begins with routine placement of a percutaneous endoscopic gastrostomy (PEG) tube (see Chapter 6).
2 Next, a snare is passed through the PEG tube and opened within the stomach.
3 The endoscope is advanced from the mouth and into the stomach, through the snare (in right lateral recumbency), across the pylorus (in left lateral recumbency) and into the duodenum or jejunum.
4 A 0.035 in (0.89 mm) 270 cm HGW[17] is advanced through the working channel of the scope and well into the jejunum.
5 The endoscope is then withdrawn over the HGW leaving the HGW within the lumen of the snare.
6 Some additional length of HGW is placed into the stomach and the snare is then closed around the HGW and withdrawn back through the PEG (a "U"-shaped wire is withdrawn with one arm extending into the jejunum and the other orad).
7 The orad segment of the HGW is identified and pulled down from the mouth and exteriorized. At this point in the procedure, there is a HGW that originates externally, passes through the PEG, into the stomach, across the pylorus and into the jejunum.
8 Finally, the jejunal portion of the PEGJ tube is advanced over the HGW and into the jejunum. In the study by Jergens et al. (2007), a 24 Fr gastrostomy tube was utilized in concert with a 12 Fr jejunal segment of varying lengths depending on the size of the patient (65 or 95 cm). Utilizing this technique in dogs and cats, the ability to achieve jejunal access was 100%. Median procedural time was 45 min (range 39–57 min) in dogs and 25 min (range 22–31 min) in cats (Jergens, 2007).

The author recently described a technique for PRGJ in normal dogs (Beal et al., 2009).

1 Briefly, dogs are positioned in right lateral recumbency and the stomach is insufflated with air from an orogastric or nasogastric tube.
2 Fluoroscopy is utilized to identify a location caudal to the left, 13th rib for placement of 3 gastrointestinal suture anchors (GSA)[18] into the stomach in a triangular pattern, creating a gastropexy allowing apposition of the stomach to the left body wall during the GJ placement.
3 An 18 Ga puncture needle[19] is advanced through the center of the triangle created by the GSA and into the stomach allowing for passage of a

0.035 in, (0.889 mm) 150 cm, standard stiffness, hydrophilic guide wire with a straight, flexible tip.[20]

4 A 5 Fr angled guiding catheter[18] is then passed over the HGW and used to direct the HGW across the pylorus and duodenum and into the jejunum. This portion of the procedure is performed in sternal or left-sternal recumbency. The latter positioning allows air to fill and outline the pylorus, however, manipulation of the devices entering the insertion site is challenging.

5 Serial, over-the-wire dilation[18] of the body wall facilities placement of an 18 Fr peel-away introducer[18] through which an 18 Fr/8 Fr 58 cm dual-lumen GJ tube[21] is advanced over the HGW and into the stomach and jejunum.

6 The intragastric balloon retention mechanism is then inflated and used in concert with the external bolster to help prevent migration (Figures 8.5 and 8.6).

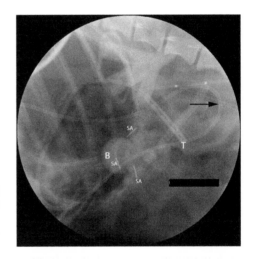

Figure 8.5 Lateral radiograph illustrating suture anchors (SA), intragastric balloon retention mechanism (B) and extension of the jejunal segment of the GJ tube past the caudal duodenal flexure (arrow) with the tip of the tube (T) terminating in the jejunum. (Weisse 2015. Reproduced with permission of Wiley & Sons.).

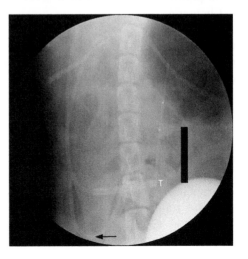

Figure 8.6 Ventrodorsal radiograph illustrating the extension of the jejunal segment of a GJ tube past the caudal duodenal flexure (arrow) with the tip of the tube (T) terminating in the jejunum. (Weisse 2015. Reproduced with permission of Wiley & Sons.).

In a pilot study that allowed development of this technique, jejunal access was accomplished in all dogs. Median time to traversing the pylorus with the HGW was 23.5 min (range 14–93 min). Median total procedural time was 53 min (range 42–126 min). Challenges encountered with the PRGJ technique included identifying and successfully traversing the pylorus as well as serial dilation of the gastrostomy site (Beal et al., 2009).

Depending on the GJ system utilized, the jejunal segment of the feeding tube may be able to be removed when the patient is eating or no longer has contraindications to or intolerance of gastric feeding. The gastric portion of GJ tubes placed using minimally invasive techniques should remain in place for approximately 2 weeks to allow the ostomy time to mature. In severely debilitated animals, due to poor healing, the tube may need to remain in place for a significantly longer period of time. Septic peritonitis has developed after tube removal in dogs and cats up to 4 weeks after placement (Armstrong and Hardie, 1990; Salinardi et al., 2006).

Monitoring

When utilizing the PRGJ techniques, the exact location of the tube is always known because the procedure is performed with fluoroscopic guidance. PEGJ techniques will require post-procedural radiography to confirm tube placement. The author routinely infuses 2–3mL of a sterile, iodine-based contrast agent[14] into the jejunal and gastric ports of GJ tubes to confirm intraluminal placement during final imaging. Additional monitoring of tube location is probably unnecessary unless the patient dislodges the jejunal segment from the gastric tube (based on the type of GJ system utilized) or demonstrates signs suggestive of intolerance of feeding, such as vomiting of the enteral diet (suggesting orad migration), abdominal pain or other clinical signs that could be referable to the procedure. GJ tubes should be maintained according to the standards described in Chapter 6. Patients with GJ tubes should be monitored closely for evidence of ostomy infection (redness, swelling, discharge, fever) or septic peritonitis (acute abdomen, fever, shock, anorexia, vomiting) as described in Chapter 6.

Complications

Procedural complications are uncommon in both the PEGJ and PRGJ techniques and, much like NJ techniques, migration of the tube and removal of the tube by the patient are the most common post-procedural complications in dogs (Jergens et al., 2007, Beal et al., 2009). In the study by Jergens et al. (2007), orad migration was a problem when the jejunal segment of the tube was duodenal in position because it was too short (65 cm). This problem was mitigated when a 95 cm jejunal segment was used. In this study, two dogs also removed their tubes prematurely (Jergens et al., 2007). Additional minor complications reported in this study in dogs included ostomy infection, and diarrhea. In cats, soft stool, transient fever, and pain at the ostomy site were noted. In the study by Beal et al. (2009), mild redness and discharge were noted at the ostomy site in all dogs. Although not seen in the aforementioned studies, failure of the ostomy site with development of septic peritonitis is a recognized complication of gastrostomy tube placement (Salinardi et al., 2006). The utilization of GSA may help relieve tension on the tube and thus help maintain the ostomy, thus making it less likely to fail. Additional investigation into the utilization of these devices in the future is warranted.

Esophagojejunal tube placement

Perhaps the procedure that provides the optimal blend of the advantages of both NJ and GJ procedures while mitigating the complications of both is the esophago-jejunal (EJ) tube. This is minimally irritating to the patient (in contrast to the NJ tube) and is unlikely to trigger the sneezing that together predispose to prema-ture dislodgement or removal of an NJ tube. In addition, in contrast to the GJ tube, if an EJ tube becomes dislodged prematurely, the ostomy will usually close without a major risk of life-threatening infection. Lastly, in comparison to the NJ tube in large dogs in which the length of the feeding tube sometimes precludes insertion well into the jejunum, the EJ tube places the insertion site approxi-mately 10–20 cm closer to the jejunum.

Technique description
The technique for fluoroscopic EJ placement is similar to that for fluoroscopic NJ placement.
1 An esophagostomy (E) tube is placed routinely (See Chapter 5) and a 0.035 in (0.89 mm) 260 cm standard stiffness, straight tip, hydrophilic guide wire[4] is introduced through the esophagostomy tube and advanced into the stomach. Esophagostomy is best performed on the left side, but can be performed on the right if there are contraindications to placement on the left (such as prox-imity to a pre-existing central venous catheter).
2 The esophagostomy tube is removed over the HGW and a 10 Fr peel-away introducer[22] placed over it.
3 The patient is rotated to left lateral recumbency allowing air to fill the pyloric antrum. Draping should be utilized to attempt to maintain cleanliness at the insertion site.
4 The 5 Fr 100 cm Berenstein[5] catheter is introduced over the HGW via the peel-away sheath introducer and is used to direct the HGW across the pylorus.
5 The remainder of the procedure proceeds as it would for the FWNJ tube.
6 Once the EJ tube is in place, the peel-away sheath is exteriorized and peeled-away and the tube is secured in place using 3-0 nylon[i] in a purse-string / finger trap pattern.
7 A sterile dressing is placed at the insertion site.
   Removal of the EJ tube or conversion to an E tube can be accomplished when the patient no longer demonstrates intolerance of or contraindications to gastric feeding. Conversion to an E tube can be accomplished by removal of the

finger trap that secured the tube at the insertion site and backing the tube out until it is positioned within the stomach or distal esophagus as desired. If a larger diameter E tube is desired, then a 0.035 in (0.889 mm), 260 cm, stiff guide wire[6] can be introduced down the EJ tube and the EJ tube can be removed. A peel-away introducer large enough to accommodate the size of the E-tube can then be introduced over the PTFE guide wire into the esophagus. The E tube is fed over the wire, through the peel-away sheath and the peel-away sheath is withdrawn and peeled away. The HGW is then removed. The E tube is then secured.

Monitoring

The author routinely infuses 2–3 mL of a sterile, iodine-based contrast agent[14] into the EJ to confirm intraluminal placement during final imaging. Additional monitoring of tube location is probably unnecessary unless the patient exteriorizes a portion of the tube from the ostomy site (suggesting migration) or demonstrates signs suggestive of intolerance of feeding, such as vomiting of the enteral diet (suggesting orad migration), abdominal pain or other clinical signs that could be referable to the procedure. The ostomy site should be evaluated and maintained as described in Chapter 5.

Complications

Procedural complications associated with EJ tube placement are usually referable to those associated with the esophagostomy phase of the procedure. Please see Chapter 5 for additional discussion. Occasional challenges are encountered when attempting to traverse the pylorus. The author has not experienced significant orad migration associated with EJ tube placement when the terminal portion of the tube was positioned within the jejunum.

Postpyloric tube feeding diets

A liquid diet is the only formulation that will easily flow through the 8 Fr jejunal feeding tubes described above. Feeding is most often accomplished via a constant rate infusion because the small bowel is not a "reservoir" organ like the stomach. Veterinary polymeric diets[23] are routinely utilized in veterinary medicine in animals with postpyloric feeding tubes. Elemental diets may not be necessary if gastrointestinal function is relatively normal. For additional discussion of tube feeding diets, please see Chapter 9.

Summary

Postpyloric (NJ, GJ, EJ) feeding tubes can be placed utilizing minimally-invasive techniques and allow the provision of enteral nutritional support in small animal patients with intolerance of or contraindications to gastric feeding.

KEY POINTS

* Veterinary patients with critical illness may be intolerant of, or have contraindications to esophageal or gastric feeding.

* Minimally invasive postpyloric feeding techniques provide enteral nutritional support while mitigating much of the invasiveness associated with surgical jejunostomy.

* Nasojejunal tube placement techniques utilizing endoscopic or fluoroscopic guidance are well established and relatively easy to perform.

* Gastrojejunal tube placement techniques utilizing endoscopic or fluoroscopic guidance have been described and provide access for a combination of postpyloric feeding and gastric decompression.

* Esophagojejunal tube placement utilizing fluoroscopic guidance may take advantage of the simplicity and minimal risk of the nasojejunal tube and the tolerance of the gastrojejunal tube.

Notes

1   Dobbhoff, 8 French 55 in. (139.7 cm); Sherwood Davis & Geck. St. Louis, MO.
2   Entriflex, 8 French, 42 in. (107 cm); Kendall (Tyco Healthcare Group). Mansfield, MA.
3   Feeding Tube and Urethral Catheter (8 Fr); Tyco Healthcare Group LP. Mansfield, MA.
4   Weasel Wire Guide wire 260 cm × 0.035 in (0.889 mm), straight regular taper tip; Infiniti Medical LLC. Menlo Park, CA.
5   Performa 5 French, 100 cm Berenstein 1; Merit Medical Systems Inc. South Jordan, UT.
6   Merit H_2O Hydrophilic Stiff Guidewire 260 cm × 0.035 in (0.889 mm), straight regular taper tip; Merit Medical Systems Inc. South Jordan, UT.
7   Nasogastric Feeding Tube 8 French × 55 in (140 cm); Mila International Inc. Erlanger, KY.
8   Bavarian Wire 'soft'; Medi-Globe GmbH. Achenmuhle, Germany.
9   LE, 702; Borsodchem Viniplast Ltd. Budapest, Hungary.
10 2.4 mm rat tooth grasping forcep; ESS. Brewster, NY.
11 2.4 mm forked jaw grasping forcep; ESS. Brewster, NY.
12 3-0 Ethilon; Ethicon LLC. San Lorenzo, PR.
13 Lidocaine Injectable 2%; Sparhawk Laboratories Inc. Lenexa, KS.
14 Omnipaque 300; GE Healthcare Inc. Princeton, NJ.
15 Metoclopramide Inj.; Hospira Inc. Lake Forest, IL.
16 Gastro-Jejunal feeding tube; Wilson-Cook Medical Inc. Winston-Salem, NC.
17 Radifocus Glidewire; Boston Scientific Corp. Watertown, MA.
18 MIC-KEY-J-TJ Introducer Kit; Kimberly-Clark Worldwide Inc. Roswell, GA.
19 Merit Advance Angiographic Needles; Merit Medical Systems Inc. South Jordan, UT.
20 Weasel Wire 150 cm × 0.035 in (0.889 mm), straight regular taper tip; Infiniti Medical LLC. Menlo Park, CA.
21 MIC Gastro Enteric Feeding Tube; Kimberly-Clark Healthcare. Roswell, GA.
22 Peel-Away Sheath Introducer Set; Cook Medical Inc. Bloomington, IN.
23 Clinicare Canine / Feline Liquid Diet; Abbott Laboratories. Abbott Park, IL.

References

Abood, S.K. and Buffington, C.A. (1992) Enteral feeding of dogs and cats: 51 cases (1989–1991). *Journal of the American Veterinary Medical Association*, **201**, 619–622.
Altintas, N.D., Aydin, K., Turkoglu, M.A. et al. (2011) Effect of enteral versus parenteral nutrition on outcome of medical patients requiring mechanical ventilation. *Nutrition in Clinical Practice*, **26**, 322–329.

Armstrong, P.J. and Hardie, E.M. (1990) Percutaneous gastrostomy; a retrospective study of 54 clinical cases in dogs and cats. *Journal of Veterinary Internal Medicine*, **4**, 202–206.

Beal, M.W., Jutkowitz, L.A. and Brown, A.J. (2007) Development of a novel method for fluoroscopically-guided nasojejunal feeding tube placement in dogs (abstr). *Journal of Veterinary Emergency and Critical Care*, **17**, S1.

Beal, M.W., Mehler, S.J., Staiger, B.A. et al. (2009) Technique for percutaneous radiologic gastrojejunostomy in the dog (abstr). *Journal of Veterinary Internal Medicine*, **23**, 713.

Beal, M.W. and Brown, M.A. (2011) Clinical experience utilizing a novel fluoroscopic technique for wire-guided nasojejunal tube placement in the dog: 26 cases (2006–2010). *Journal of Veterinary Emergency and Critical Care*, **21**, 151–157.

Campbell, J.A., Jutkowitz, L.A., Santoro, K.A. et al. (2010) Continuous versus intermittent delivery of nutrition via nasoenteric feeding tubes in hospitalized canine and feline patients: 91 patients (2002–2007). *Journal of Veterinary Emergency and Critical Care*, **20**, 232–236.

Campbell, S.A. and Daley, C.A. (2011) Endoscopically assisted nasojejunal feeding tube placement: technique and results in five dogs. *Journal of the American Animal Hospital Association*, **47**, e50–e55.

Cavanaugh, R.P., Kovak, J.R., Fischetti, A.J. et al. (2008) Evaluation of surgically placed gastrojejunostomy feeding tubes in critically ill dogs. *Journal of the American Veterinary Medical Association*, **232**, 380–388.

Chan, D.L. and Freeman, L.M. (2006) Nutrition in critical illness. *Veterinary Clinics of North America Small Animal Practice*, **36**, 1225–1241.

Chan, D.L. (2004) Nutritional requirements of the critically ill patient. *Clinical Techniques in Small Animal Practice*, **19**, 1–5.

Crowe, D.T. and Devey, J.J. (1997) Clinical experience with jejunostomy feeding tubes in 47 small animal patients. *Journal of Veterinary Emergency and Critical Care*, **7**, 7–19.

Gramlich, L., Kichian, K., Pinilla, J. et al. (2004) Does enteral nutrition compared to parenteral nutrition result in better outcomes in critically ill adult patients? A systematic review of the literature. *Nutrition*, **20**, 843–848.

Han, E. (2004) Esophageal and gastric feeding tubes in icu patients. *Clinical Techniques in Small Animal Practice*, **19**, 22–31.

Heuter, K. (2004) Placement of jejunal feeding tubes for post-gastric feeding. *Clinical Techniques in Small Animal Practice*, **19**, 32–42.

Hewitt, S.A., Brisson, B.A., Sinclair, M.D. et al. (2004) Evaluation of laparoscopic-assisted placement of jejunostomy feeding tubes in dogs. *Journal of the American Veterinary Medical Association*, **225**, 65–71.

Heyland, D.K., Dhaliwal, R., Drover, J.W. et al. (2003) Canadian clinical practice guidelines for nutrition support in mechanically ventilated, critically ill adult patients. *Journal of Parenteral and Enteral Nutrition*, **27**, 355–373.

Holahan, M., Abood, S., Hauptman, J. et al. (2010) Intermittent and continuous enteral nutrition in critically ill dogs: a prospective randomized trial. *Journal of Veterinary Internal Medicine*, **24**, 520–526.

Jennings, M., Center, S.A., Barr, S.C. et al. (2001) Successful treatment of feline pancreatitis using an endoscopically placed gastrojejunostomy tube. *Journal of the American Animal Hospital Association*, **37**, 145–152.

Jergens, A.E., Morrison, J.A., Miles, K.G. et al. (2007) Percutaneous endoscopic gastrojejunostomy tube placement in healthy dogs and cats. *Journal of Veterinary Internal Medicine*, **21**, 18–24.

Michel, K.E. and Higgins, C. (2006) Investigation of the percentage of prescribed enteral nutrition actually delivered to hospitalized companion animals. *Journal of Veterinary Emergency and Critical Care*, **16**, S2–S6.

Papa, K., Psader, R., Sterczer, A. et al. (2009) Endoscopically guided nasojejunal tube placement in dogs for short-term postduodenal feeding. *Journal of Veterinary Emergency and Critical Care*, **19**, 554–563.

Peter, J.V., Moran, J.L. and Phillips-Hughes, J. (2005) A metaanalysis of treatment outcomes of early enteral versus early parenteral nutrition in hospitalized patients. *Critical Care Medicine*, **33**, 213–220.

Remillard, R.L., Darden, D.E., Michel, K.E. et al. (2001) An investigation of the relationship between caloric intake and outcome in hospitalized dogs. *Veterinary Therapeutics: Research in Applied Veterinary Medicine*, **2**, 301–310.

Salinardi, B.J., Harkin, K.R., Bulmer, B.J. et al. (2006) Comparison of complications of percutaneous endoscopic versus surgically placed gastrostomy tubes in 42 dogs and 52 cats. *Journal of the American Animal Hospital Association*, **42**, 51–56.

Swann, H.M., Sweet, D.C. and Michel, K.E. (1997) Complications associated with use of jejunostomy tubes in dogs and cats: 40 cases (1989–1994). *Journal of the American Veterinary Medical Association*, **210**, 1764–1767.

Waddell, L.S. and Michel, K.E. (1998) Critical care nutrition: routes of feeding. *Clinical Techniques in Small Animal Practice*, **13**, 197–203.

Weisse, C. and Berent, A. (2015) Veterinary Image-Guided Interventions, Wiley-Blackwell.

Wohl, J.S. (2006) Nasojejunal feeding tube placement using fluoroscopic guidance: technique and clinical experience in dogs. *Journal of Veterinary Emergency and Critical Care*, **16**, S27–S33.

Yagil-Kelmer, E., Wagner-Mann, C. and Mann, F.A. (2006) Postoperative complications associated with jejunostomy tube placement using the interlocking box technique compared with other jejunopexy methods in dogs and cats:76 cases (1999–2003). *Journal of Veterinary Emergency and Critical Care*, **16**, S14–S20.

CHAPTER 9

Tube feeding in small animals: diet selection and preparation

Iveta Becvarova

Academic Affairs, Hill's Pet Nutrition Manufacturing, Czech Republic

Introduction

Diet selection for tube feeding is made based on careful consideration of the nutritional assessment of the patient (Freeman et al., 2011). Diets for tube feeding of hospitalized veterinary patients should be energy and nutrient dense (1–2 kcal/mL) and highly digestible, allowing lower feeding volumes to be used. Feeding smaller volumes of high-energy dense diet may help prevent gastric distention, and may alleviate gastrointestinal (GI) discomfort and stress on the respiratory system (i.e., pressure on the diaphragm). Diets for tube feeding should be easy to administer with syringe or enteral infusion pumps and should be specifically formulated for dogs and cats. There are multiple commercial products for tube feeding of dogs and cats with different nutrient profiles, energy densities, moisture contents and viscosities. Factors to consider when selecting an enteral diet are listed in Table 9.1.

Diets for tube feeding

Commercial enteral diets designed for tube feeding of small animal patients include 'recovery-type diets' (usually semi-liquid canned diets) and veterinary liquid diets. Semi-liquid diets can also be prepared by blenderizing canned foods with water or with liquid diet using a kitchen blender (Figure 9.1). A number of commercial human liquid diets are also available from pharmacies and grocery stores. These diets are typically less expensive but they are nutritionally inadequate and may contain inappropriate ingredients for dogs and cats, such as cocoa powder, a source of toxic methylxanthines (Kovalkovicova et al., 2009). While canine patients tolerate short-term feeding of human liquid diets without adverse effects, their use is inappropriate for cats because they are too low in protein and lack adequate taurine and arginine.

Nutritional Management of Hospitalized Small Animals, First Edition. Edited by Daniel L. Chan.

Table 9.1 Factors to consider when choosing an enteral diet.

Is the gastrointestinal tract functioning and safe for use?

What is the caloric density and protein content of the diet or liquid formula?

What is the type of protein, fat, carbohydrate and fiber in the diet/liquid formula and is the patient able to digest and absorb nutrients in this form?

Is the diet/liquid formula complete and balanced for dog or cat? Is it meeting the patient's nutrient requirements? Is the liquid formula for cats supplemented with taurine?

Is the sodium, potassium, phosphorus and magnesium content of the diet/liquid formula appropriate, especially for patients with cardiopulmonary, renal, or hepatic failure?

What is the viscosity (thickness) of the food relative to the tube size and method of feeding?

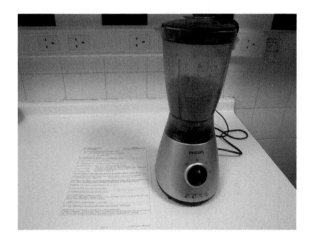

Figure 9.1 Canned diets can be blenderized in a kitchen blender enabling them to be used for tube feeding.

Commercial veterinary 'recovery diets'[1-3] consist of more typical pet food ingredients (e.g., meats and organ meats, animal fats, vegetable oils, cereal grains, fiber sources, vitamin-mineral supplements) with textures designed to allow easy administration through syringe and feeding tubes. In general, 'recovery diets' are highly digestible, low-fiber, high-protein, high-fat and low-digestible carbohydrate formulas with variable mineral and electrolyte contents. These diets require digestion with pancreatic and intestinal enzymes, and are indicated for patients with normal GI function. 'Recovery diets' are formulated to meet nutrient requirements of adult dogs and cats when fed in adequate volumes. When feeding an immature patient, the clinician should review the nutritional adequacy statement on the food label to determine whether the diet is suitable for growth. 'Recovery diets' do not usually require dilution and can generally be used with feeding tubes ≥ 10 French in diameter. Some selected products can be used for smaller tube sizes (e.g., 8 French) (see Table 9.2). These foods can be administered via 'luer-slip' syringes with catheter adapters (Figure 9.2) or via catheter tip syringes (Figure 9.3). However, in order to prevent inadvertent feeding into intravenous catheters, special enteral safety devices[4] (See Chapter 5) which do not use luer-type connections can be used to prevent accidental misconnections.

Table 9.2 Diet options for tube feeding.

	Animal species	Water added to make a gruel with a blender (mL)	Volume of the can (mL)	8 Fr tube	10 Fr tube	>10 Fr tube	Energy density (kcal/mL)
Severe stress / trauma (high-protein, high-fat, low-carbohydrate; fortified with glutamine, EPA, DHA, arginine)							
'Recovery diet'							
Royal Canin Recovery RST™ [1]	Canine / Feline	–	160	Yes	Yes	Yes	1.1
Hill's a/d® [2]	Canine / Feline	–	160	No	Yes	Yes	1.1
IAMS™ Maximum-Calorie™ [3]	Canine / Feline	–	160	No	No	Yes	2.1
Liquid diet							
CliniCare® [5] Canine/Feline	Canine / Feline	–	237	Yes	Yes	Yes	1.0
Liquid Diet							
Renal failure (low-protein, high-fat, low-phosphorus, low-sodium)							
Blenderized gruel							
Royal Canin Renal LP®	Canine	100	360	Yes	Yes	Yes	1.4
Modified Canine[11] (385g can)							
Royal Canin Renal LP®	Feline	20	65	Yes	Yes	Yes	1.0
Modified Morsels in Gravy							
Feline[12] (70g can)							
Liquid diet							
CliniCare® RF Feline	Feline	–	237	Yes	Yes	Yes	1.0
Liquid Diet[6]							
Hepatoencephalopathy (restricted-low-protein, high-fat, restricted-low-sodium)							
Blenderized gruel							
Hill's l/d® Canine[13] (370g can)	Canine	150	370	Yes	Yes	Yes	1.0
Hill's l/d® Feline[14] (156g can)	Feline	20	160	No	Yes	Yes	1.0
		40	160	No	Yes	Yes	0.9

Table 9.2 (*Continued*)

	Animal species	Water added to make a gruel with a blender (mL)	Volume of the can (mL)	8 Fr tube	10 Fr tube	>10 Fr tube	Energy density (kcal/mL)
Royal Canin Renal LP® Modified Canine[11] (385g can)	Canine	100	360	Yes	Yes	Yes	1.4
Royal Canin Renal LP® Modified Morsels in Gravy Feline[12] (70g can)	Feline	20	65	Yes	Yes	Yes	1.0
Liquid diet							
CliniCare® RF Feline Liquid Diet[6]	Feline	–	237	Yes	Yes	Yes	1.0
Cardiopulmonary disease (high-fat, low-carbohydrate, restricted-sodium [<100 mg/100 kcal])							
IAMS Maximum-Calorie™ [3]	Canine / Feline	–	160	No	No	Yes	2.1
CliniCare® Canine/Feline Liquid Diet[5]	Canine / Feline	–	237	Yes	Yes	Yes	1.0
CliniCare® RF Feline Liquid Diet[6]	Feline	–	237	Yes	Yes	Yes	1.0
Fat intolerance (moderate-protein, low-fat, low-fibre, highly-digestible)							
Blenderized gruel							
Royal Canin Gastrointestinal™ Low Fat LF™[15] (386 g can)	Canine	150	360	Yes	Yes	Yes	0.7
IAMS™ Low-Residue™ Feline[16] (170 g can)	Feline	50	160	No	Yes	Yes	0.9

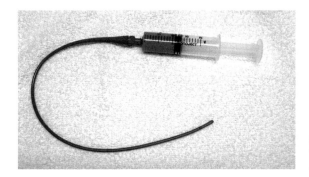

Figure 9.2 Luer slip syringe with catheter adapter for food administration via feeding tube.

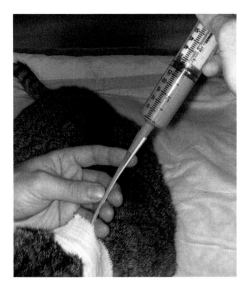

Figure 9.3 Administration of blenderized canned food by catheter syringe via esophagostomy feeding tube with flared end.

Commercial veterinary liquid diets are polymeric products that contain intact milk proteins (e.g., casein, sodium caseinate, whey protein), animal fats, vegetable oils, digestible carbohydrates (e.g., maltodextrins), soluble fibres, vitamins and minerals. Some products have added taurine, L-arginine, fish oil and L-carnitine. Liquid diets are appropriate for all feeding tube sizes and can be administered via special enteral infusion pumps (Figure 9.4).

Enteral diet composition
Osmolality
The nutrient composition of the enteral diet is the major determinant of total osmolality. Liquid formulas that contain intact proteins and glucose polymers (i.e., polymeric diets) have a lower osmolality than formulas with free amino acids, peptides, mono- and di-saccharides (i.e., monomeric diets). Canine and feline polymeric diets have osmolality approximating that of plasma (~235 – 310 mOsm/kg water)[5,6] while human monomeric formulas are hypertonic

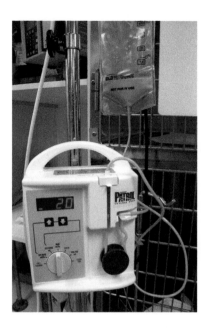

Figure 9.4 Liquid diet administration via enteral pump.

(650 mOsm/kg water).[7,8] Previously, it was assumed that hypertonic diets drew water into the GI lumen inducing an osmotic diarrhea. However, studies in people have identified that the GI tract possesses several mechanisms to maintain osmotic regulation within the lumen when hypertonic formulas are fed, regardless of the site of administration (e.g., stomach vs. small intestine) (Keohane et al., 1984; Zarling et al., 1986). Similarly to human patients, the author's experience is that hypertonic solutions (i.e., monomeric diets) do not cause diarrhea in patients with functional GI tract and their dilution to isotonicity is not required when fed as a constant rate infusion into the small intestine. Formula dilution can be instituted when there is a need for increased water intake or for patients with impaired GI function.

Water content

Daily maintenance fluid needs of hospitalized patients are generally estimated as 60 mL/kg body weight. Special attention to dietary water intake should be paid in patients with alterations in fluid balance (i.e., cardiopulmonary and renal disease). Liquid diets, 'recovery diets' and diet blends with ≥1 kcal/mL contain approximately 80% moisture (i.e., 800 mL of 'free' water in each litre of diet) which does not meet maintenance fluid requirement when fed in an amount equivalent to the estimated resting energy requirement (RER). Diet formulations that provide more than 1 kcal/mL contain less water, while formulas with less than 1 kcal/mL provide more water. Additional water to meet patient's fluid needs is typically provided as tube flushes (Figure 9.5) and with dissolved medications. Therefore, it is important to monitor patient's hydration status and subtract enterally administered fluids (e.g., 'free' water in the diet, water for flushing, water administered with medications) from intravenously administered fluids. Additional water can be administered through the feeding tube between main meals as needed. The

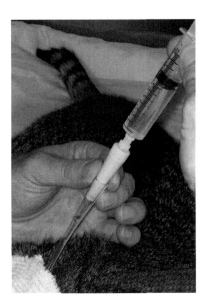

Figure 9.5 Administration of water via esophagostomy feeding tube.

moisture content of commercial canine and feline diets is listed on the guaranteed or on the typical analysis of the product label.

Protein content

The percentage of total calories provided from protein in liquid formulas and 'recovery diets' varies from 22 to 41%, depending on the condition for which the product was designed. Standard canine and feline formulas contain highly-digestible biologically intact proteins, such as sodium and calcium caseinate, whey protein, dried egg whites, liver or whole meats. Human monomeric diets contain protein fragments, peptides and amino acids that are derived from hydrolysis of casein, whey, lactalbumin or soy, which improves digestibility but contributes to higher osmolality of the solution. Provision of intact proteins requires a functional intestinal tract for digestion and absorption. The brush border of the small intestine is capable of absorbing single amino acids as well as di- and tri-peptides, therefore, diets containing protein hydrolysates rich in small peptides might be of benefit for patients with impaired GI function.

Critically ill patients require sufficient intake of essential amino acids for maintenance, healing, tissue repair, immune cell function, albumin synthesis and correction of protein losses. Feline diets should always be sufficient in taurine. Glutamine may become conditionally essential during critical illness (Weitzel and Wischmeyer, 2010). Glutamine is the primary carrier of nitrogen from the skeletal muscle, provides energy to immune cells and enterocytes and is precursor for the antioxidant glutathione (Weitzel and Wischmeyer, 2010). Arginine has immune enhancing and vasoactive properties, and excessive supplementation could be harmful in sepsis due to its vasodilative action (Gough et al., 2011). Essential branched-chain amino acids (BCAAs), leucine, isoleucine and valine, are mobilized from the skeletal muscle during injury and are important dietary protein components for muscle anabolism during recovery

(Kadowaki and Kanazawa, 2003). A number of 'recovery diets' are fortified with BCAAs in an amount of 8.9–13.3 g/1000 kcal metabolizable energy (ME). Their efficacy for alleviating hepatic encephalopathy in humans, dogs and cats is controversial (Charlton, 2006; Meyer et al., 1999). Presently, the utility of including BCAAs in veterinary critical care diets is unknown.

Diets with high protein content are contraindicated in patients with acute and chronic renal failure, azotemia and hepatic encephalopathy. Special diets for protein intolerant patients are listed in Table 9.2.

Fats and oils content

Fats and oils are a concentrated source of energy and supply essential fatty acids. Liquid diets and 'recovery diets' for dogs and cats are high in fat with approximately 45–57% and 55–68% calories from fat, respectively. Dietary lipids are isotonic (~260 mOsm/kg) and are not water soluble. In liquid diets, lipids are emulsified to be incorporated into the aqueous phase of the solution. The sources of lipid in liquid and 'recovery' diets are vegetable oils and animal fats. These include soybean oil, chicken fat and various fish oils. Soybean oil is an excellent source of essential polyunsaturated fatty acids (PUFA), linoleic (n-6 PUFA) and alpha-linolenic (n-3 PUFA) acid. Chicken fat is a source of monounsaturated, saturated and polyunsaturated fat with 47%, 31% and 22% of total fat, respectively.[9] The n-6:n-3 PUFA ratio of the chicken fat is 20:1, the major PUFA is linoleic acid and main n-3 PUFA is alpha-linolenic acid.[9] Fish oils (e.g., menhaden oil, sardine oil), are concentrated sources of n-3 PUFA, such as eicosapentaenoic (EPA) and docosahexaenoic (DHA) fatty acid with n-6:n-3 PUFA ratio of 0.1:1.[9]

Linoleic acid serves as a precursor of arachidonic acid in dogs, while cats require preformed arachidonic acid from animal sources in their diet (Rivers, Sinclair and Craqford, 1975). Arachidonic acid is associated with increased inflammation and immunosupression in critically ill patients through production of inflammatory eicosanoids (Ricciotti and Fitzgerald, 2011; Sardesai, 1992). While the need for essential linoleic acid is well recognized, critically ill patients may benefit from a decreased ratio of n-6:n-3 in their diet to alleviate the inflammatory process and modify hemodynamic functions, although results of human clinical studies are contradictory (Martin and Stapleton, 2010). The clinical use of fish oil in critically ill patients appears to be safe but more studies are needed to determine the optimal dose. Alpha-linolenic acid from animal fat (e.g., chicken fat) or vegetable oils (e.g., flaxseed oil, soybean oil, canola oil) serves as a precursor for EPA and DHA in many species; however, this conversion is deficient in dogs and minimal in cats (Bauer, Dunbar and Bigley, 1998; Pawlosky, Barnes and Salem, 1994). Addition of fish oil derived EPA and DHA product to the diet can efficiently lower the total n-6:n-3 ratio.

Typical dietary fat sources require intact digestive and absorptive capacity, as well as normal function of the intestinal lymphatic system. Selected human liquid diets contain medium-chain triglycerides[10] (MCT, 6-12 carbon-chain- length) from the coconut oil that by-passes lymphatics to a great extent and are directly delivered to the liver through the portal system where they serve as a direct source of energy through beta-oxidation (Ramirez, Amate and Gil, 2001). Medium-chain triglycerides are not a source of essential fatty acids but they provide extra calories to patients with fat malabsorptive disorders.

Feeding diets with a high fat content (i.e., canine and feline liquid diets, 'recovery diets') are considered contraindicated in patients with fat malabsorptive diseases, pancreatitis, hyperlipidemia, lymphangiectasia or chylothorax. These patients require preparation of special low-fat formulas (Table 9.2). Human liquid diets ultra-low in fat (3–6% of the total calories) can be used as short-term diet alternatives.[7,8]

Digestible carbohydrates

The percentage of total calories from digestible (hydrolysable) carbohydrates in the liquid enteral diets for dogs and cats is typically restricted to 21 to25%.[5,6] Lowering the calories from carbohydrates is beneficial for patients with insulin resistance, hyperglycemia and respiratory distress as a result of decreased CO_2 production from carbohydrate metabolism. Diets with low carbohydrate content are also useful in prevention of 'Refeeding Syndrome' (See Chapter 16) in patients with a history of long-term suboptimal caloric intakes. Carbohydrate sources used in liquid diets are maltodextrins (D-glucose units connected in chains of variable length) and glucose. Formulas that contain sucrose (disaccharide derived from glucose and fructose) should be avoided in feline patients since cats have low intestinal sucrase activity (Kienzle, 1993) and possibly lack fructokinase activity (Kienzle, 1994). Formulas that contain lactose (milk sugar; disaccharide derived from glucose and galactose), such as milk replacers, should be avoided in adult dogs and cats due to the lack of intestinal lactase activity in adulthood (Hore and Messer, 1968). Formulas high in digestible carbohydrates or with smaller carbohydrate molecules tend to have higher osmolality when compared to formulas with high-fat and high-protein content.

Digestible carbohydrate sources in 'recovery diets' are present in low amount (1.8–12% ME), and come from cereal grains, such as cornflour or rice.

Prebiotic fibers and probiotics

Interest is increasing in inclusion of prebiotic fibers and probiotic bacteria in enteral diets for veterinary patients. Probiotics are products with a single strain or a combination of multiple strains of bioactive lactic acid bacteria. Prebiotic fibers (e.g., fructooligosaccharides, mannanoligosaccharides, inulin, vegetable gums) resist hydrolysis in the small intestine, promote intestinal fermentation, support healthy colonic microflora, increase short-chain fatty acid synthesis, foster absorption of water and sodium in the large bowel and improve the immunological status of intestinal mucosa and gut barrier function (Manzanares and Hardy, 2008). Probiotics work synergistically with prebiotics by breaking them down by the action of bacterial enzymes. Some human studies show that addition of guar gum decreases the duration and severity of diarrhea (Rushdi, Pichard and Khater, 2004; Spapen et al., 2001), while other studies report that the use of fibers in enteral formulas (i.e., fructooligosaccharides, inulin) to treat GI symptoms in acutely ill patients is controversial (Bosscher, Van Loo and Franck, 2006; Whelan, 2007). In general, canine and feline liquid and 'recovery diets' have very low total dietary fiber (TDF) content. The crude fiber concentration on the diet label represents the insoluble fraction of the TDF and is generally very low at 3–6.9 g/1000 kcal and 1.2 g/1000 kcal in 'recovery diets' and liquid diets, respectively. Whenever desirable, non-thickening soluble fibers (i.e., wheat dextrin) can be gradually added into liquid diets or 'recovery diets' in an attempt to manage diarrhea. The optimal doses of probiotics for dogs and cats are uncertain but it is safe to follow product dosing recommendations. Canine and feline probiotic supplements can be blenderized with the canned food for the tube feeding but these products do not readily dissolve in liquid diets.

Minerals and vitamins

Canine and feline enteral diets are designed to meet or exceed vitamin and mineral requirements of adult or growing patients, assuming that sufficient amount of the diet is consumed. Special consideration for diet of choice is needed in patients with renal failure that require diets with low phosphorus, restricted sodium and chloride, and high B-complex vitamin concentration, or in patients with cardiac disease, systemic or portal hypertension that require restricted intake of sodium and chloride (Table 9.2). Conversely, patients with a history of anorexia, exudation/transudation, high rates of intravenous fluid administration, vomiting and diarrhea can be depleted of minerals and vitamins and require a diet fortified with electrolytes and water-soluble vitamins. Evidence is increasing for inclusion of antioxidant supplements in diets for hospitalized patients because critical illness is associated with deficits in circulating antioxidants in people (Berger and Chiolero, 2007). The antioxidant defence system includes enzymes (i.e., superoxide dismutase, glutathione peroxidase), trace elements (e.g., selenium, zinc), vitamins (i.e., vitamin C, E, beta-carotene), sulfhydryl group donors (i.e., glutathione), and glutamine. 'Recovery diets' and liquid diets are fortified with variable concentrations of antioxidant nutrients, such as vitamin E, vitamin A, vitamin C, taurine, zinc, selenium and folic acid. The clinical utility of including antioxidants in diets designed for dogs and cats is currently unknown.

Specialized diets for tube feeding

Patients with renal failure, liver disease with hepatic encephalopathy, cardiopulmonary disease or fat intolerance require special consideration. While there is a commercially available liquid diet for cats with renal failure available,[6] there are no other specialized formulas for tube feeding on the market. These patients will require enteral diets that are prepared by blenderizing special canned foods in a kitchen blender (See Figure 9.1).

KEY POINTS

- Choosing a diet for tube feeding is performed after careful consideration of the nutritional assessment of the patient.
- The suitability of a diet for tube feeding in a dog or cat is determined based on:
  - the functional status of the patient's gastrointestinal tract.
  - the size and location of the feeding tube.

- ○ the physical characteristics of the diet, such as osmolality and viscosity.
- ○ the energy and nutrient composition of the diet
- ○ the digestive and absorptive capability of the patient
- ○ other patient parameters such as hydration status, electrolyte and acid base abnormalities, and organ function
- Diets for tube feeding of hospitalized veterinary patients should be energy and nutrient dense and highly digestible.
- Diets for tube feeding should be easy to administer with a syringe or enteral infusion pumps and should be specifically formulated for dogs and cats.
- While there is a commercially available liquid diet for cats with renal failure available, there are no other specialized formulas for tube feeding on the market.

Notes

1 Royal Canin Veterinary Diet® Recovery RS™, Royal Canin USA, Inc., St. Charles, MO.
2 Hill's a/d Prescription Diet, Hill's Pet Nutrition, Inc., Topeka, KS.
3 IAMS™ Veterinary Formulas, Maximum-Calorie™, P&G Pet Care, Dayton, OH.
4 BD Enteral syringe, UniVia. BD, Franklin Lakes, NJ.
5 CliniCare® Canine/Feline Liquid Diet, Abbott Animal Health, Abbott Park, IL.
6 CliniCare® RF Feline Liquid Diet, Abbott Animal Health, Abbott Park, IL.
7 Vivonex® TEN, Nestlé Nutrition, Highland Park, MI.
8 Vivonex® Plus, Nestlé Nutrition, Highland Park, MI.
9 Portagen® Powder, Mead Johnson Pediatric Nutrition, Evansville, IN.
10 http://nutritiondata.self.com (accessed December, 2012).
11 Royal Canin Veterinary Diet® Renal LP® Modified Canine, Royal Canin USA, Inc., St. Charles, MO.
12 Royal Canin Veterinary Diet® Renal LP® Modified Morsels in Gravy Feline, Royal Canin USA, Inc., St. Charles, MO.
13 Hill's Prescription Diet® l/d® Canine, Hill's Pet Nutrition, Inc., Topeka, KS.
14 Hill's Prescription Diet® l/d® Feline, Hill's Pet Nutrition, Inc., Topeka, KS.
15 Royal Canin Veterinary Diet® Gastrointestinal™ Low Fat LF™.
16 IAMS™ Veterinary Formulas, Intestinal Low-Residue™/Feline, P&G Pet Care, Dayton, OH.

References

Bauer, J. E., Dunbar, B. L. and Bigley, K. E. (1998) Dietary flaxseed in dogs results in differential transport and metabolism of (n-3) polyunsaturated fatty acids. *Journal of Nutrition*, **128**, 2641S–2644S.

Berger, M. M. and Chiolero, R. L. (2007) Antioxidant supplementation in sepsis and systemic inflammatory response syndrome. *Critical Care Medicine*, **35 (**suppl**)**, S584–590.

Bosscher, D., Van Loo, J. and Franck, A. (2006) Inulin and oligofructose as prebiotics in the prevention of intestinal infections and diseases. *Nutrition Research Review*, **19**, 216–226.

Charlton, M. (2006) Branched-chain amino acid enriched supplements as therapy for liver disease. *Journal of Nutrition*, **136**, 295S–298S.

Freeman, L., Becvarova, I., Cave, N. et al. (2011) WSAVA Nutritional Assessment Guidelines. *Journal of Small Animal Practice*, **52**, 385–396.

Gough, M. S., Morgan, M. A., Mack, C. M. et al. (2011) The ratio of arginine to dimethylarginines is reduced and predicts outcomes in patients with severe sepsis. *Critical Care Medicine*, **39**(6), 1351–1358.

Hore, P. and Messer, M. (1968) Studies on disaccharidase activities of the small intestine of the domestic cat and other carnivorous mammals. *Comparative Biochemical Physiology* **24**, 717–725.

Kadowaki, M. and Kanazawa, T. (2003) Amino acids as regulators of proteolysis. *Journal of Nutrition* **133**, 2052S–2056S.

Keohane, P. P., Attrill, H., Love, M. et al. (1984) Relation between osmolality of diet and gastro-intestinal side effects in enteral nutrition. *British Medical Journal (Clinical Research Education)* **288**, 678–680.

Kienzle, E. (1993) Carbohydrate-Metabolism of the Cat .4. Activity of Maltase, Isomaltase, Sucrase and Lactase in the Gastrointestinal-Tract in Relation to Age and Diet. *Journal of Animal Physiology and Animal Nutrition-Zeitschrift Fur Tierphysiologie Tierernahrung Und Futtermittelkunde* **70**, 89–96.

Kienzle, E. (1994) Blood sugar levels and renal sugar excretion after the intake of high carbo-hydrate diets in cats. *Journal Nutrition* **124**, 2563S–2567S.

Kovalkovicova, N., Sutiakova, I., Pistl, J. et al. (2009) Some food toxic for pets. *Interdisciplinary Toxicology* **2**, 169–176.

Manzanares, W. and Hardy, G. (2008) The role of prebiotics and synbiotics in critically ill patients. *Current Opinion Clinical Nutrition Metabolic Care* **11**, 782–789.

Martin, J. M. and Stapleton, R. D. (2010) Omega-3 fatty acids in critical illness. *Nutritional Reviews* **68**, 531–541.

Meyer, H. P., Chamuleau, R. A., Legemate, D. A. et al. (1999) Effects of a branched-chain amino acid-enriched diet on chronic hepatic encephalopathy in dogs. *Metabolic Brain Diseases* **14**, 103–115.

Pawlosky, R., Barnes, A. and Salem, N., Jr. (1994) Essential fatty acid metabolism in the feline: relationship between liver and brain production of long-chain polyunsaturated fatty acids. *Journal Lipid Research* **35**, 2032–2040.

Ramirez, M., Amate, L. and Gil, A. (2001) Absorption and distribution of dietary fatty acids from different sources. *Early Human Development* **65** Suppl, S95–S101.

Ricciotti, E. and Fitzgerald, G. A. (2011) Prostaglandins and inflammation. *Arteriosclerosis Thrombosis Vascular Biology* **31**, 986–1000.

Rivers, J. P., Sinclair, A. J. and Craqford, M. A. (1975) Inability of the cat to desaturate essential fatty acids. *Nature* **258**, 171–173.

Rushdi, T. A., Pichard, C. and Khater, Y. H. (2004) Control of diarrhea by fiber-enriched diet in ICU patients on enteral nutrition: a prospective randomized controlled trial. *Clinical Nutrition* **23**, 1344–1352.

Sardesai, V. M. (1992) The essential fatty acids. *Nutrition Clinical Practice* **7**, 179–186.

Spapen, H., Diltoer, M., Van Malderen, C. et al. (2001) Soluble fiber reduces the incidence of diarrhea in septic patients receiving total enteral nutrition: a prospective, double-blind, ran-domized, and controlled trial. *Clinical Nutrition* **20**, 301–305.

Weitzel, L. R. and Wischmeyer, P. E. (2010) Glutamine in critical illness: the time has come, the time is now. *Critical Care Clinics* **26**, 515-525, ix–x.

Whelan, K. (2007) Enteral-tube-feeding diarrhoea: manipulating the colonic microbiota with probiotics and prebiotics. *Proceedings Nutrition Society* **66**, 299–306.

Zarling, E. J., Parmar, J. R., Mobarhan, S. et al. (1986) Effect of enteral formula infusion rate, osmolality, and chemical composition upon clinical tolerance and carbohydrate absorption in normal subjects. *Journal Parenteral Enteral Nutrition* **10**, 588–590.

CHAPTER 10

Intravenous access for parenteral nutrition in small animals

Sophie Adamantos

Langford Veterinary Services, University of Bristol, UK

Introduction

Obtaining appropriate intravenous access is vital for the successful implementation of parenteral nutrition (PN). Parenteral nutrition in both animals and people is associated with increased catheter complication rates, including thrombotic events, catheter-related infections and sepsis (Chan et al., 2002; Lippert, Fulton and Parr, 1993; Ryan et al., 1974). Although septic and infectious complications are most concerning, mechanical complications are more common than infection in animals receiving PN (Reuter et al., 1998) and these can be frustrating as these complications will frequently result in the loss of the catheter.

Parenteral nutrition can be administered via a number of routes in dogs and cats including central venous catheters (most commonly placed in the jugular vein), peripheral venous catheters (e.g., cephalic, saphenous vein) and also peripherally inserted central catheters accessing for example the caudal vena cava via the femoral vein. Generally speaking central venous access is used more commonly in dogs and cats for the administration of PN. The insertion and use of central venous catheters is associated with complications, even when not being used for PN (Adamantos, Brodbelt and Moores, 2010). As such, it is important that catheters are placed aseptically and monitored for complications carefully during their use. Furthermore, it is recommended that catheters placed for this purpose are retained for the sole use of the administration of the PN solution and that disconnection is avoided to reduce the risk of introducing infection.

Guidelines for PN in people recommend that high osmolarity solutions (i.e., >1200 mOsm/L) should be administered through central venous catheters as these solutions are irritating to the endothelium and believed to increase the risk of thrombophlebitis. This is somewhat controversial as a number of studies demonstrate conflicting results. A study in people administered PN centrally found no increased risk of thrombophlebitis when PN solutions with an osmolarity of 1700 mOsm/L were compared with solutions with 1200 mOsm/L (Kane et al., 1996). In dogs, the use of a PN solution administered peripherally with an osmolarity of 840 mOsm/L reported similar rates of thrombophlebitis as those seen in people, possibly suggesting that osmolarity alone may not be the only

Nutritional Management of Hospitalized Small Animals, First Edition. Edited by Daniel L. Chan.
© 2015 John Wiley & Sons, Ltd. Published 2015 by John Wiley & Sons, Ltd.

factor influencing thrombophlebitis (Chandler and Payne-James, 2006). A more recent study evaluating the use of a high osmolarity solution (1350 mOsm/L) in dogs administered peripherally reported a high rate of mechanical complications, which included thrombophlebitis (Gajanayake and Chan, 2013). The adminis-tration of high osmolarity PN solutions peripherally has also been associated with an increased rate of thrombosis in people (Turcotte, Dubé and Beauchamp, 2006). Given these results, it would be prudent to recommend that PN solu-tions should have osmolarities <850 mOsm/L when administered peripherally. (Singer et al., 2009).

Indications for catheter placement

All patients requiring PN administration should have a dedicated catheter placed for this sole purpose. As previously mentioned, patients that require high osmolar-ity PN solutions should have a central venous catheter placed. Patients receiving lower osmolarity solutions can receive the solution through a peripheral catheter (Singer et al., 2009). In patients requiring high osmolarity solutions where central venous catheterization is contraindicated (e.g., due to coagulopathy), peripherally inserted central catheters may be considered although there is an increased risk of loss of the catheter due to mechanical complications (e.g., thrombosis). Where PN is likely to be used for >7 days central venous access is recommended. Once the catheter is no longer required it should be removed as soon as possible.

General guidelines for placement of catheters for parenteral nutrition

As there is an increased risk of thrombosis and infection associated with the use of catheters for PN it is vitally important that catheters are placed aseptically. In people, ensuring appropriate placement technique is associated with a reduction in infection rates associated with central catheterization; this involves using a strict aseptic technique, empowering nurses to prevent violations in protocol and utilizing an evidence-based approach for catheter placement (Berenholtz et al., 2004). It is likely that using a similar approach to prevent breaches of asepsis in veterinary patients will be associated with a similar risk reduction in infection rate although this has not been evaluated. As patients receiving PN are typically critically ill and therefore are already at risk of other associated morbidities, including nosocomial infection, it is probably prudent to utilize a similar approach in veterinary patients and clinicians should take every precaution to prevent introduction of infection at the time of catheter placement.

When placing catheters the patient should be adequately restrained to pre-vent movement that may lead to irritation of the vessel at the time of placement or increase the risk of introducing infection. If the patient is unlikely to allow placement with gentle restraint the use of sedation or anesthesia should be con-sidered if the patient's cardiovascular status allows. The site of catheter place-ment should be prepared surgically using a chlorhexidine solution.

Catheter material choice is also important. Polyurethane and silicone catheters are less thrombogenic than other materials and are recommended. Many central catheters are made from these materials; however, over the needle catheters typically used for peripheral access are frequently made from other materials and so should be checked prior to use.

There is limited evidence in veterinary patients that the use of antimicrobial or silver impregnated catheters is associated with a reduced risk of infection although this has been shown in people. Risk benefit and cost considerations should be considered when choosing whether to use antimicrobial or silver impregnated catheters. Recommendations in people include that antimicrobial or silver impregnated catheters are used only in high-risk patients (O'Grady et al., 2002). Similarly there is limited evidence to recommend the use of anti-septic ointment as a means to prevent catheter-related infections, and the use of this has been associated with fungal infections and antimicrobial resistance (O'Grady et al., 2002).

Placement of catheters for parenteral nutrition

Placement of peripheral catheters is well described elsewhere and will not be further discussed here. Central venous access is recommended for high osmolality solutions and the modified Seldinger technique is recommended for placement in people as it is associated with a lower complication rate compared with other techniques for central venous access (Jauch et al., 2009). This evidence is lacking in veterinary patients, however, it is recommended that the tip of the catheter lie in the vena cava and therefore a long catheter is required. The modified-Seldinger technique allows any length catheter to be placed over a wire and therefore is a useful technique for catheter placement for PN use. Multiple lumen central catheters that can be used for PN administration are commercially available as kits and greatly facilitate the procedure (Figure 10.1)

Placement of central catheters by any method is not recommended in animals with coagulopathies. Furthermore, placement of central venous catheters for administration of PN is not recommended in bacteremic patients or those that are clinically hypercoagulable due to the higher risk of thrombosis and infection in animals receiving PN.

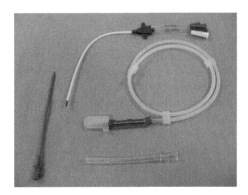

Figure 10.1 Multi-lumen catheter kits greatly facilitate placement. These catheters are placed using a modified-Seldinger technique.

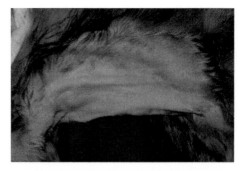

Figure 10.2 To ensure aseptic technique for catheter placement, a large area over the jugular vein should be clipped and prepared with an antimicrobial scrub and surgical alcohol.

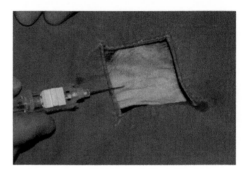

Figure 10.3 A large through-the needle catheter is inserted into a distended vein. Making a small skin incision with a no. 11 blade facilitates this step.

Placement of a central catheter by the modified- Seldinger technique:

1 The patient should be restrained and placed in lateral recumbency by one or two assistants. This can be facilitated by using light sedation.
2 A large area over the jugular vein should be clipped and prepared with an antimicrobial scrub and surgical alcohol (Figure 10.2).
3 Sterile gloves should be worn.
4 A sterile drape should be placed over the site.
5 A small skin incision should be made using a no. 11 blade to facilitate venopuncture.
6 The vein is occluded under the drape by an assistant to facilitate visualization.
7 A large through-the-needle catheter is inserted into the vein (Figure 10.3).
8 The stylet is removed and a long wire is inserted through the catheter into the vein (Figure 10.4). The wire should be fed far enough to ensure that accidental displacement does not occur during the subsequent steps. Enough wire should remain outside the animal to allow a catheter to be placed over it and the wire grasped out of one of the catheter ports before the catheter passes through the skin (approximately 20–30 cm, depending on the length of the catheter).
9 The catheter is removed leaving the wire in place (Figure 10.5).
10 A dilator is passed over the wire into the vein (Figure 10.6). The wire should be held still and the dilator advanced over it. A twisting motion assists passage through the skin into the vein
11 The dilator is removed, leaving the wire in place
12 The catheter is passed over the wire into the vein; again, a twisting motion can facilitate catheter passage (Figure 10.7).

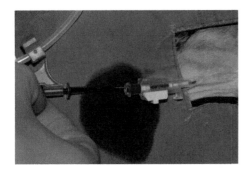

Figure 10.4 The stylet is removed and a long wire is inserted through the catheter.

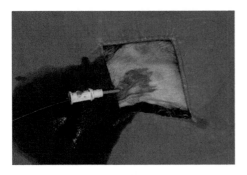

Figure 10.5 The catheter is removed leaving the wire in place.

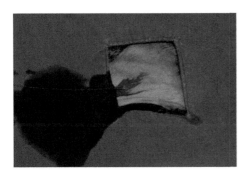

Figure 10.6 A dilator is passed over the wire into the vein. The wire should be held still and the dilator advanced over it. A twisting motion assists passage through the skin into the vein.

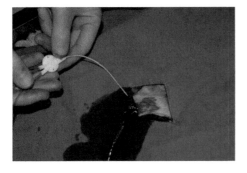

Figure 10.7 The catheter is passed over the wire into the vein; again, a twisting motion can facilitate catheter passage.

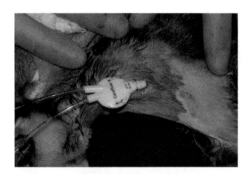

Figure 10.8 The wire is removed leaving the catheter in place.

13 The wire is removed leaving the catheter in place (Figure 10.8).
14 The catheter ports are capped promptly to prevent air embolization.
15 The ports should be aspirated to obtain blood and any air from the catheter before flushing with heparin saline.
16 The catheter is secured in place with 3-0 metric suture material.
17 A light bandage wrap is applied to prevent contamination of the area and prevent accidental dislodgement.

Complications and monitoring of catheters used for PN

The two main complications identified in patients receiving PN are thrombosis and phlebitis. This risk is higher in patients receiving PN compared with those receiving other solutions and therefore catheters should be monitored very closely and if there is any concern with the catheter it should be removed. There is no limit as to the duration of time a catheter can be used for PN as long as no complications are observed.

Catheters should be maintained and monitored as is done for any catheter. They should be covered with a sterile permeable dressing, such as gauze, and bandaged in place securely to prevent patient interference and contamination. The catheter should be examined at least once daily for signs of redness, tenderness, swelling or discharge (Figure 10.9). It is recommended that lines for administration of PN solutions are changed every 48 hours. Systemic signs that may be attributable to catheter-related sepsis (e.g., pyrexia and left-shifted neutrophilia) with no other explanation should prompt evaluation including bacterial blood culture and removal and culture of the catheter tip. Systemic intravenous broad-spectrum antimicrobials should be initiated once samples have been collected.

Catheters should be maintained for exclusive use of PN and disconnection should be avoided, hence flushing of the catheter is not required. Catheters should also not be used for blood sampling. As many of these patients are critically ill use of multi-lumen catheters is useful although there is a higher risk of infection with multi-lumen versus single lumen catheters in people (McCarthy et al., 1987). If these are used for administration of PN the other lumen may be used for administration of other solutions, however, strict asepsis should be used when handling the catheter to prevent contamination and infection and one

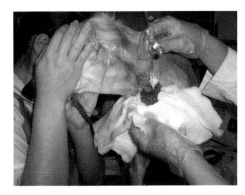

Figure 10.9 Catheters used for parenteral nutrition administration should be examined at least once daily for signs of redness, tenderness, swelling or discharge. The amount of discharge shown in this picture should prompt catheter removal.

port should be dedicated for administration of PN. In order to minimize the risks of using multi-lumen catheters use of the other port for blood sampling, administration of blood products or central venous blood pressure monitoring is not recommended as there may be an increased risk of bacterial contamination (Johnson and Rypins, 1990).

Thrombosis will result in the loss of use of the catheter and will require removal of the catheter. This should be done at the earliest opportunity. Some authors have recommended the use of heparin in the PN solutions or by administering it as a continuous rate infusion (Dollery et al., 1994); however, there is limited evidence that this reduces the risk of thrombosis (Shah and Shah, 2001).

Summary

Intravenous catheterization is essential for administration of PN. Catheters should be placed and monitored extremely carefully to minimize the risks of infection and thrombosis. Catheters should be maintained for exclusive use of PN and disconnections prevented to reduce the risk of contamination and potential infection. Central catheterization using catheters of low thrombogenicity is extremely useful in these patients and clinicians should consider placement using the modified-Seldinger technique to ensure accurate placement within the vena cava.

KEY POINTS

- Animals receiving PN have a risk of thrombosis and catheter-related infections.
- Catheters should be minimally thrombogenic (e.g., silicone or polyurethane).
- Central venous catheterization should be utilized for administration of high osmolarity PN solutions (> 850 mOsm/L) and only lower osmolarity solutions should be administered peripherally.
- Catheters should be maintained for sole use of PN and disconnections should be avoided.
- Catheters should be monitored carefully for complications of thrombosis and infection and they should be immediately removed if there is any concern of these complications.

References

Adamantos, S., Brodbelt, D. and Moores, A.L. (2010) Prospective evaluation of complications associated with jugular venous catheter use in a veterinary hospital. *Journal of Small Animal Practice*, **51**, 254–257.

Berenholtz, S.M., Pronovost, P.J., Lipsett, P.A. et al. (2004) Eliminating catheter-related bloodstream infections in the intensive care unit. *Critical Care Medicine*, **32**, 2014–2020.

Chan, D.L., Freeman, L.M., Labato, M.A. et al. (2002) Retrospective Evaluation of Partial Parenteral Nutrition in Dogs and Cats *Journal of Veterinary Internal Medicine*, **16**, 440–445.

Chandler, M.L. and Payne-James, J.J. (2006) Prospective evaluation of a peripherally administered three-in-one parenteral nutrition product in dogs. *Journal of Small Animal Practice*, **47**, 518–523.

Dollery, C.M., Sullivan, I.D., Bauraind, O. et al. (1994) Thrombosis and embolism in long-term central venous access for parenteral nutrition. *Lancet*, **344**, 1043–1045.

Gajanayake, I. and Chan, D.L. (2013) Clinical experience using a lipid-free, ready-made parenteral nutrition solution in 70 dogs. *Journal of Veterinary Emergency and Critical Care*, **23**(3), 305–313.

Jauch, K.W., Schregl, W., Stanga, Z. et al. (2009) Working group for developing the guidelines for parenteral nutrition of The German Association for Nutritional Medicine. Access technique and its problems in parenteral nutrition- Guidelines on Parenteral Nutrition. *German Medical Science*, 7, Doc 19.

Johnson, B.H. and Rypins, E.B. (1990) Single lumen vs double lumen catheters for total parenteral nutrition. A randomized, prospective trial. *Archives of Surgery*, **125**, 990–992.

Kane, K.F., Cologiovanni, L., McKiernan, J. et al. (1996) High osmolality feedings do not increase the incidence of thrombophlebitis during peripherally i.v. nutrition. *Journal Parenteral and Enteral Nutrition*, **20**, 194–197.

Lippert A.C., Fulton R.B. Jr. and Parr A.M. (1993) A Retrospective Study of the Use of Total Parenteral Nutrition in Dogs and Cats, *Journal of Veterinary Internal Medicine*, **7**, 52–64.

McCarthy, M.C., Shives, J.K., Robison, R.J. et al. (1987) Prospective evaluation of single and triple lumen catheters in total parenteral nutrition. *Journal of Parenteral and Enteral Nutrition*, **11**, 259–262.

O'Grady, N.P., Alexander, M., Dellinger, E.P. et al. (2002) Control and Prevention Guidelines for the prevention of intravascular catheter-related infections. *Pediatrics*, **110**, e51.

Reuter, J.D., Marks, S.L., Rogers, Q.R. et al. (1998) Use of Parenteral Nutrition in Dogs: 209 Cases (1988–1995). *Journal of Veterinary Emergency and Critical Care*, **8**, 201–213.

Ryan, J.A., Jr, Abel, R.M., Abbott, W.M. et al. (1974) Catheter Complications in Total Parenteral Nutrition – A Prospective Study of 200 Consecutive Patients. *New England Journal of Medicine*, **290**, 757–761.

Shah, P. and Shah, V. (2010) Continuous heparin infusion to prevent thrombosis and catheter occlusion in neonates with peripherally placed percutaneous central venous catheters in neonates. *Cochrane Database* of *Systematic Reviews*: CD002772.

Singer, P., Berger, M.M., Van de Berge, G. et al. (2009) ESPEN Guidelines on Parenteral Nutrition: Intensive Care. *Clinical Nutrition*, **28**, 387–400.

Turcotte, S., Dubé, S. and Beauchamp, G. (2006) Peripherally inserted central venous catheters are not superior to central venous catheters in the acute care of surgical patients on the ward. *World Journal of Surgery*, **30**, 1605–1619.

CHAPTER 11

Parenteral nutrition in small animals

Daniel L. Chan[1] and Lisa M. Freeman[2]

[1] Department of Veterinary Clinical Sciences and Services, The Royal Veterinary College, University of London, UK
[2] Department of Clinical Sciences, Tufts Cummings School of Veterinary Medicine, North Grafton, MA, USA

Introduction

The provision of nutrition to animals via the parenteral route is an important therapeutic modality for hospitalized animals that cannot tolerate enteral nutrition (EN). Although parenteral nutrition (PN) can be an effective means of providing animals with calories, protein and other nutrients, there are a number of possible complications associated with its use that requires careful patient selection, appropriate formulation, safe and effective administration practices, and close patient monitoring. In most cases hospitalized patients that do not consume adequate quantities of food voluntarily should be supported with EN as it is the safest, most convenient, most physiologically sound and least expensive method of nutritional support (see Chapter 3). While EN support is the preferred method of nutritional support in hospitalized patients, PN is the established method of providing nutritional support to patients whose gastrointestinal tracts cannot tolerate enteral feedings (Barton, 1994; Braunschweig et al., 2001; Biffl et al., 2002).

While the use of PN support has certainly increased in recent years, there is a perception that this technique is technically difficult, associated with many complications and limited to university hospitals and major referral centers. In reality, PN support can be adopted in many practices and complications can be significantly reduced with proper and meticulous care. The goals of this chapter are to outline the proper identification of patients most likely to benefit from PN, to review the process of formulating, implementing, and monitoring parenteral nutritional support, and discuss how PN can be incorporated into many practices.

Indications for PN support

Studies in people have shown that the use of PN in some patient populations actually increases the risk of complications and worsens outcome (Braunschweig et al., 2001; Gramlich et al., 2004; Simpson and Doig, 2005). Moreover, some

Nutritional Management of Hospitalized Small Animals, First Edition. Edited by Daniel L. Chan.
© 2015 John Wiley & Sons, Ltd. Published 2015 by John Wiley & Sons, Ltd.

studies have demonstrated worse morbidity (e.g., increased risk of infectious complications, greater dependence on mechanical ventilation) in intensive care unit (ICU) patients when PN was initiated within the first 48 hours of ICU admission compared with delayed initiation of PN until day 8 of ICU admission. (Casaer and et al., 2011). The increase in complications may be related to early initiation of PN in well-nourished ICU patients and, therefore, careful patient selection may be particularly important when considering implementing PN (Lee et al., 2014). However, there are conflicting reports on the subject regarding the impact of PN on ICU outcome. A recent large prospective controlled study found that early PN in critically ill patients with relative contraindications to early EN was not associated with any negative impact on survival and in fact identified decreased dependence on mechanical ventilation and better preservation of lean muscle mass (Doig et al., 2013). Furthermore, a new study compared initiation of EN or PN within 36 hours of ICU admission and found significant reductions in rates of hypoglycemia and vomiting in the PN group and no differences in the rates of infectious complications, 30- or 90-day mortality or rates of 14 other secondary endpoints (Harvey et al., 2014). In light of these conflicting findings, perhaps the sensible first step in considering patients for nutritional support is to perform a nutritional assessment (see Chapter 1). Following the nutritional assessment of the patient, the most appropriate route of nutritional support should be selected. The indications for PN support include situations in which malnourished animals cannot voluntarily or safely consume food (i.e., animals unable to protect their airways) or those that cannot tolerate EN despite attempts to improve tolerance to EN. Persistent hyporexia or anorexia is not sufficient justification for PN and should be considered an inappropriate use of PN. In patients that require nutritional support but have contraindications for placement of feeding tubes (e.g., coagulopathic, presence of cardiovascular or cardiopulmonary instability), short term (e.g., <3 days) administration of PN may be considered.

Parenteral nutrition

The terminology used to describe the use of PN in veterinary patients has evolved and so it is worth reviewing the current terminology. Total parenteral nutrition (TPN) was previously defined as the provision of all of the patient's protein, calorie and micronutrient requirements intravenously, whereas partial parenteral nutrition (PPN) was defined as the provision of only a part of this requirement (typically 40–70% of the energy requirement) (Chan and Freeman, 2012). More recently, there has been a shift away from describing PN in terms of 'meeting energy and nutrient requirements' as they remain largely unknown in animals and so recent recommendations emphasize categorizing PN by the mode of delivery such that PN delivered into a central vein is described as 'central PN' and PN delivered into a peripheral vein is described as 'peripheral PN. (Queau et al., 2011; Perea, 2012). For the purposes of this chapter, 'PPN' will refer to peripheral PN.

To enable safe administration of PN solutions using peripheral veins the osmolarity of the solutions is decreased because osmolarity is believed to be one of the main contributing factors for the development of thrombophlebitis. A recent study in paediatric human patients found that PN solutions with osmolarity >1000 mOsm/L was associated with greater risk of phlebitis and infiltration of PN as compared with solutions <1000 mOsm/L when administered via a peripheral vein (Dugan, Le and Jew, 2014). Although similar studies in animals have not been reported, a recent veterinary study evaluated the administration of a PN product with an osmolarity of 1350 mOsm/L to dogs and the authors did not report high rates of phlebitis or infiltration of PN (Gajanayake, Wylie and Chan, 2013). Interestingly, the majority of dogs (66% of 70 dogs) received this high-osmolarity solution peripherally, with a single occurrence of thrombophlebitis and only two incidents of infiltration noted in this study. Nevertheless, some authors recommend that PN solutions administered peripherally should have osmolarities <950 mOsm/L. In order to achieve these lower osmolarities (e.g., <1000 mOsm/L), the concentrations of amino acids and dextrose are reduced and this also decreases the caloric density of these solutions. As such, because PPN only provides a portion of the patient's RER, it should be used for short-term nutritional support in non-debilitated patients with average nutritional requirements.

The administration of PN always requires a dedicated catheter that is newly placed using an aseptic technique (see Chapter 10). Once placed, this catheter should not be used for anything other than PN administration. The use of long catheters composed of silicone or polyurethane is recommended for use with PN to reduce the risk of thrombophlebitis. Multi-lumen catheters are often recommended for PN because they can remain in place for longer periods of time (as compared with normal jugular catheters) and provide other ports for blood sampling and administration of additional fluids and IV medications.

Components of parenteral nutrition

Amino acids

Most PN solutions are composed of amino acids, a carbohydrate source (dextrose or glycerol) and lipids. Amino acid solutions vary from 3–10% concentrations. The most commonly cited concentration of amino acids used in veterinary patients is 8.5%, with an energy density of 0.34 kcal/ml and osmolarity of approximately 880 mOsm/L. Amino acid solutions are typically available with and without added electrolytes. The amino acid profile of these solutions is intended to meet the essential amino acid requirements in people. Currently, there are no amino acid solutions made specifically for dogs or cats and, therefore, these solutions do not meet all amino acid requirements in these species. However, when used for short-term nutritional support, their use is unlikely to result in clinically relevant deficiencies. The minimal protein requirement of healthy dogs supported via parenteral nutrition has been estimated to be 3 g/100 kcal (Mauldin et al., 2001). While the protein requirement of ill veterinary patients has not been extensively investigated, in order to support hospitalized animals with PN the standard recommendations for protein provision are 4–6 g/100 kcal (15–25% of total energy requirements) for dogs and 6–8 g/100 kcal

(25–35%) for cats (Michel and Eirmann, 2014; Chan and Freeman, 2012; Chan, 2012). The presumed increase in protein requirements in ill animals relates to inadequate food intake that accompanies many diseases, increased protein losses and altered metabolic and inflammatory pathways (Michel, King and Ostro, 1997; Chan, 2004).

Given the risk of protein malnutrition in hospitalized animals, the goal of PN support should be to provide sufficient amino acids to minimize muscle protein breakdown and maintain lean body mass. Whereas healthy animals that are deprived of food can adapt to conserve muscle mass and use stored fat for energy (simple starvation), critically ill animals that are malnourished may have accelerated muscle catabolism (stressed starvation) for generation of amino acids used for gluconeogenesis and synthesis of acute phase proteins. (Biolo et al., 1997; Chan, 2004). However, not all animals require increased protein during nutritional support; animals with protein intolerance (e.g., patients with hepatic encephalopathy, severe kidney failure) should be supported with reduced levels of protein (e.g., 3 g protein/100 kcal)

Carbohydrates

For provision of carbohydrate calories, dextrose solutions ranging from 5 to 50% are typically used for PN solutions. In CPN, 50% dextrose is the most commonly used concentration of dextrose, with an osmolarity of 2523 mOsm/L and providing 1.7 kcal/ml. For PPN the typical dextrose solution used is 5% dextrose, which corresponds to 0.17 kcal/ml and an osmolarity of 250 mOsm/L. The proportion of calories provided with carbohydrates depends on the patient's individual circumstances (e.g., protein, carbohydrate, lipid intolerance) but is typically half of the non-protein calories. The ratio of calories provided by carbohydrate and lipid can be adjusted as dictated by the patient's needs. As dextrose infusion rates exceeding 4 mg/kg/min have been associated with the development of hyperglycemia in non-diabetic human patients, the authors recommend limiting the amount of dextrose provided in PN to this amount (Rosmarin, Wardlaw and Mirtallo, 1996) When formulating PN for diabetic patients, a greater proportion of calories should be provided from amino acids and lipids. In some patients, insulin therapy may be necessary to control the degree of hyperglycemia.

Lipids

Lipid emulsions are used in PN to provide energy and essential fatty acids. The most commonly used lipid emulsion is a 20% solution, providing 2 kcal/ml with an osmolarity of 260 mOsm/L. Commercial lipid emulsions in the United States are usually based on soybean or safflower oil. They also include egg yolk phospholipids, glycerin and water. As the principal type of lipid used for PN is composed primarily of n-6 fatty acids, there are concerns on its affect on the inflammatory response. *In vivo* studies in people have shown an exaggerated inflammatory response to endotoxin following a long-chain triglyceride infusion (Krogh-Madsen et al., 2008). There have also been concerns raised with regards to possible effects of n-6 fatty acids on immune function, oxidative stress and negative hemodynamic effects, as well as an increased risk for hyperlipidemia, lipid embolization and microbial contamination (Grimes and Abel, 1979; Wiernik, Jarstrand and Julander, 1983; Mirtallo et al., 2004; Kang and Yang, 2008; Calder et al., 2010; Kuwahara et al., 2010). In order to reduce these effects, different lipid emulsions containing n-3 fatty acids, n-9 fatty acids, medium-chain triglycerides or structured lipids have been developed but are not currently available in the United States (Wanten and Calder, 2007; Sala-Vila, Barbosa and Calder, 2007). Until these different types of lipids are evaluated in dogs and cats and demonstrated to have clinical benefits, the authors recommend limiting the typical n-6-based lipid emulsion dosage in dogs and cats to 2 g/kg/day (30–40% of total calories provided) to decrease the risk of lipemia and possible immunosuppression. Animals with pre-existing lipemia may also require lower doses of lipid or PN formulations without lipids. A recent study evaluated the use of a lipid-free PN formulation in dogs, and so this may be an option for some animals (Gajanayake and others 2013.

Electrolytes and trace minerals

Parenteral nutrition can be formulated with or without electrolytes depending on patient needs. The most commonly adjusted electrolyte in PN solution is potassium and most formulations contain 20 to 30 mmol/L (20 to 30 mEq/L) potassium. Potassium chloride and potassium phosphate can be used to adjust potassium content. In patients requiring additional phosphorus (e.g., patient with hypophosphatemia), the authors recommend supplementing phosphate as a separate infusion as requirements may change frequently and there may be an increased risk of mineral precipitation with addition of minerals to PN solutions. Adjusting electrolytes separately allows greater flexibility.

Trace minerals are sometimes added to PN solutions but the majority of veterinary patients receive PN without the addition of trace minerals. In patients that require prolonged PN support (e.g., >10 days) or are severely malnourished, the addition of zinc, copper, manganese and chromium may be considered. The authors have used a commercial trace element preparation[1] containing (per 5 mL) 4 mg zinc, 1 mg copper, 0.8 mg manganese and 10 μg chromium at a dosage of 0.2 to 0.3 ml/100 kcal of solution.

Vitamins

As many hospitalized animals requiring PN may already have a degree of malnutrition, supplementation of PN with B vitamins may be of benefit. As some B vitamins are light sensitive (e.g., riboflavin) it may be best to add B vitamins immediately before administration and dose it so that the dose is administered within the first 6 hours of infusion. Commercial vitamin B formulations[2] containing thiamine, niacin, pyridoxine, panthothenic acid, riboflavin and cyanocobalamin may be sufficient in most cases. The dosages that have been recommended for these B vitamins in PN formulation (per 1000 kcal of PN solution) include: 0.29 mg thiamine, 0.63 mg riboflavin, 3.3 mg niacin, 2.9 mg pantothenic acid, 0.29 mg pyridoxine and 6 μg cyanocobalamin (Perea, 2012).

Formulation of parenteral nutrition solutions

Using parenteral nutrient admixtures that include amino acids, dextrose and lipids in a single bag is preferred over single nutrient solutions. The authors use the calculations in Box 11.1 to formulate PN. The first step is to determine the animal's calorie requirements. As discussed in Chapter 2, a sensible starting point in estimating energy requirements of most hospitalized animals is to calculate the resting energy requirement (RER). The authors do not apply illness energy factors in determining the target calories to be administered due to concerns over overfeeding and its associated complications. It is worth noting that

Box 11.1 Worksheet for calculating parenteral nutrition using commonly available components.

---

1 Resting energy requirement (RER)

$70 \times$ (current body weight in kg)$^{0.75}$ = kcal/day or for animals 3–25 kg, can also use:
[$30 \times$ (current body weight in kg)] + 70 = kcal/day
RER = _____kcal/day. This caloric target can be adjusted down (e.g., 70% RER) if necessary.

2 Protein requirements

	Canine (g/100 kcal)	Feline (g/100 kcal)
Standard	4–5	6
Decreased requirements (hepatic/renal failure)	2–3	4–5
Increased requirements (protein-losing conditions)	5–6	6–8

(RER ÷ 100) × _____g/100 kcal = _____g protein required/day (protein required)

3 Volumes of nutrient solutions required each day

a. 8.5% amino acid solution = 0.085 g protein/mL
   _____g protein required/day ÷ 0.085 g/mL = _____mL of amino acids/day
b. Nonprotein calories:
   The calories supplied by protein (4 kcal/g) are subtracted from the RER to get total nonprotein calories needed:
   _____g protein required/day × 4 kcal/g = _____kcal provided by protein
   RER – kcal provided by protein = _____nonprotein kcal needed/day
c. Nonprotein calories are usually provided as a 50:50 mixture of lipid and dextrose. However, if the patient has a preexisting condition (e.g., diabetes, hypertriglyceridemia), this ratio may need to be adjusted:
   *20% lipid solution = 2 kcal/mL
   To supply 50% of nonprotein kcal:
   _____lipid kcal required ÷ 2 kcal/mL = _____mL of lipid
   *50% dextrose solution = 1.7 kcal/mL
   To supply 50% of nonprotein kcal:
   _____dextrose kcal required ÷ 1.7 kcal/mL = _____mL dextrose

4 Total daily requirements
   _____mL 8.5% amino acid solution
   _____mL 20% lipid solution
   _____mL 50% dextrose solution
   _____mL total volume of PN solution

---

the method of calculating the distribution of energy from carbohydrate, amino acids and lipids used in this chapter includes the contribution of energy provided by the amino acid solution. Some authors meet the target energy requirement with only the carbohydrate and lipid component, arguing that this results in a "protein sparring effect," whereby the amino acids are solely used for protein synthesis when all the energy needs are met by the other components. However, this strategy risks overfeeding so the authors and the calculations used in the worksheet do account for the calories provided by the amino acids (i.e., protein calories). As a final check, the estimated osmolarity of the final solution can be determined by the following formula: final osmolarity = [(mL of amino acids × osmolarity of solution) + (mL of dextrose × osmolarity of solution) + (mL of dextrose x osmolarity of solution) + (mL of additional fluids × osmolarity of solution)]/ total volume of parenteral admixture.

Compounding

To compound the PN admixtures aseptic conditions are required. Ideally, only individuals with the expertise and facilities who can ensure accurate and sterile preparation should compound PN solutions. This usually entails the use of automated compounders (Figure 11.1) within sterile environments (Figure 11.2). However, these compounders are not widely available, are expensive and usually

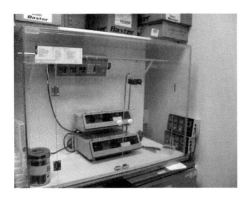

Figure 11.1 An automated parenteral nutrition compounder can facilitate accurate and safe compounding of admixtures.

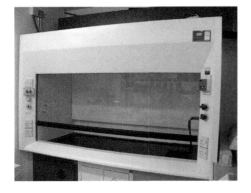

Figure 11.2 In situations where manual parenteral nutrition compounding is required, sterile environments such as a positive air-pressure hood is required.

are not cost-effective unless PN is used frequently. For this reason, it may be preferable for veterinary practices that infrequently use PN to obtain solutions from hospitals or home-care companies that can compound PN to the required specifications for the patient. If this is not feasible, a less ideal option is to manually compound solutions using a "3-in-1" bag system. These bags have three attached leads that can be connected using an aseptic technique to bags of dextrose, amino acids and lipids, respectively. The components then are added to the recipient bag in a closed system by gravity. To make this system more accurate, the recipient bag should be weighed to ensure that an accurate amount of each solution is added, especially in very small animals. Many hospitals that do not use PN frequently do not find this method to be time- or cost-effective. The sequence for mixing the PN admixture should be to mix the amino acid solution with the dextrose solution, followed by any crystalloid fluid if required and finally, the lipid emulsion. If any other additive is required e.g., potassium, trace mineral, this is done last. The reason for this sequence is that lipids may destabilize if mixed with the amino acid solution.

Alternatives to compounding parenteral nutrition admixtures

In practices that do not have compounding capabilities or access to facilties that can provide PN, there are a number of combination products commercially available that could be used in practice. Some products have multi-chambered sealed bags that keep the components (e.g., amino acids, dextrose, lipids) separate until the seals are broken by squeezing the bag and mixing the contents. (Figure 11.3a–c). There are also products that have premixed amino acids and a carbohydrate source. The advantages of these commercial combination products are their availability and the fact that they require no special compounding. There are several different formulations of the dextrose/amino acid solutions. Box 11.2 provides calculations for the use of a commonly used product (ProcalAmine)[3] available in the United States. There are two retrospective studies reporting the use of these combination products and findings are not dissimilar to studies reporting the use of partial PN (Gajanayake et al., 2013; Olan and Prittie, 2015). The major disadvantage of these products is that they do not allow the proportions of different components to be adjusted to suit the needs of the patient. The use of these ready-made products is a compromise that enables some form of nutritional support for patients requiring PN in practices that cannot provide individualized PN formulation.

Administering parenteral nutrition

The procedure described for formulation of PN in this chapter yields an admixture that is intended to last 24 hours when administered as a constant-rate infusion. Current recommendations are that bags of PN admixtures should not be at room temperature for more than 24 hours. The bag should be administered

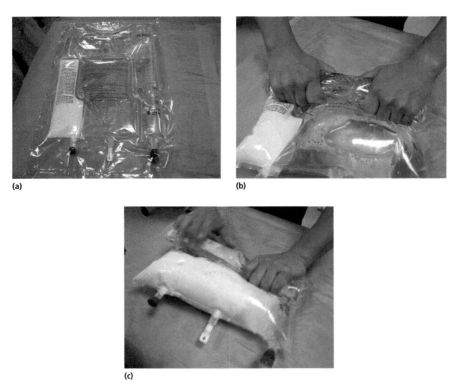

(a)

(b)

(c)

Figure 11.3 a) Commercially available 3-in-1 parenteral nutrition products are available which allow fixed-formulation admixtures to be used in facilities unable to compound parenteral nutrition. Components (dextrose, amino acids, lipids) are held in separate compartments until solution is prepared for administration. **b**) For mixing the various components, the bag is rolled from the top and the pressure opens the internal seals, first between the dextrose and amino acids and then the lipid compartment. **c**) After all the internal seals are opened, the bag is gently inverted to ensure complete mixing. The bag is now ready for set up and administration.

during the 24-hour period via a fluid infusion pump (Figure 11.4). During this time, the lines should not be disconnected from the bag or the patient (i.e., it should remain a closed system). At the end of each 24-hour period, the infusion should be complete, and the empty bag, along with the lines, can be changed using an aseptic technique and a new bag and lines substituted (Figure 11.5). Some studies have reported the use of PN administered for only part of the day (i.e., 10–12 hour infusions), which is termed "cyclic PN" (Zentek et al., 2003; Chandler and Payne-Jones, 2006). Although this may be appealing for practices without 24 hour care, this increases the risk of cathether contamination and is not recommended by the authors. All PN should be administered through a 1.2-μm in-line filter. The filter can help to prevent lipid globules or precipitates (particularly calcium phosphate) from being introduced to the patient.

Parenteral nutrition should be instituted gradually over 48 to 72 hours. Most animals tolerate receiving 50% of total requirements on the first day and 100%

Box 11.2 Worksheet for calculating parenteral nutrition using ProcalAmine®

1 Calculate resting energy requirement (RER):

RER = 70 × (current body weight in kg)$^{0.75}$
or for animals weighing between 2 and 30 kg:
RER = (30 × current body weight in kg) + 70
RER = _____ kcal/day

2 Calculate protein requirement:

	Canine (g/100 kcal)	Feline (g/100 kcal)
*Standard	4	6
*Reduced (hepatic/renal disease)	2–3	3–4
*Increased (excessive protein losses)	6	7–8

(RER÷100) × _____ g/100 kcal protein requirement = _____ g protein required/day

3 Calculate rate of administration for *ProcalAmine*®:

ProcalAmine® is a 3 % amino acid solution thus it has 0.03 g protein /mL
Rate of administration required = _____ g of protein/day ÷ 0.03 g prot /mL ÷ 24 h
= _____ mL/h of ProcalAmine®

Make sure this rate of infusion is acceptable for this patient.

4 Calculate proportion of RER provided at this rate:

ProcalAmine® has 0.25 kcal/mL of energy
Energy provided = 0.25 kcal/mL × _____ mL/h × 24 h = _____ kcal/d
Proportion of energy met = _____ PPN energy ÷ _____ RER x 100 = _____ %

5 Calculate rate of glucose infusion at calculated PPN rate:

ProcalAmine® has 3% glycerol (dextrose equivalent) i.e. 30 mg/ml
Glucose infusion rate = _____ ml/hr PPN ÷ 60 mins × 30 mg/ml ÷ kg body weight.
= _____ mg/kg/min glucose.

Glucose infusion rate should not exceed 4 mg/kg/min as it may cause hyperglycemia. May need to decrease infusion rate and recalculate.

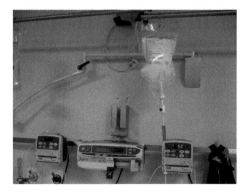

Figure 11.4 It is recommended that parenteral nutrition admixtures should be administered continuously over 24 hours with automated fluid infusion pumps and that the system remain closed until infusion is complete.

on the second day. Animals that have been without food for long periods may require slower introduction (i.e., 33% on the first day, 66% on the second day, and 100% on the third day). It is important to adjust the animal's other intravenous fluids when initiating PN support to avoid fluid volume overload.

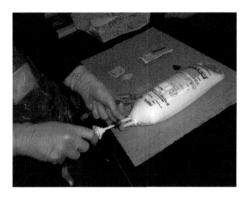

Figure 11.5 Set up of parenteral nutrition requires strict adherence to an aseptic technique which includes use of disposable protective clothing, sterile gloves and new infusion sets.

Monitoring

The other critical aspect in reducing the risk of complications is vigilant monitoring. Checking the catheter site daily can identify malpositioning of the catheter and phlebitis or cellulitis early, before serious problems develop. Body weight should be monitored daily in animals receiving PN. Fluid shifts can also explain rapid changes in weight during hospitalization, emphasizing the need for continued nutritional assessment. Use of the RER as the patient's caloric requirement is merely a starting point. The number of calories provided may need to be increased to prevent weight loss or to keep up with the patient's changing needs. To avoid complications with PN, the patient should be monitored carefully and frequently. General attitude, body weight, temperature, blood glucose concentration, total plasma protein (also checking the serum for presence of gross lipemia or hemolysis) and serum electrolyte concentrations should be assessed daily, or more frequently if indicated. Pulse and respiratory rates should be recorded several times a day. Metabolic complications can occur frequently in animals receiving PN and monitoring is crucial to detect and address them early, if necessary. The clinical situation should dictate the frequency and spectrum of monitoring required because some patients will need more intensive monitoring. The development of metabolic abnormalities usually does not require discontinuation of PN but may require reformulation (e.g., a reduction in the lipid content for animals that develop hypertriglyceridemia). Other parameters to monitor include gastrointestinal signs and appetite so that enteral nutrition or oral intake can be initiated as soon as possible. Finally, the overall nutritional plan should be reassessed on a regular basis so that it can be adjusted to meet the animal's changing needs.

Complications

Metabolic complications

A number of possible complications can be associated with PN and these generally are grouped into one of three categories. Metabolic complications are the most common, with hyperglycemia typically seen most frequently (Lippert,

Fulton and Parr, 1993; Reuter et al., 1998; Chan et al., 2002; Pyle et al., 2004; Crabb et al., 2006; Queau et al., 2011). Despite being the most commonly encountered complication, hyperglycemia was only associated with a poorer survival in cats in the Pyle study (2004). In that study, cats that developed hyperglycemia after the first 24 hours of PN had a fivefold increase in mortality risk. It is worth noting that many of the cats in that study were fed in excess of RER. Although the development of hyperglycemia following PN administration may not necessarily worsen outcome, it may still be prudent to avoid this complication. Using conservative energy targets (i.e., initial target of RER), slowly increasing PN infusion rates during first day, close monitoring of patients receiving PN are recommended for minimizing the risks for development of hyperglycemia.

Hyperlipidemia is also a commonly reported metabolic complication in dogs and cats receiving PN (Lippert et al., 1993; Chan et al., 2002; Crabb et al., 2006), although in two studies some animals experienced a resolution of hyperlipidemia following initiation of PN (Reuter et al., 1998; Pyle et al., 2004). The rates of hyperlipidemia appear to be decreasing from almost 70% in the Lippert study reported in 1993, to <20% in more recent studies (Reuter et al., 1998; Chan et al., 2002; Pyle et al., 2004, Crabb et al., 2006). A decrease in overall energy targets and decrease in the proportion of energy provided via lipids in more recent studies are likely reasons for improvement for this complication.

Electrolyte disturbances can develop either after instituting nutritional support or may worsen in animals with preexisting abnormalities. Hyponatremia, hypokalemia, hypocalcemia, hypophosphatemia and hypochloremia have been reported in various studies although these complications were not associated with non-survival, (Lippert et al., 1993; Reuter et al., 1998; Chan et al., 2002; Pyle et al., 2004; Crabb et al., 2006; Queau et al., 2011). In contrast, a recent report, Gajanayake et al., (2013) reported that hyperkalemia occurred in approximately 24% of dogs receiving a commercially available amino acid and dextrose solution and that this complication was associated with a decrease in survival.

Refeeding syndrome (see Chapter 16) is rarely reported in companion animals but can be difficult to manage when it occurs (Armitage-Chan, O'Toole and Chan, 2006; Brenner, KuKanich and Smee, 2011). Refeeding syndrome refers to a potentially fatal complication secondary to reintroduction of feeding in severely malnourished patients (Solomon and Kirby, 1990; Crook, Hally and Pantelli, 2001). It includes the development of hypophosphatemia with or without hypokalemia, hypomagnesemia, thiamine deficiency, and fluid shifts (Solomon and Kirby, 1990; Crook et al., 2001). It can develop when nutritional support, either parenteral or enteral, is initiated in a severely malnourished animal (particularly those that have not eaten for a prolonged period). The glucose provided stimulates insulin secretion that drives extracellular ions (e.g., phosphorus, potassium, magnesium) intracellularly and stimulates protein synthesis. The result may be clinically significant hypophosphatemia, hypokalemia, and hypomagnesemia. The shift to carbohydrate metabolism increases demands for important cofactors such as thiamine, which may already be depleted in malnourished patients, and neurological manifestations of thiamine deficiency may occur (Solomon and Kirby, 1990; Crook et al., 2001; Armitage-Chan et al., 2006; Brenner et al., 2011). Congestive heart failure also can occur secondary to fluid shifts. It is important, particularly in animals with prolonged anorexia, to initiate parenteral nutrition slowly, to supplement vitamins (particularly thiamine), and to monitor serum electrolytes for the first 3 to 4 days after initiation.

Other metabolic complications that have been reported in association with PN in animals include hyperbilirubinemia and azotemia. Hyperbilirubenemia is a more significant complication in infants as cholestasis and fatty infiltration of the liver are of particular concern. It is unknown if the development of hyperbilirubinemia in animals following PN administration is due to similar liver pathology. The rates of azotemia reported in dogs receiving PN range from 1 to 17% (Lippert et al., 1993; Reuter et al., 1998; Chan et al., 2002; Queau et al., 2011). The development of azotemia associated with PN administration may be due to increased turnover of amino acids due to influx of amino acids in the PN admixture, progression of endogenous muscle catabolism or onset of acute kidney injury. In the study by Queau et al. (2011), azotemia was the only metabolic complication associated with mortality.

Mechanical complications

The most commonly reported mechanical complications reported in association with PN include catheter dislodgement, catheter disconnection, catheter occlusion, chewed lines, occluded lines and thrombophlebitis. Mechanical complications appear to be more common in dogs compared with cats, with chewed lines and catheter disconnection occuring more frequently. (Lippert et al., 1993; Reuter et al. 1998; Chan et al., 2002). In the study by Gajanayake et al. (2013) there was a particularly high rate of catheter dislodgement (40%) and this was mostly encountered in peripherally inserted catheters. As most other studies of PN in animals had predominantly used central catheters, it is difficult to draw conclusions whether the high rate of complication was related to PN administration, the formulation of PN (dextrose/amino acid combination) or no different if compared to peripheral catheters where PN was not used.

Septic complications

Although potentially the most devastating, septic complications appear to be uncommon in animals receiving PN. In all studies to date, septic complication has been described in < 7% of animals receiving PN (Lippert et al., 1993; Reuter et al., 1998; Chan et al., 2002; Pyle et al., 2004; Crabb et al., 2006; Queau et al., 2011; Gajanayake et al., 2013). Catheter-related infections are the main concern in this patient population and many patients respond with removal of the intravenous catheter. Although contamination of PN admixture is said to pose a particular risk, especially if the admixture contains lipids, to date, there are no reports of a positive bacterial culture of PN admixture in any of the studies in animals. The low rates of septic complications may be due to insistance on strict aseptic techniques during catheter placement, PN compounding and handling of PN bags and infusing sets.

Preventative measures

The most important factor in reducing the risk of complications is institution of preventative measures and protocols. Careful attention to catheter placement and catheter and line care will reduce the risk of problems. Placement of catheters by experienced personnel has been shown to reduce mechanical and septic complications (O'Grady et al., 2002). Elizabethan collars should be used for any animal that shows a propensity to chew lines. Protocols for catheter placement, handling catheters and line with an aseptic technique and maintaining dedicated catheters also are beneficial in minimizing the incidence of sepsis. If there is a suspicion of the development of a septic complication, the catheter must be investigated or removed. Submission of the catheter tip or of any discharge from around the catheter site, a sample of the PN admixture, or a blood culture for bacteriological cultures should be considered in all patients that develop pyrexia or an unexplained left-shifted neutrophilia following institution of PN, especially if this is not believed to be directly related to underlying disease.

Transitioning to enteral nutrition

Animals receiving PN should be transitioned to enteral feeding as soon as it is feasible. Unless there are specific contraindications to enteral feeding (e.g., intractable vomiting or regurgitation) animals receiving PN should be offered food and water on a daily basis. Some authors have recommended reducing the rate of PN infusion when tempting animals to eat voluntarily as there is some thought that PN administration in itself can suppress appetite via peptide YY and neuropeptide Y receptor-mediated events (Lee et al., 1997; Perea, 2012). The effectiveness of this technique has not been further evaluated but can be trialed and PN administration can be restored to the previous infusion rate if the animal continues to be intolerant of enteral feeding. The use of antiemetic and prokinetic therapy may be of further benefit in such patients.

Summary

The provision of nutritional support in patients intolerant of enteral nutrition can be challenging due to technical, logistical and management issues. As many hospitalized animals may already have a degree of malnutrition present or are at high risk of becoming malnourished, being able to implement PN support is an important technique in such cases. Proper identification of patients that will benefit from PN as well as the ability to formulate and compound PN safely are critical for successful management of these cases. As the patient population that requires PN support is usually afflicted with serious conditions, avoiding and minimizing complications is also important. Despite some of the technical challenges associated with the compounding and administration of PN in animals, this form of nutritional support can be successfully adopted in many practice settings and play an important role in the recovery of critically ill animals.

> **KEY POINTS**
>
> - Parenteral nutrition may be an important mode of nutritional support for hospitalized patients intolerant of enteral nutrition.
> - Before initiation of PN support, nutritional assessment should be carried out to assess the need for PN, identify complicating factors and devise a plan for commencing PN.
> - Formulation of PN requires calculation of energy and protein needs and facilities for safe compounding techniques.
> - The safe provision of PN requires special attention to the placement and maintenance of intravenous catheters, the aseptic technique in compounding and handling of PN and vigilant patient monitoring.
> - Potential complications associated with PN include metabolic, mechanical and septic complications.
> - With appropriate protocols and safeguards in place, the use of PN can be successfully incorporated in the care of critically ill patients in many practice settings.
> - Transitioning to enteral nutrition should occur as soon as it is feasible.

Notes

1 4 Trace Elements, Abbott Laboratories, North Chicago, Ill.
2 B vitamin complex, Veterinary Laboratories, Lenexa, KS.
3 ProcalAmine. B. Braun Medical Inc, Irvine, CA.

References

Armitage-Chan, E.A., O'Toole, T. and Chan, D.L. (2006) Management of prolonged food deprivation, hypothermia and refeeding syndrome in a cat. *Journal of Veterinary Emergency and Critical Care*, **16**, S34–S41.

Barton, R.G. Nutrition support in critical illness. (1994) *Nutrition Clinical Practice*, **9**, 127–139.

Biffl, W.L., Moore, E.E., Haenel, J.B. et al. (2002) Nutritional support of the trauma patient. *Nutrition*, **18**, 960–965.

Biolo G, Toigo G, Ciocchi B et al. (1997) Metabolic response to injury and sepsis: Changes in protein metabolism. *Nutrition*, **13**, 52S–57S.

Braunschweig, C.L., Lecy, P., Sheean, P.M. et al. (2001) Enteral compared with parenteral nutrition: a meta-analysis. *American Journal of Clinical Nutrition*, **74**, 534–542.

Brenner, K., KuKanich, K.S. and Smee, N.M. (2011) Refeeding syndrome in a cat with hepatic lipidosis. *Journal of Feline Medicine and Surgery*, **13**, 614–617.

Casaer, M.P., Mesotten, D., Hermans, G. et al. (2011) Early versus late parenteral nutrition in critically ill adults. *New England Journal of Medicine*, **365**, 506–517.

Calder P.C., Jensen G.L., Koletzko B.V. et al. (2010) Lipid emulsions in parenteral nutrition of intensive care patients: current thinking and future directions. *Intensive Care Medicine*, **36**, 735–749.

Chan, D.L. (2004) Nutritional requirements of the critically ill patient. *Clinical Techniques in Small Animal Practice*, **19**(1), 1–5.

Chan, D.L. (2012) Nutrition in critical care. in *Kirk's Current Veterinary Therapy*, 15th edn (eds J.D. Bonagura and D.C. Twedt) Elsevier Saunders, St Louis, pp. 38–43.

Chan D.L. and Freeman L.M. (2012) Parenteral nutrition. in *Fluid, Electrolyte, and Acid–Base Disorders in Small Animal Practice*. 4th edn (ed. S.P. DiBartola) Saunders Elsevier, St Louis, pp. 605–622.

Chan, D.L., Freeman, L.M., Labato, M.A. et al. (2002) Retrospective evaluation of partial parenteral nutrition in dogs and cats. *Journal of Veterinary Internal Medicine*, **16**, 440–445.

Crabb, S.E., Chan, D.L., Freeman, L.M. et al. (2006) Retrospective evaluation of total parenteral nutrition in cats: 40 cases (1991-2003). *Journal of Veterinary Emergency and Critical Care*, **16**, S21–S26.

Crook, M.A., Hally, V. and Pantelli, J.V. (2001) The importance of the refeeding syndrome. *Nutrition*, **17**, 632–637.

Chandler, M. L. and Payne-Jones, J. (2006) Prospective evaluation of a peripherally administered three-in-one parenteral nutrition product in dogs. *Journal of Small Animal Practice*, **47**, 518–523.

Doig, G.S., Simpson, F., Sweetman, E.A. et al. (2013) Early parenteral nutrition in critically ill patients with short-term relative contraindications to early enteral nutrition in a randomized controlled trial. *Journal of the American Medical Association*, **309**, 2130–2138.

Dugan, S., Le, J. and Jew, R.K. (2014) Maximum tolerated osmolarity for peripheral administration of parenteral nutrition in pediatric patients. *Journal of Parenteral and Enteral Nutrition*, **38**, 847–851.

Gajanayake, I., Wylie, C.E. and Chan, D.L. (2013) Clinical experience using a lipid-free, ready-made parenteral nutrition solution in dogs: 70 cases (2006–2012). *Journal of Veterinary Emergency and Critical Care*, **23**, 305–313.

Gramlich, L., Kichian, K., Pinilla, J. el al. (2004) Does enteral nutrition compared to parental nutrition result in better outcomes in critically ill adult patients? A systematic review of the literature. *Nutrition*, **20**, 843–848.

Grimes, J.B. and Abel, R.M. (1979) Acute hemodynamic effects of intravenous fat emulsion in dogs. *Journal of Parenteral Enteral Nutrition*, **3**, 40–44.

Harvey, S.E., Parrott, F., Harrison, D.A., et al. (2014) Trial of the route of early nutritional support in critically ill adults. *The New England Journal of Medicine*, **371**(18), 1673–1684.

Kang, J.H. and Yang, M.P. (2008) Effect of a short-term infusion with soybean oil-based lipid emulsion on phagocytic responses of canine peripheral blood polymorphonuclear neutrophilic leukocytes. *Journal of Veterinary Internal Medicine*, **22**, 1166–1173.

Krogh-Madsen, R., Plomgaard, P., Akerstrom, T. et al. (2008) Effect of short-term intralipid infusion on the immune response during low-dose endotoxaemia in humans. *American Journal of Physiology Endocrinology and Metabolism*, **94**, E371–E379.

Kuwahara, T., Kaneda, S., Shimono, K. et al. (2010) Growth of microorganisms in total parenteral nutrition solutions without lipid. *International Journal of Medical Science*, **7**, 43–47.

Lee, H., Chung, K.S., Parl, M.S. et al. (2014) Relationship of delayed parenteral nutrition protocol with the clinical outcomes in a medical intensive care unit. *Clinical Nutrition Research*, **3**, 33–38.

Lee, M.C., Mannon, P.J., Grand, J.P. et al. (1997) Total parenteral nutrition alters NPY / PYY receptor levels in the rat brain. *Physiology and Behavior*, **62**, 1219–1223.

Lippert, A.C., Fulton, R.B. and Parr, A.M. (1993) A retrospective study of the use of total parenteral nutrition in dogs and cats. *Journal of Veterinary Internal Medicine*, **7**, 52–64.

Mauldin, G.E., Reynolds, A.J., Mauldin, N. et al. (2001) Nitrogen balance in clinically normal dogs receiving parenteral nutrition solutions. *American Journal of Veterinary Research*, **62**, 912–920.

Michel, K.E. and Eirmann, L. (2014) Parenteral nutrition. in *Small Animal Critical Care Medicine*, 2nd edn, (eds D.C. Silverstein and K. Hopper), Elsevier Saunders, St Louis, pp. 687–690.

Michel, K.E., King, L.G. and Ostro, E. (1997) Measurement of urinary urea nitrogen content as an estimate of the amount of total urinary nitrogen loss in dogs in intensive care units. *Journal of the American Veterinary Medical Association*, **210**, 356–359.

Mirtallo, J., Canada, T., Johnson, D. et al. (2004) Task force for the revision of safe practices for parenteral nutrition. Safe practices for parenteral nutrition. *Journal of Parenteral and Enteral Nutrition*, **28**, S39–S70.

O'Grady, N.P., Alexander, M., Dellinger, E.P. et al. (2002) Guidelines for the prevention of intravascular catheter-related infections. *Infection Control Hospital Epidemiology*, **23**, 759–769.

Olan, N.V. and Prittie, J. (2015) Retrospective evaluation of ProcalAmine administration in a population of hospitalized ICU dogs: 36 cases (2010–2013). *Journal of Veterinary Emergency and Critical Care*, (in press)

Perea, S. C. (2012) Parenteral nutrition. in *Applied Veterinary Clinical Nutrition*, 1st edn (eds A.J. Fascetti and S.J. Delaney) Saunders Elsevier, St. Louis, pp. 353–373.

Pyle, S.C., Marks, S.L., Kass, P.H. et al. (2004) Evaluation of complication and prognostic factors associated with administration of parenteral nutrition in cats: 75 cases (1994–2001). *Journal of the American Veterinary Medical Association*, **225**, 242–250.

Queau, Y., Larsen, J.A., Kass, P.H., et al. (2011) Factors associated with adverse outcomes during parenteral nutrition administration in dogs and cats. *Journal of Veterinary Internal Medicine*, **25**, 446–452.

Reuter, J.D., Marks, S.L., Rogers, Q. R. et al. (1998) Use of total parenteral nutrition in dogs: 209 cases (1988–1995). *Journal of Veterinary Emergency and Critical Care*, **8**, 201–213.

Rosmarin D.K., Wardlaw G.M. and Mirtallo J. (1996) Hyperglycemia associated with high, continuous infusion rates of total parenteral nutrition dextrose. *Nutrition Clinical Practice*, **11**, 151–156.

Sala-Vila, A., Barbosa V.M. and Calder P.C. (2007) Olive oil in parenteral nutrition. *Current Opinion in Clinical Nutrition and Metabolic Care*, **10**, 165–174.

Simpson, F. and Doig, G.S. (2005) Parenteral vs. enteral nutrition in the critically ill patient A meta-anlysis of trials using the intention to treat principle. *Intensive Care Medicine*, **31**, 12–23.

Solomon, S.M. and Kirby, D. F. (1990) The refeeding syndrome: a review. *Journal of Parenteral and Enteral Nutrition*, **14**, 90–97.

Wanten G.J.A. and Calder P.C. (2007) Immune modulation by parenteral lipid emulsion. *American Journal of Clinical Nutrition*, **85**, 1171–1184.

Wiernik, A., Jarstrand, C. and Julander, I. (1983) The effect of Intralipid on mononuclear and polymorphonuclear phagocytes. *American Journal of Clinical Nutrition*, **37**, 256–261.

Zentek, J., Stephan, I., Kramer, S. et al. (2003) Response of dogs to short-term infusions of carbohydrate- or lipid-based parenteral nutrition. *Journal of Veterinary Medicine, A Physiology Pathology Clinical Medicine*, **50**, 313–21.

CHAPTER 12

Pathophysiology and clinical approach to malnutrition in dogs and cats

Jason W. Gagne[1] and Joseph J. Wakshlag[2]

[1] Nestle Purina Incorporated, St Louis, MO, USA

[2] Cornell University College of Veterinary Medicine, Ithaca, NY, USA

Introduction

Malnutrition can be defined as a state of suboptimal nutritional status due to inadequate, unbalanced, or excessive consumption of nutrients that leads to physical and mental compromise of the host. Given that malnutrition may increase morbidity and mortality in critically ill patients, it is imperative that clinicians understand its consequences and know when and how to initiate nutritional interventions that may mitigate the deleterious effects of malnutrition. This chapter will focus on undernutrition resulting from anorexia and cachexia, describe the specific pathophysiology of malnutrition and discuss the nutritional interventions and supplements that have the potential to ameliorate these disorders.

Hyporexia, although not classically defined, refers to a reduction in appetite, rather than a total loss of appetite, that can occur for numerous reasons (Delaney, 2006; Forman, 2010). This is also differentiated from the starvation patient (i.e., anorectic) and from the cachectic patient as the cachectic patient may be hyporexic or display normal eating behaviour. More importantly, the anorectic patient will lose fat when deprived of sufficient calories before catabolizing lean body mass (Chan, 2004). The cachectic patient will have equal loss of adipose and muscle tissues and this may precede a noticeable decrease in food intake. Thus, there may be progressive weight loss in the face of apparent adequate caloric intake. While anorexia may be a component of cachexia, the body composition changes observed suggest that anorexia alone is not responsible for cachexia (Costa, 1977; DeWys, 1972). This should not diminish the importance of anorexia without the presence of cachexia, as it has been reported in people that the presence of an appetite and the ability to eat are the most important factors in the physical and psychological aspects of a patient's quality of life (Padilla, 1986). The same likely holds true in companion animals.

Nutritional Management of Hospitalized Small Animals, First Edition. Edited by Daniel L. Chan.
© 2015 John Wiley & Sons, Ltd. Published 2015 by John Wiley & Sons, Ltd.

Pathophysiology of starvation and cachexia

In a healthy mammal with adequate caloric intake, exogenous dietary nutrients will be used to meet the metabolic needs of tissues, followed by replenishment of glycogen reserves in the liver and muscle. Any excess amount of macronutrients will be stored in adipose, muscle and liver tissue as triglycerides (Saker and Remillard, 2010). In the fasting or starved animal, any exogenous glucose consumed will be utilized within about 4 to 5 hours. Glycogen reserves will then be sought as glucose declines below approximately 120 mg/dL (6.6 mmol/L). At this point hepatic glycogenolysis will commence to preserve blood glucose for an additional 12 to 24 hours (Welborn and Moldawer, 1997). Insulin will also be downregulated (to further augment glucose preservation) and, consequently, decrease the conversion of thyroxine (T4) to triiodothyronine (T3) initiating a hypometabolic state. Furthermore, while glycogen stores are quickly depleted, stimulation of muscle catabolism begins to occur by glucose counterregulatory hormones, such as glucagon and endogenous glucocorticoids, and is even further exacerbated in strict carnivores such as the cat. Release of muscle alanine and glutamine undergoes gluconeogenesis in the liver and kidney, respectively (Welborn and Moldawer, 1997). In addition to stimulating muscle catabolism, glucagon stimulates fat catabolism. By day 3 of starvation, fatty acids are mobilized from adipose stores and undergo beta oxidation in the liver to produce ketone bodies. With the exception of the renal medulla and red blood cells, all tissues can utilize ketones as an energy source. The body can now spare the muscle of catabolic effects and optimize glucose usage.

In accordance with the starvation model, there is a decrease in glucose usage and a shift towards ketones utilization. However, the diseased state leads to the release of inflammatory mediators and sympathetic nervous system stimulation that may induce a hypermetabolic state typified by an increased energy expenditure and proteolysis creating a potential state of cachexia. This hypermetabolic state has been studied in multiple models including sepsis, trauma, critical illness, burn victims and cancer (Inui, 2011; Tisdale, 2000). The degree of alterations and duration of the hypometabolic and transition to hypermetabolic phases (commonly referred to as the 'ebb and flow' model) depends upon the specific illness. Though there is much debate regarding total energy expenditure in disease states (particularly in cancer), hypermetabolism may be the direct cause of weight loss in cachectic patients (Nelson, Walsh and Sheehan, 1994). Some of the factors stimulating this hypermetabolic state include tumour necrosis factor (TNF-α), Interleukin-1 (IL-β), Interleukin-6 (IL-6), Interferon-γ (INF-γ) and, if associated with cancer, additional tumour-derived factors, known as proteolysis inducing factor (PIF) and lipid mobilizing factor (LMF), may be involved (Argiles and Lopez-Soriano, 1999; Inui, 2011; Llovera et al., 1998).

Alterations in carbohydrate metabolism include hyperglycemia and insulin resistance. This results from the induction of the sympathetic nervous system inducing release of glucose counterregulatory hormones, including cortisol, glucagon, growth hormone and other adrenal corticosteroids and catecholamines. It has been hypothesized that cancer patients release lactate from their tumour(s) which is then converted to glucose in the liver (via the Cori cycle).

This additional interconversion of substrate is an energy wasting process. This metabolic shift has not been firmly recognized in any specific canine or feline neoplastic diseases (Barber, Ross and Fearon, 1999; Tisdale, 2000). In addition, lipid metabolism is disrupted by increased levels of TNF-α and IL-1β inhibiting expression of several lipogenic genes, including lipoprotein lipase (LPL). LPL is an enzyme that is responsible for triglyceride clearance from plasma, thereby inducing mild alterations in lipoprotein composition and mild hypertriglyceridemia in some cases. Additionally, unlike starvation where proteins are spared by utilization of ketones, cachectic patients continue to utilize amino acids, resulting in a negative nitrogen balance and depletion of lean body mass. In most cases of disease-related anorexia there are neuroendocrine alterations that are inducing the anorexia or hyporexia. In response, the hypothalamus will release orexigenic signals to stimulate feeding and suppress energy expenditure. Administration of TNF-α, IL-1β, IL-6, and INF-γ (in combination or solely) is capable of reducing food intake, possibly by stimulating expression or release of leptin, thereby inhibiting the normal feedback mechanisms, even in the face of decreased food intake and body weight (Inui, 2011). These cytokines also have direct effects in diminishing neuropeptide Y (potent orexigenic hormone) release from the arcuate nucleus of the hypothalamus, diminishing appetite. Injection of IL-1β into the cerebral ventricles of rats in an amount similar to pathophysiologic concentrations in the cerebrospinal fluid of rats with tumours induced anorexia (Sonti, Ilyin and Plata-Salaman, 1996a; Gayle, Ilyin and Plata-Salaman, 1997; Sonti, Ilyin and Plata-Salaman, 1996). The exact roles these neuropeptides are playing in companion animal anorexia are not well defined, but are likely influencing orexigenic behaviours. The above-mentioned macronutrient and neurohormonal alterations are depicted in Figure 12.1.

Clinical manifestation and amelioration of malnutrition

Clinicians are often faced with a hyporexia or anorexia associated weight loss or a patient that is losing weight in the face of a normal appetite. In either scenario, the patient may be malnourished. The reason may or may not be obvious. A full nutritional assessment (see Chapter 1) of the patient should be carried out. This should entail a review of the medical history to rule out environmental stressors, unpalatable food, anosmia, side effects to medications, a complete dietary history needs to be performed that includes the brand and amount of food being offered as well as how much is consumed, including treats and table foods (Buffington, Holloway and Abood, 2004). Next, the total daily caloric intake should be calculated. A thorough physical examination should be performed to further rule out respiratory, cardiovascular, neurologic, orthopaedic or oral/pharyngeal etiologies and appropriate diagnostic tests carried out to rule out disease processes. Quite possibly, no inciting cause for the hyporexia will be determined from the history and physical examination, as is the case in many geriatric patients with mild cognitive dysfunction.

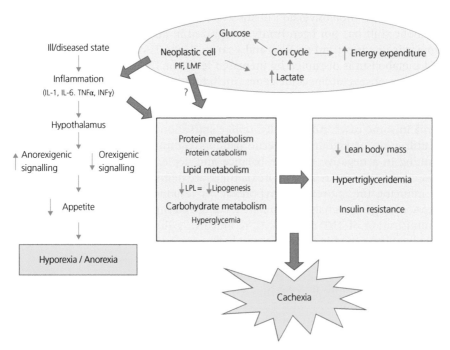

Figure 12.1 Neurohormonal influences of anorexia and cachexia. A number of hormonal and cytokine signals are thought to induce the changes related to anorexia and cachexia, including alterations in lean and fat mass distribution during various disease processes associated with chronic inflammation.

Identification of the malnourished patient (Figure 12.2a,b) is complex since there are no established criteria in companion animals. Indicators that the clinician may identify include unintentional weight loss of greater than 10% in less than 3 months, poor hair-coat quality, muscle wasting, inadequate wound healing, hypoalbuminemia, lymphopenia and coagulopathy. These abnormalities are not specific to malnutrition and often occur late in the disease process (Chan and Freeman, 2006). Hypoalbuminemia may be observed and is considered a negative prognostic indicator. This albumin deficit is thought to represent hepatic protein reprioritization towards acute phase proteins and inflammatory mediators rather than albumin synthesis (Saker and Remillard, 2010). While a trend in weight change is sometimes informative, if observed on a consistent basis, the clinician should keep in mind that hydration status (e.g., history of vomiting, diarrhea, third spacing) can significantly alter weight. Additionally, when assessing body weight the same scale should be used every time to eliminate variation in recorded body weights. While determining body condition scores (BCS) is a practical method of quantifying a patient's body composition and a way to convey an image to a colleague (Delaney, Fascetti and Elliot, 2006), BCS methods were designed to assess body fat content and not lean muscle mass. Highlighting this point, a study of 100 oncology canine patients diagnosed with 27 different forms of neoplasia, found approximately 3 times as many dogs with evidence of moderate or severe muscle wasting despite a normal or overweight

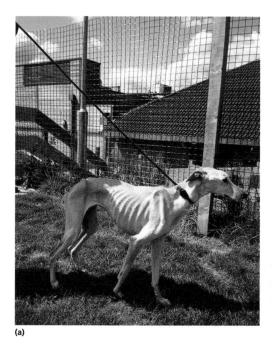
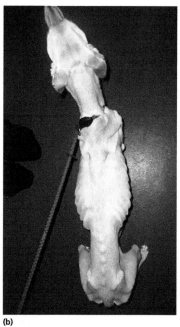

(a)   (b)

Figure 12.2 a), **b**) This dog is exhibiting advanced signs of malnutrition with overt lean muscle loss. However, not all patients with malnutrition will have overt changes in body condition as these may only manifest later in the disease process. Source: Lucy Goodwin. Reproduced with permission of Lucy Goodwin.

body condition when compared to dogs classified as underweight (Michel, Sorenmo and Shofer, 2004). Similarly, a study of 57 feline patients diagnosed with 9 different forms of neoplasia (32 of which were lymphoma) examining weight loss and muscle wasting demonstrated a significantly lower median survival time in those with a BCS <5 when using a scale of 1–9. This study concluded that not only weight loss, but loss of lean body mass may be more prevalent in cats than in dogs with cancer (Baez et al., 2007). Therefore BCS alone may not detect cachexia since loss of lean muscle mass is the hallmark sign.

Feeding the malnourished patient

Following the establishment of a diagnosis, primary treatment should be aimed at the underlying disease causing the anorexia or hyporexia, and a nutritional plan should be tailored to the disease condition(s). However, even in the absence of a definitive diagnosis, implementing a nutritional plan using assisted or unassisted enteral support should ensue.

Upon determining that nutritional intervention is required, the route of delivery needs to be assessed. The enteral route is the preferred choice for animals because it is considered more physiologically sound than parenteral feeding. Mucosal integrity will be maintained and this may reduce the risk of translocation of intestinal bacteria and subsequent sepsis with enteral support

(Michel, 1998). Voluntary oral intake is the preferred route of enteral nutrition; however, animals must be able to consume at least 85% of their calculated resting energy requirement (RER) for this method to be effective (Donaghue, 1989). Alternatively, other methods of enteral feeding include nasoesophageal, esophagostomy, nasogastric, gastrotomy and jejunostomy feeding tubes. Appropriate choice, placement procedures, maintenance and advantages/disadvantages of these devices are described in earlier chapters.

Although energy expenditure has been demonstrated to be increased in some conditions, e.g., septicemia, burns, the typical critically ill or post-operative patient does not appear to have increased energy requirements above baseline needs (Brunetto et al., 2010). Illness factors ranging from 1.1 to 2.0 times RER that have been used in the past are considered unnecessary and may actually lead to further complications (Chan, 2004). Therefore using the following allometric equation for RER of the malnourished dog or cat is appropriate: RER = 70 x (current body weight in kg)$^{0.75}$. A patient is typically fed $\frac{1}{3}-\frac{1}{2}$ of RER over day 1, $\frac{2}{3}-\frac{3}{4}$ of RER over day 2, and $\frac{3}{4}$–full RER on day 3, given that no complications are encountered. In addition to monitoring tolerance to feedings, blood work should be used to monitor electrolyte changes that may occur following feeding, for example, as seen with refeeding syndrome. This syndrome is characterized in Chapter 16.

In the malnourished state, replenishment of protein to spare further skeletal muscle proteins and to attempt to correct the negative nitrogen balance is key. A starting point of 4 g of protein per 100 kcal enterally can be used for most canine patients when their ability to handle nitrogenous waste products is not in question and there are no known extraordinary protein losses. In cats 6 g or more of protein per 100 kcal enterally is a more reasonable estimate. Fat has more metabolizable energy on a per gram basis. The choice of food should be 5 to 7.5 g fat/100 kcal or approximately 20% fat or higher on a dry matter basis, which increases caloric intake and should enhanced palatability (Wakshlag and Kallfelz, 2006). This increased fat will cause a decrease in carbohydrate which may be appropriate given insulin resistance may be a factor. Appropriate foods for feeding cachectic dogs and cats are listed in Tables 12.1 and 12.2.

Multiple substances have been added to critical care formulas and foods for treatment of malnourished patients in the hope of accelerating recovery. While most of these nutrients have not been extensively studied in small animals, some recommended dosages are listed in Table 12.3. The following is a brief overview of some common supplements employed in the management of malnourished patients, however, there is little evidence of their efficacy in companion animals. A more detailed discussion of some of these nutritional supplements can be found in Chapter 18.

Arginine

Arginine is an essential amino acid that is an intermediary in the urea cycle and when a deficiency occurs, hyperammonemia develops. Given the proteolysis that occurs in malnutrition, the urea cycle is accelerated and therefore supplementation may be warranted. Arginine-enriched diets have been associated with enhanced immune function and wound healing in rodents and people (Michel, 1998). In a

Table 12.1 High calorie globally easily accessible feline diets.

PRODUCT	Calories (kcal/ml or g)	Protein (g/100 kcal)	Fat (g/100 kcal)
Veterinary Therapeutic Diets			
Hill's a/d (5.5 oz)	1.2	9.2	6.3
Eukanuba Max Cal (6 oz)	2.0	7.2	6.4
Royal Canin Recovery RS (6 oz)	1.0	10.0	7.0
Purina DM (dry)	1.3 (4.1)	11.1 (12.9)	6.8 (4.0)
Hill's m/d (dry)	1.0 (4.0)	13.1 (12.3)	4.8 (5.2)
Feline High Calorie Kitten Diets			
Purina Proplan Kitten Formula (dry)	1.16 (4.4)	12.1 (10.1)	6.7 (4.2)
Eukanuba Kitten formula (dry only)	(4.7)	(8.5)	(5.3)
Hill's Science Diet Kitten (dry)	1.3 (4.5)	10.4 (8.3)	5.1 (5.9)
Royal Canin Feline DD Growth (dry)	1.1 (4.2)	10.8 (8.1)	5.4 (4.8)

Table 12.2 High calorie globally easily accessible canine diets.

	Calories (kcal/ml or g)	Protein (g/100 kcal)	Fat (g/100 kcal)
Veterinary Therapeutic Diets			
Hill's a/d (5.5 oz)	1.2	9.2	6.3
Eukanuba Max Cal (6 oz)	2.0	7.2	6.4
Royal Canin Recovery RS (6 oz)	1.0	10.0	7.0
Purina JM (dry)	1.1 (3.8)	9.6 (7.9)	4.9 (3.3)
Hill's n/d	1.6	7.0	6.1
Hill's j/d (dry)	1.3 (3.7)	4.7 (5.4)	4.6 (3.9)
Canine Performance Diets			
Impact (2 oz scoop; 56 gr.)	2.6	9.6	6.0
Proplan Chicken and rice Entrée or (Performance-dry)	1.2 (4.4)	8.4 (7.1)	7.3 (4.8)

study of 48 critically ill dogs higher concentrations of arginine (amongst other amino acids) were shown to be higher in survivors ($n = 28$) compared to non-survivors ($n = 20$) (Chan, Rozanski and Freeman, 2009). However, in one study, beagles with induced septic shock received arginine supplementation parenterally at doses lower than that supplied in standard dog food, resulting in lower blood pressure, evidence of organ injury and decreased survival (Kalil et al., 2006). Therefore arginine supplementation at this time is questionable.

Glutamine

Glutamine is considered a conditionally essential amino acid during times of stress and is involved in protein synthesis, acts as an energy source for enterocytes and lymphocytes, and is an essential precursor for nucleotide biosynthesis. A glutamine-enriched enteral diet was shown to have positive effects on protein

Table 12.3 Recommended dosages for nutritional supplements for use in malnourished dogs and cats.

Supplement	Recommended dosage
Arginine	2% of dietary protein on a dry matter basis[a]
Glutamine	500 mg/100 kcal of enteral diet[b]
Branched-chain amino acids	100–150 mg/kg[c]
Fish oils (EPA/DHA)	1–0.5:1 (omega 6: omega 3) in dogs[c]
	2:1 (omega 6:omega 3) in cats[c]
Vitamin E	5 IU per gram of omega 3 supplement[d]

[a] Olgivie et al., 2000.
[b] Saker and Remillard, 2010,
[c] Wakshlag and Kallfelz, 2006,
[d] Foods approved by AAFCO should provide sufficient quantities of Vitamin E to account for this recommendation. Consideration should be given to home-prepared diets.

metabolism, intestinal and pancreatic repair and regeneration, nutrient absorption, gut barrier function, systemic and intestinal immune function, and animal survival (Ziegler, 1997). Glutamine is unstable in solution and may be cost prohibitive in the long run. Most high protein enteral support supplies adequate glutamine therefore the benefits of its addition are also questionable.

Branched-chain amino acids

The branched-chain amino acids (BCAA), leucine, isoleucine and valine, are used with the goal of improving nitrogen balance and may spare muscle protein in malnourished patients. BCAA may counteract anorexia/cachexia by competing for tryptophan (precursor of serotonin) across the blood brain barrier, thus blocking increased hypothalamic activity of serotonin. Oral and parenteral administration of BCAA decreased the severity of anorexia and improved protein accretion and albumin synthesis in human cancer patients (Cangiano et al., 1996). Leucine administered solely has had a positive effect on protein synthesis in skeletal muscle in comparison to increases in other amino acids, shifting the balance towards anabolism rather than catabolism (Anthony et al., 2000; Nakashima et al., 2005). Currently there is no evidence of any benefits in canine and feline patients on high protein diets.

Fish oils

Fatty acids in the form of marine fish oils are a rich source of omega-3 fatty acids, particularly eicosopentaenoic acid (EPA) and docosohexaenoic acid (DHA). Omega-3 fatty acids are thought to (i) displace arachidonic acid from cell membranes, (ii) produce the inert 3-series prostaglandins and 5-series leukotrienes (differential production of prostaglandin E_2 (PGE2) and leukotriene B4) and (iii) downregulate IL-1β, IL-6, TNF-α, synthesis in inflammatory cells. Some dog foods have been supplemented to achieve a 10:1–5:1 ratio of omega-6 to omega-3 fatty acids. A study examining cardiac cachexia suggested that additional fish oil to provide 27 mg/kg EPA and 18 mg/kg DHA in the daily diet showed decreased inflammatory cytokine production and improved body mass indices (Freeman et al., 1998). Another canine study using a 0.3:1 ratio showed increased survival times and disease free intervals in dogs with lymphoma with no discernible side effects (Ogilvie et al., 2000), while other studies have demonstrated when ratios lower than 1:1 have been used, they result in increased clotting times and decreased vitamin E concentrations within cellular membranes in other species (Davidson and Haggan, 1990; Bright et al., 1994, Saker et al., 1998, Hendricks et al., 2002).

Vitamins

B-vitamins are coenzymes that are required for the Kreb's Cycle. Therefore, they are required for glucose, protein, and fat metabolism. Most pet foods contain adequate amounts of B-vitamins, however, if the patient is not eating, B-vitamins should be supplemented. Fat soluble vitamins are stored in the liver and fat stores. However, if a patient has not been eating for an extended amount of time (weeks) and has excessive loss of fat stores, parenteral supplementation should be considered.

Summary

Management of anorexia and cachexia requires a multimodal approach, which may include pharmacologic agents (see Chapter 13) and is best started early in the disease process. The enteral route of nutritional supplementation is preferable to parenteral nutrition in the majority of cases. Improvement may not be possible, at which point the clinician must attempt to stabilize cachexia and prevent further decline. Many patients present with very substantial weight losses and these may be very difficult to reverse. There is no one single or combined treatment regime that is known to be successful, but the above mentioned approaches are used to counteract the hypermetabolism and lean body wasting associated with malnutrition.

KEY POINTS

- Given that malnutrition may increase morbidity and mortality in critically ill patients, it is imperative that clinicians understand its consequences and know when and how to initiate nutritional interventions that may mitigate the deleterious effects of malnutrition.

- In diseased states characterized by the release of inflammatory mediators and sympathetic nervous system stimulation there may be an induced state of hypermetabolism typified by an in increased energy expenditure and proteolysis creating a potential state of cachexia.

- Anorectic patients will lose fat when deprived of sufficient calories before catabolizing lean body mass whereas cachectic patients will have equal loss of adipose and muscle tissues.

- The identification of the malnourished patient is complex since there are no established criteria in companion animals. Common indicators that the clinician may use to identify these patients include unintentional weight loss of greater than 10% in less than 3 months, poor hair-coat quality, muscle wasting, inadequate wound healing and hypoalbuminemia.

- Following identification of malnourished patients, primary treatment should be aimed at the underlying disease causing the anorexia or hyporexia, and a nutritional plan should be tailored to the disease condition. However, even in the absence of a definitive diagnosis, implementing a nutritional plan using assisted or unassisted enteral support should ensue.

- In the malnourished state, replenishment of protein to spare further skeletal muscle proteins and to attempt to correct the negative nitrogen balance is key.

- Management of anorexia and cachexia requires a multimodal approach, which may include pharmacologic agents and is best initiated early in the disease process.

References

Anthony, J.C., Anthony, T.G., Kimball, S.R. et al. (2000) Orally administered leucine stimulates protein synthesis in skeletal muscle of post absorptive rats in association with increased eIF4F formation. *Journal of Nutrition*, **130**(2), 139–145.

Argiles, J.M. & Lopez-Soriano F.J. (1999) The role of cytokines in cancer cachexia. *Medicinal Research Reviews*, **19**, 223–248.

Barber, M.D., Ross, J.A. and Fearon, K.C. (1999) Cancer Cachexia. *Surgical Oncology*, **8**, 133–141.

Baez, J.L., Michel, K.E., Soremon, K. et al. (2007) A prospective investigation of the prevalence and prognostic significance of weight loss and changes in body condition in feline cancer patients. (Abstr) *Journal of Feline Medicine and Surgery*, **9**, 526.

Bright, J.M., Sullivan, P.S., Melton, S.L. et al. (1994) The effects of n-3 fatty acid supplementation on bleeding time, plasma fatty acid composition, and in vitro platelet aggregation in cats. *Journal of Veterinary Internal Medicine*, **8**(4), 247–252.

Brunetto, M.A., Gomes, M.O.S., Andre, M.R. et al. (2010) Effects of nutritional support on hospital outcome in dogs and cats. *Journal of Veterinary Emergency and Critical Care*, **20**(2), 224–231.

Buffington, T., Holloway C. and Abood A. (2004) Nutritional assessment. in *Manual of Veterinary Dietetics* (eds T. Buffington, C. Holloway and S. Abood) W.B. Saunders, St. Louis. pp.1–7.

Cangiano, C., Laviano, A., Meguid, M.N. et al. (1996) Effects of administration of oral branched-chain amino acids on anorexia and caloric intake in cancer patients. *Journal of the National Cancer Institute*, **88**(8), 550–552.

Chan, Daniel (2004) Nutritional requirements of the critically ill patient. *Clinical Techniques in Small Animal Practice*, **19**, 1–5.

Chan, D. and Freeman, L. (2006) Nutrition in critical illness, *The Veterinary Clinics of North America Small Animal Practice*, **36**, 1225–1241.

Chan, D.L., Rozanski, E.A. and Freeman, L.M. (2009) Relationship among plasma amino acids, C-reactive protein, illness severity, and outcome in critically ill dogs. *Journal of Veterinary Internal Medicine*, **23**(3), 559–563.

Costa G. (1977) Cachexia, the metabolic component of neoplastic diseases. *Cancer Research*, **37**, 2327–2335.

Davidson, B.C. & Haggan, J. (1990) Dietary polyenoic fatty acids change the response of cat blood platelets to inductions of aggregation by ADP. *Prostaglandins, Leukotrienes, and Essential Fatty Acids*, **39**(1), 31–37.

Delaney, S.J. (2006) Management of anorexia in dogs and cats. *The Veterinary Clinics of North America Small Animal Practice*, **36**, 1243–1249.

Delaney, S.J., Fascetti, A.J. and Elliot, D.A. (2006) Nutritional status of dogs with cancer: dietetic evaluation and recommendations. in *Encyclopedia of Canine Clinical Nutrition*, Aniwa SAS, Aimargues, France. pp. 426–450.

DeWys W.D. (1972) Anorexia as a general effect of cancer. *Cancer*, **45**, 2013–2019.

Donaghue, S. (1989) Nutritional support of hospitalized patients. *The Veterinary Clinics of North America Small Animal Practice*, **19**, 475–493.

Forman, M. (2010) Anorexia. in *Textbook of Veterinary Internal Medicine*, 7th edn (eds S.J. Ettinger and E.C. Feldman) Saunders Elsevier, St. Louis. pp. 172–173.

Freeman, L.M., Rush, E., Kehayias, J.J., et al. (1998) Nutritional alterations and the effect of fish oil supplementation in dogs with heart failure. *Journal of Veterinary Internal Medicine*, **12**(6), 440–448.

Gayle, D., Ilyin S.E. and Plata-Salaman C.R. (1997) Central nervous system IL-1β system and Neuropeptide Y mRNA during IL-1β induced anorexia in rats. *Brain Research Bulletin*, **44**, 311–317.

Hendricks, W.H., Wu, Y.B., Shields, R.G. et al. (2002) Vitamin E requirement of adult cats increases slightly with high dietary intake of polyunsaturated fatty acids. *The Journal of Nutrition*, **132**, 1613S–1615S.

Inui, Akio (2011) Cancer anorexia-cachexia syndrome: Current issues in research and management. *CA A Cancer Journal for Clinicians*, **52**, 72–91.

Kalil, A.C., Sevransky J.E., Myers, D.E. et al. (2006) Preclinical trial of L-arginine monotherapy alone or with N-acetylcysteine in septic shock. *Critical Care Medicine*, **34**(11), 2719–2728.

Llovera, M., Garcia-Martinez, C., Lopez-Soriano, J. et al. (1998) Role of TNF receptor1 in protein turnover during cancer cachexia using gene knockout mice. *Molecular Cell Endocrinology*, **142**, 183–189.

Michel, K.E. (1998) Interventional nutrition for the critical care patient: Optimal diets. *Clinical Techniques in Small Animal Practice*, **13**, 204–210.

Michel, K.E., Sorenmo, K. and Shofer, F.S. (2004) Evaluation of body condition and weight loss in dogs presented to a veterinary oncology service. *Journal of Veterinary Internal Medicine*, **18**, 692–695.

Nakashima, K., Ishida, A., Yamazaki, M. et al. (2005) Leucine suppresses myofibrillar proteolysis by down-regulating ubiquitin- proteasome pathway in chick skeletal muscles. *Biochemical and Biophysical Research Communications*, **336**(2), 660–666.

Nelson, K.A., Walsh, D. and Shehann F.A. The cancer anorexia-cachexia syndrome. *Journal of Clinical Oncology*, **12**, 213–225.

Ogilvie, G.K., Fettman, M.J., Mallinckrodt, C.H. et al. (2000) Effect of fish oil, arginine, and doxorubicin chemotherapy on remission and survival time for dogs with lymphoma: a double-blind, randomized placebo-controlled study. *Cancer*, **88**(8), 1916–1928.

Padilla, G.V. (1986) Psychological aspects of nutrition and cancer. *Surgical Clinics of North America*, **66**, 1121–1135.

Saker, K.E., Eddy, A.L., Thatcher, C.D. et al. (1998) Manipulation of ietary (n-6) and (n-3) fatty acids alters platelet function in cats. *The Journal of Nutrition*, **128**(12), 26455–26475.

Saker, K. and Remillard, R. (2010) Critical care nutrition and enteral-assisted feeding. in *Small Animal Clinical Nutrition*, 5th edn (eds M.S. Hand, C.D. Thatcher, R.L. Remillard, et al.) Mark Morris Institute, Topeka. pp. 439–476.

Sonti, G., Ilyin S.E. and Plata-Salaman C.R. (1996a) Neuropeptide Y blocks and reverses interleukin-1β-induced anorexia in rats. *Peptides*, **17**, 517–520.

Sonti, G., Ilyin S.E. and Plata-Salaman C.R. (1996b) Anorexia induced by cytokine interactions at pathophysiological concentrations. *American Journal of Physiology*, **270**, 1349–1402.

Tisdale, M.J. (2000) Metabolic abnormalities in cachexia and anorexia. *Nutrition*, **16**, 1013–1014.

Tisdale, M.J. (2001) Cancer anorexia and cachexia. *Nutrition*, **17**, 438–442.

Wakshlag, J. and Kallfelz, F. (2006) Nutritional status of dogs with cancer: dietetic evaluation and recommendations. in *Encyclopedia of Canine Clinical Nutrition*, Aniwa SAS, Aimargues, France. pp. 408–425.

Welborn, M.B. and Moldawer, L.L. (1997) Glucose metabolism. in *Clinical Nutrition Enteral and Tube Feeding*, 3rd edn (eds J.L. Rombeau and R.H. Rolandelli) W.B. Saunders, Philadelphia. pp. 61–80.

Ziegler, T.R. and Young, L.S. (1997) Therapeutic effects of specific nutrients. in *Clinical Nutrition Enteral and Tube Feeding*, 3rd edn (eds J.L. Rombeau and R.H. Rolandelli) W.B. Saunders, Philadelphia, pp. 112–137.

CHAPTER 13

Appetite stimulants in dogs and cats

Lisa P. Weeth

Weeth Nutrition Services, Edinburgh, Scotland, UK

Introduction

Appetite is the manifestation of hunger and is a normal adaptive response to periods of decreased energy intake, while anorexia is a maladaptive response that results in the absence of food intake despite inadequate energy consumption. Left untreated, prolonged anorexia can result in generalized wasting, delayed wound healing, impaired immune function, altered drug metabolism, and is known to increase morbidity and mortality in human patients (Donohoe, Ryan and Reynolds, 2011). The behavioral expression of appetite is complex and can be modified by altered sense of taste and smell, dysphagia, pain and learned food aversions, as well as alteration in hormone and cytokine levels within the body. A change in any one of these parameters can result in the outward appearance of anorexia.

Loss of appetite can occur with a variety of medical conditions in dogs and cats including kidney disease, cardiovascular disease, pancreatitis, neoplasia, gastrointestinal diseases and dental disease. Since appetite is also viewed as a "quality of life" indicator by pet owners, pharmacological appetite stimulants may be more effective at managing the caregiver's perception of health rather than stopping or reversing anorexia.

Meeting nutritional needs of patients with anorexia can be challenging. In patients that are not already exhibiting signs of malnutrition (e.g., severe lean muscle loss) nutritional management should involve addressing the primary underlying disorder, coaxing the animal to eat by modifying the diet to increase palatability, addressing pain and nausea (Figure 13.1). If these measures are not effective, consideration should be given to using pharmacological agents to stimulate appetite. Although there are various agents that have been used to stimulate appetite in animals, it is worth noting that there is a paucity of data evaluating the effectiveness of appetite stimulants in clinical patients. It is also important to understand the pathophysiology of anorexia and how pharmacological agents may interact with various signals in the body to potentially increase food intake.

Nutritional Management of Hospitalized Small Animals, First Edition. Edited by Daniel L. Chan.
© 2015 John Wiley & Sons, Ltd. Published 2015 by John Wiley & Sons, Ltd.

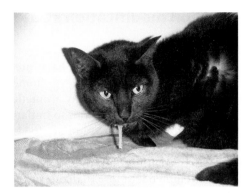

Figure 13.1 The cat depicted is exhibiting pronounced hypersalivation, which is common sign of nausea and may explain reluctance to eat.

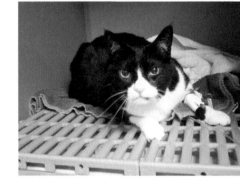

Figure 13.2 Example of an at-risk patient that may benefit from short-term use of appetite stimulants. A 13-year-old obese female spayed domestic shorthaired cat with history of weight loss associated with recent diet change and dental extractions due to multiple tooth root abscesses. Photo courtesy of L.P. Weeth.

Pathophysiology of anorexia

Whether a potential food item is appealing to an individual will depend on a number of external stimuli, such as past experiences (e.g., learned food aversions or preferences), environmental triggers (e.g., location of food, other animals or people nearby), and food characteristics (e.g., aroma, texture and temperature). Animals that experience mouth pain, pain related to chewing or swallowing, or that experience maldigestion associated with food consumption (whether related to a primary disease or a side effect of treatment) may refuse to eat to avoid real or anticipated pain or discomfort (Figure 13.2).

An animal's desire to eat is also in part controlled by the balance of hormones, such as insulin, glucagon and leptin (a polypeptide produced by adipocytes), and cytokines such as interleukin-6 (IL-6), tumour necrosis factor a (TNFα), and prostaglandin E_2α (PGE2α). Systemic increases in IL-6, TNFα, and PGE2α concentrations can occur with chronic medical conditions and can suppress appetite despite the individual being in a negative energy balance (Perboni and Inui, 2006; Braun and Marks, 2010). Even in the absence of chronic conditions, the 'anorexia of aging' has been described in older people and laboratory animals (Morley, 2001) and involves age related declines in the sense of taste and olfaction; decreased renal clearance of hormones, such as cholecystokinin (CCK), as well as IL-6, TNFα, and PGE_2α, which can suppress appetite; and poor dietary intake of certain essential nutrients, such as zinc, that can alter taste perception.

Nutrition modification strategies

Diet characteristics

Individual cats and dogs may have preferences for or aversions to certain textures (e.g., dry vs. canned vs. home-prepared foods) and aromas (e.g., strongly aromatic vs. minimally aromatic) that can impact that animal's willingness to eat voluntarily. Prior to initiating pharmacological intervention the initial step to stimulating voluntary food intake should be aimed at modifying the food itself to increase palatability, if possible. This approach may be counterproductive with certain conditions (e.g., feline hepatic lipidosis) and should not be attempted for more than one or two days before more direct nutritional support is initiated.

Long-chain omega-3 fatty acids

While currently used for chronic inflammatory conditions such as osteoarthritis, neoplasia and cardiovascular disease, the use of fish oil as a means of improving appetite and lean body mass in cachexic and inappetant dogs and cats has not been extensively evaluated. However, in one study, the use of omega-3 fatty acids was associated with reduction in IL-1 concentrations and improved cachexia scores in a group of 28 dogs with heart failure (Freeman et al., 1998). When taken by people with cancer-associated cachexia in conjunction with appetite stimulants, supplementation with fish oil was shown to decrease circulating IL-6 concentrations, improve lean body mass and increase food intake more than when either fish oils or appetite stimulants were given alone (Mantovani et al., 2010). Given the current lack of data regarding the concurrent use of omega-3 fatty acids and appetite stimulants in animals, further research in this area is warranted.

Pharmacological agents

Various agents have been used as appetite stimulants in dogs and cats (Tables 13.1 and 13.2). In many instances, the effect on appetite is a side-effect rather than its main effect. Nevertheless, understanding the purported mechanism of how these agents affect appetite may allow the clinician to choose the most appropriate agent or to forgo their use and implement more effective means of nutritional support such as feeding tubes.

Prednisone/prednisolone

These agents are not used as an appetite stimulant *per se*, but perhaps more for their palliative effects. Glucocorticoids are typically used to decrease inflammation associated with primary underlying diseases. However, glucocorticoids also have a series of side-effects and an increase in appetite is well appreciated as a common consequence. Other systemic side effects of this medication include increased muscle catabolism and gastrointestinal ulceration. Given these sequelae, glucocorticoids are not a good first choice for appetite stimulation in dogs and cats.

Table 13.1 Appetite stimulants for use in cats. Adapted from Plumb, 2011.

Drug	Dosage	Considerations
Cyproheptadine	2–4 mg/cat PO daily to twice daily	Can cause excess sedation, behavioural changes and aggression.
Diazepam	0.05–0.15 mg/kg IV or 1 mg/cat/day PO	Associated with hepatic failure with repeated usage; can cause excessive sedation.
	0.05–0.4 mg/kg IV, IM or PO	
Oxazapam	2 mg/cat PO twice daily	Use with caution, similar to diazepam.
Mirtazapine	3–4 mg/cat PO every 3 days	Hepatic metabolism via glucuronidation, delayed metabolism relative to dogs. Can cause sedation. May be weak anti-emetic.

Table 13.2 Appetite stimulants for use in dogs. Mirtazapine information adapted from Plumb, 2011; megestrol acetate information adapted from Kuehn, 2008.

Drug	Dosage	Considerations
Mirtazapine	0.6 mg/kg PO q 24h, not to exceed 30 mg/day	Can cause sedation. May be weak anti-emetic.
Megestrol acetate	<20 kg: 2.5 mg PO q24h x 5 days; then 2.5 mg PO q48h	Dosages extrapolated from human usage.
	>20 kg: 5 mg PO q24h x 5 days; then 5 mg PO q48h	

Cyproheptadine

Cyproheptadine is a serotonin receptor antagonist as well as an H_1-receptor antagonist. Published clinical studies as to the use and efficacy of cyproheptadine as an appetite stimulant in veterinary medicine are lacking, though clinically a short-term increase in food intake can be seen in anorexic cats after oral administration. This is not an effective appetite stimulant in dogs due to a more rapid metabolism and clearance of this medication in this species. Undesired effects include aggression, vocalization and altered behaviour. These signs tend to resolve with either dose reduction or discontinuation of use.

Benzodiazepine derivatives

Diazepam or midazolam given intravenously or diazepam and oxazepam given orally have been used as appetite stimulants in dogs and cats, but limitations in patient selection (i.e., cannot be given to debilitated or critically ill animals due to sedative and hypotensive affects) (Figure 13.3), lack of efficacy in dogs, and risk of hepatic failure in cats with repeated administration (Center et al., 1996) limit the use of benzodiazepine derivatives as appetite stimulants.

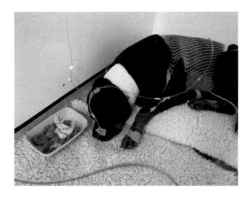

Figure 13.3 The dog depicted is debilitated and has a dull mentation and the use of appetite stimulants, which have sedation or hypotension as possible side-effects, are not recommended.

Megestrol acetate

Megestrol acetate is a synthetic progestin that has been used to suppress estrus and treat pseudo-pregnancy in female dogs as well as benign prostatic hypertrophy in male dogs. In human medicine, megestrol acetate has been used to improve appetite, promote weight gain and improve quality of life indicators in people undergoing cancer treatments (Loprinzi et al., 1990; Loprinzi et al., 1993). Though it is important to note that the weight gain shown in these studies was related to increased water retention or increased body fat mass, or both, and not improvement in lean body mass. Megestrol acetate may help minimize signs of anorexia and reported nausea and improve quality of life parameters in people (Berenstein and Ortiz, 2009) though there are no published studies to data demonstrating efficacy for the use of megestrol acetate to treat anorexia in dogs. Clinically, modest increases in food intake can be seen in anorexic dogs with repeated oral administration of megestrol acetate. Megestrol acetate should not be used in cats due to adrenocortical suppression and hepatic toxicity associated with oral administration of this medication (Plumb, 2011).

Mirtazapine

Mirtazapine is a tricyclic antidepressant used to treat clinical depression in people but has gained popularity in both human and veterinary medicine in recent years as an appetite stimulant. Mirtazapine acts as a serotonin receptor antagonist, H_1-receptor antagonist and enhances norepinephrine release in people. Its effects on appetite are thought to be mediated both through serotonin receptor inhibition as well as norepinephrine's effect on promoting food intake. It has also been used as an anti-nausea medication and appetite stimulant in people with cancer-associated cachexia (Riechelmann et al., 2010) as well as sarcopenia of aging (Fox et al., 2009) and use in veterinary medicine is largely extrapolated from human studies. Recent pharmacokinetics studies in healthy dogs (Giorgi and Yun, 2012) and cats with renal disease (Quimby, Gustafson and Lunn, 2011) show mirtazapine to be absorbed, metabolized and excreted in these species similarly to people. Hepatic metabolism is primarily via glucuronidation and long-term safety studies of mirtazapine administration in cats are lacking. A recent abstract detailing a prospective observational study attempted to quantify food intake subsequent to administration of mirtazapine to hospitalized dogs and cats

(Casmian-Sorrosal and Warman, 2010). The study suggested that mirtazapine stimulated food intake in 86% of dogs and 83% of cats. However, as this study has not been published in the peer reviewed literature, definitive conclusions about the efficacy of mirtazapine cannot be drawn. However, it does appear that mirtazapine can increase short-term food intake in dogs and cats similar to other appetite stimulants.

Monitoring and complications

The goal of therapy in anorectic patients is to improve total energy intake and ultimately resolve anorexia, to improve lean body mass and to improve quality of life. The use of appetite stimulants as either the primary or sole means of improving food intake is not recommended. Consideration for the use of appetite stimulants after the primary disease process has been addressed and the animal is recovering and beginning to exhibit interest in eating may be useful. Body weight and lean body mass should be evaluated daily, either in the clinic or at home by the pet owner. Additionally, daily food consumption logs should be recorded and reviewed daily to ensure adequate energy intake and response to medical intervention. Animals that are persistently anorexic or hyporexic (i.e., energy intake below daily energy requirements) for more than three days are candidates for either modification of overall medical treatment or consideration for more directed nutritional support via an indwelling feeding tube. Patients treated on an out-patient basis should also be evaluated by the veterinarian at least weekly to monitor for efficacy of treatment as well as specific adverse effects of medications (see Tables 13.1 and 13.2).

Summary

It is important to remember that anorexia is a symptom of disease and not a disease itself and, as such, the primary medical treatment should be aimed at addressing the causes of food refusal. For animals with reduced but not absent food intakes, those where the duration of anorexia is expected to be less than one week, or for those whose owners are reluctant to place an indwelling feeding tube, short-term use (i.e., less than one week) of appetite stimulants can be considered. In animals that experience persistent anorexia for more than three days despite medical management of the underlying disease state or those requiring longer-term nutritional support (i.e., expected anorexia for more than one week), placement of an indwelling feeding tube should be considered (see Chapter 3).

Clinical trials of the use of appetite stimulants in people have shown mixed results, with improvement in quality of life indicators but no change in median survival time or improvement in lean body mass. Appetite stimulants for dogs and cats may improve the owner's perception of food intake though there is a lack of evidence that they will reverse anorexia. In veterinarian medicine where the perceived quality of life may determine whether a pet owner continues treatment or not, managing the caregiver's perception of the animal's overall "wellness" may be just as valuable as addressing the patient's medical and nutritional needs.

KEY POINTS

- Appetite stimulants can be considered for short-term administration once the primary disease process has been addressed.
- It is important to recognize that symptomatic treatment of anorexia does not correct the underlying reason for food refusal.
- Side effects, such as hypotension, encountered with some appetite stimulants limit use in critically ill or debilitated patients.
- The use of appetite stimulants may address pet owners' perception of "quality of life".
- Animals being treated with appetite stimulants should be closely monitored and continued lack of adequate food intake should be addressed by altering either the medical or nutritional plan.

References

Berenstein, G. and Ortiz, Z. (2005) Megestrol acetate for the treatment of anorexia-cachexia syndrome. *Cochrane Database of Systemic Reviews*, Issue 2, No.: CD004310.

Braun, T.P. and Marks, D.L. (2010) Pathophysiology and treatment of inflammatory anorexia in chronic disease. *Journal of Cachexia, Sarcopenia and Muscle*, **1**, 135–145.

Casmian-Sorrosal, D. and Warman, S. (2010) The use of mirtazapine as an appetite stimulant in dogs and cats: a prospective observational study (Abstract). Proceedings of 53rd British Small Animal Veterinary Association Annual Congress. April 8 to 11, Birmingham, UK, p. 420.

Center, S.A., Elston, T.H., Rowland, P.H. et al. (1996) Fulminant hepatic failure associated with oral administration of diazepam in 11 cats. *Journal of the American Veterinary Medical Association*, **209**, 618–625.

Donohoe, C.L., Ryan, A.M. and Reynolds, J.V. (2011) Cancer cachexia: mechanisms and clinical implications. *Gastroenterology Research and Practice*, **60**, 14–34.

Fox, C.B., Treadway, A.K., Blaszczyk, A.T. et al. (2009) Megestrol acetate and mirtazapine for the treatment of unplanned weight loss in the elderly. *Pharmacotherapy*, **29**, 383–397.

Freeman, L.M., Rush, J.E., Kehayias, J.J. et al. (1998) Nutritional alterations and the effect of fish oil supplementation in dogs with heart failure. *Journal of Veterinary Internal Medicine*, **12**, 440–448.

Giorgi, M. and Yun, H. (2012) Pharmacokinetics of mirtazapine and its main metabolites in beagle dogs: a pilot study. *The Veterinary Journal*, **192**, 239–241.

Kuehn, N. (2008) *North American Companion Animal Formulary*, 8th edn, North American Compendiums.

Loprinzi, C.L., Ellison, N.M., Schaid, D.J. et al. (1990) Controlled trial of megestrol acetate for the treatment of cancer anorexia and cachexia. *Journal of the National Cancer Institute*, **82**, 1127–1132.

Loprinzi, C.L., Schaid, D.J., Dose, A.M. et al. (1993) Body composition changes in patients who gain weight while receiving megestrol acetate. *Journal of Clinical Oncology*, **11**, 152–154.

Morley, J.E. (2001) Anorexia, sarcopenia, and aging. *Nutrition*, **17**, 660–663.

Mantovani, G., Maccio, A., Madeddu, C. et al. (2010) Randomized phase III clinical trial of five different arms of treatment in 332 patients with cancer cachexia. *The Oncologist*, **15**, 200–211.

Perboni, S. and Inui, A. (2006) Anorexia in cancer: role of feeding regulatory peptides. *Philosophical Transactions of the Royal Society London Biological Sciences*, **361**, 1281–1289.

Plumb, D.C. (2011) *Plumb's Veterinary Drug Handbook*. 7th edn, Wiley-Blackwell Publishing.

Quimby, J.M., Gustafson, D.L. and Lunn, K.F. (2011) The pharmacokinetics of mirtazapine in cats with chronic kidney disease and in age-matched control cats. *Journal of Veterinary Internal Medicine*, **25**, 985–989.

Riechelmann, R.P. Burman, D. Tannock, I.F. et al. (2010) Phase II trial of mirtazapine for cancer-related cachexia and anorexia. *American Journal of Hospice and Palliative Care*, **27**, 106–110.

CHAPTER 14

Adverse food reactions in small animals

Cecilia Villaverde and Marta Hervera

Servei de Dietètica i Nutrició, Fundació Hospital Clínic Veterinari, Universitat Autònoma de Barcelona, Bellaterra, Spain

Introduction

An adverse food reaction (AFR) refers to an abnormal response to ingested food components. Reactions involving immune-mediated mechanisms are defined as a food allergy (FA) whereas in all other cases they are defined as food intolerances (Gaschen and Merchant, 2011). Food intolerance can be further categorized into metabolic, pharmacologic, toxic and idiosyncratic reactions (see Table 14.1).

The prevalence in dogs and cats of AFR is unknown, in part due to the difficulty in diagnosing and the variety in clinical signs. The most frequent clinical signs associated with AFR are dermatological (i.e., cutaneous adverse food reactions (CAFRs) and gastrointestinal (Verlinden et al., 2006; Gaschen and Merchant, 2011). The most common dermatological sign is non-seasonal pruritus, which can be generalized or localized (Bryan and Frank, 2010; Hensel, 2010). Common skin lesions include erythema, papules, excoriations, pododermatitis and otitis externa in dogs (Watson, 1998; Hensel, 2010) (see Figure 14.1) and military dermatitis, eosinophilic plaques, self-induced symmetrical alopecia, and head and neck excoriations in cats (Hobi et al., 2011). Gastrointestinal signs include vomiting, diarrhea and abdominal pain (Guilford et al., 2001; Verlinden et al., 2006). The coexistence of skin and gastrointestinal signs, usually reported as 10–15% of the cases (Guilford et al., 1998: Chesney, 2002), is considered very suggestive of AFR, at least in cats (Guilford et al., 2001). There is no age, sex, or breed predilection described, although clinical signs often arise before 1 year in dogs, and Siamese cats have been suggested to be at higher risk (Verlinden et al., 2006).

Nutritional Management of Hospitalized Small Animals, First Edition. Edited by Daniel L. Chan.
© 2015 John Wiley & Sons, Ltd. Published 2015 by John Wiley & Sons, Ltd.

Table 14.1 Classification of adverse food reactions (adapted from Verlinden et al., 2006 and Gaschen and Merchant, 2011).

Adverse Food reactions					
Food Allergy		**Food Intolerance**			
Ig E-mediated (immediate and intermediate hypersensitivity)	Non-IgE mediated (delayed hypersensitivity)	Idiosyncratic (idiopathic)	Metabolic (e.g. lactase deficiency)	Pharmacological (e.g. theobromine, caffeine)	Toxic (e.g. bacterial and fungal toxins)

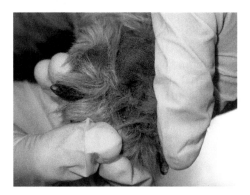

Figure 14.1 Pododermatitis in a West Highland White Terrier diagnosed with food allergy.

Pathophysiology

The term AFR includes multiple pathophysiological mechanisms that result in similar clinical signs for both FA and food intolerance. The pathophysiology of FA in dogs and cats is poorly understood, although it is assumed that there is an alteration in the normal processing of food antigens and the development of oral tolerance, as reviewed by Verlinden et al. (2006) and Gaschen and Merchant (2011). Although there are little data, both IgE- and non-IgE-mediated mechanisms are believed to exist in companion animals. Dietary antigens are commonly glycoproteins that require a minimum size to trigger a reaction. This size has been defined in human medicine as 10–70 kD, but there are no data available for dogs or cats to make a similar assertion (Cave, 2006). As for food intolerance, the pathophysiology mechanism varies depending on the particular reaction. In these cases, other non-protein ingredients can be responsible for the clinical signs (such as food additives).

It has been suggested that an intestinal inflammatory environment is capable of playing a role in the genesis of FA (Philpott et al., 1998). Thus, it could be hypothesized that patients with inflammatory bowel disease (IBD) might be predisposed to the development of FA. Several authors believe that a subset of patients with IBD respond to diet changes and it could be considered a form of AFR (Cave, 2006; Fogle and Bissett, 2007). There are some specific syndromes, such as gluten-sensitive enteropathy of Irish Setters and protein losing enteropathy–protein losing nephropathy of the Soft Coated Wheaten Terrier that are also considered AFRs (Verlinden et al., 2006).

Nutritional management strategies

The management of AFR consists in avoiding the ingredients to which the patient shows a negative response. The offending ingredients have to be identified first, and this is accomplished through an elimination-challenge process (reviewed by Verlinden et al., 2006; Bryan and Frank, 2010) after other diseases have been ruled out, such as flea allergy dermatitis, parasitic dermatitis, pyoderma and parasitic diarrhea (see Figure 14.2). The elimination part consists in exclusively feeding a diet with ingredients that the patient has never been exposed to. Other antigen sources should be eliminated (e.g., treats, flavored medication, flavoured toothpaste, unmonitored sources of food). The duration of this trial should be 8–12 weeks for CAFR and 2–4 weeks for enteropathies. The elimination trial can give false results if the ingredients used were not really novel to the patient, so at least two different elimination diets should be tested before ruling out AFR.

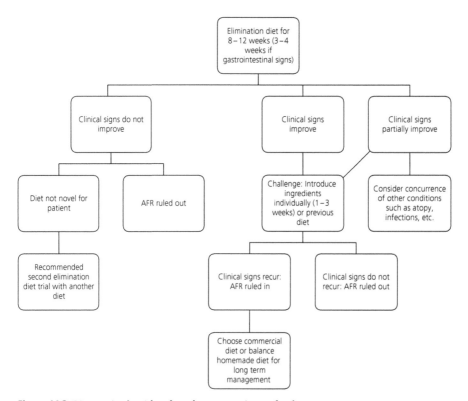

Figure 14.2 Diagnostic algorithm for adverse reaction to foods.

Animals that improve clinically to the elimination phase should then be challenged with individual ingredients suspected of eliciting the adverse reaction for 1–3 weeks. It is also possible to challenge with the previous diet, but then the individual offender might never be identified. If the clinical signs recur the patient is then diagnosed with AFR. A high percentage of dogs (35%) may react to more than one ingredient (Paterson, 1995). Patients whose clinical signs do not recur with the challenge cannot be diagnosed with AFR. In one study it was reported that 20% of cats with chronic diarrhea responded to elimination but not to the challenge (Guilford et al., 2001). The authors hypothesized that the offending ingredient might not have been correctly identified, the challenge phase might have been too short, the disease might have spontaneously resolved or other aspects of the elimination diet might be responsible for the improvement, such as digestibility or fat content.

Other diagnostic procedures have been proposed, due to the complexity of the elimination-challenge test. Specific IgE measurement in serum has very poor sensitivity (Jeffers, Shanley and Meyer, 1991) and other techniques such as gastroscopic and colonoscopic food testing have not been sufficiently evaluated (Mandigers and German, 2010).

Elimination Diets
Diet characteristics
The source and form of protein in food is the key nutritional factor in patients with suspected AFR. The ingredients most frequently implied as culprits are beef, dairy, wheat, egg, chicken, lamb and soy in dogs; and beef, dairy, fish and poultry in cats (Verlinden et al., 2006). These ingredients are routinely avoided in elimination diets. However, it is believed that these ingredients are often implicated due to their high frequency of use in pet foods in the past years, so the animals are repeatedly exposed to them, and not due to some inherent "allergenicity" (Cave, 2006). Cross reactivity between antigens of related species may exist (Garcia and Lizaso, 2011) but it has not been demonstrated in veterinary medicine as yet.

Digestibility can be considered theoretically an important characteristic to minimize the time and presence of undigested large peptides in the gut lumen, which could trigger an abnormal reaction.

There are two types of elimination diets: diets that use uncommon ingredients (to maximize the likelihood of the patient being unexposed to them) and diets that use hydrolyzed proteins.

Diets with uncommon ingredients
Finding a diet with ingredients the patient has never eaten previously can be difficult, especially with the growing number of pet foods that include exotic protein sources (e.g., bison, salmon or venison) in their formulation. There are two dietary options we can choose from: commercial or homemade. Both approaches have pros and cons which should be considered before choosing (see Table 14.2).

Homemade foods usually include a combination of a single protein source and a single carbohydrate source. The ingredients should be novel to the patient (carbohydrate sources contain some protein as well), which will restrict choices to ingredients that may be expensive and hard to find. Many authors propose

Table 14.2 Pros and cons of diets used in the diagnosis and treatment of adverse food reactions.

Homemade diets
Pros
• Do not contain food additives
• Low risk of new antigen formation during processing
• Allows the owners' involvement in patient management
• Highly digestible
Cons
• Expensive
• Time consuming
• Ingredients may be difficult to source for the owners
• Requires considerable commitment by the owner
• They are usually nutritionally unbalanced unless formulated by a veterinary nutritionist
Commercial diets with uncommon ingredients
Pros
• Generally they are the cheapest option
• Complete and balanced, can be fed long-term
• Some products are adequate for growth
• Easily available to the owner
Cons
• Contain pet food additives
• There is a risk of new antigen formation during processing
• Can contain traces of other ingredients (if not manufactured in a dedicated line)
Hydrolyzed protein source diets
Pros
• Useful in animals with a complex diet history that have been exposed to multiple ingredients
• Complete and balanced, can be fed long-term
• Some products are adequate for growth
Cons
• Contain pet food additives
• There is a risk of new antigen formation during processing
• A number of patients sensitive to the "original" protein may still be sensitive to the hydrolyzed counterpart

that homemade diets are superior as elimination diets because they do not include food additives (which are suggested as a possible cause of AFR) and they are processed at lower temperatures (Jeffers et al., 1991, Harvey, 1993). The high temperatures of pet food processing have been proposed to form new antigens that might trigger AFR (Cave and Marks, 2004). However, most of the homemade foods recommended for initial management of dogs and cats with suspected AFR were nutritionally inadequate (Roudebush and Cowell, 1992). Such diets should not be fed for longer than the elimination trial and never to growing animals. If a long term diet is required a nutritionally adequate and complete recipe must be formulated by a veterinary nutritionist. Other problems of homemade foods include cost and time.

There are several complete and balanced commercial therapeutic foods with uncommon ingredients in the market that use a single protein source and a single carbohydrate source, since not one commercial diet will work for all

Table 14.3 Lists of uncommon ingredients in canine and feline prescription products in US and Europe.

Uncommon ingredients list in canine prescription diets in US					
Producer	**Product**	**Form**	**Protein source**	**Carbohydrate source**	**Fat source**
Royal Canin	Hypoallergenic selected protein PD	Dry	Duck by-product meal/ potato protein	Potato	Coconut oil / vegetable oil / fish oil
Royal Canin	Hypoallergenic selected protein PD	Canned	Duck / duck by-product meal	Potato	Fish oil
Royal Canin	Hypoallergenic selected protein PR	Dry	Rabbit meal / potato protein	Potato	Coconut oil / vegetable oil / fish oil
Royal Canin	Hypoallergenic selected protein PR	Canned	Rabbit meal / potato protein	Potato	Vegetable oil / fish oil
Royal Canin	Hypoallergenic selected protein PV	Dry	Venison meal / potato protein	Potato	Coconut oil / vegetable oil / fish oil
Royal Canin	Hypoallergenic selected protein PV	Canned	Venison / venison meal / potato protein	Potato	Vegetable oil / fish oil
Royal Canin	Hypoallergenic selected protein PW	Dry	Whitefish meal / potato protein	Potato	Coconut oil / vegetable oil
Royal Canin	Hypoallergenic selected protein PW	Canned	Whitefish / potato protein	Potato	Vegetable oil
Royal Canin	Hypoallergenic selected protein PW moderate calorie	Dry	Whitefish meal / potato protein	Potato	Coconut oil / vegetable oil
Hill's	d/d skin support duck formula	Canned	Duck	Potato / potato starch	Soybean oil / fish oil
Hill's	d/d skin support venison formula	Canned	Lamb	Rice flour	Soybean oil / fish oil
Hill's	d/d skin support salmon formula	Canned	Salmon	Potato / potato starch	Soybean oil / fish oil
Hill's	d/d skin support venison formula	Canned	Venison / potato protein	Potato / potato starch	Soybean oil / fish oil
Hill's	d/d skin support potato & duck formula	Dry	Duck / potato protein / duck by-product meal	Potato / potato starch	Pork fat / soybean oil / fish oil
Hill's	d/d skin support potato & salmon formula	Dry	Salmon / potato protein / fish meal	Potato / potato starch	Pork fat / soybean oil / fish oil
Hill's	d/d skin support potato & venison formula	Dry	Venison / potato protein / venison meal	Potato / potato starch	Pork fat / soybean oil / fish oil
Hill's	d/d skin support rice & egg formula	Dry	Dried egg product	Brewers rice	Pork fat / soybean oil / fish oil

(Continued)

Table 14.3 (*Continued*)

Uncommon ingredients list in canine prescription diets in US

Producer	Product	Form	Protein source	Carbohydrate source	Fat source
Eukanuba	Iams veterinary formula skin & coat response FP	Canned	Catfish	Modified potato starch	Herring meal / corn oil
Eukanuba	Iams veterinary formula skin & coat response FP	Dry	Catfish	Potato	Herring meal / animal fat
Eukanuba	Iams veterinary formula skin & coat response KO	Dry	Kangaroo	Oat flour	Animal fat / fish oil
Purina	DRM dermatologic management	Dry	Salmon meal / trout	Brewers rice	Animal fat

Canine Hydrolyzed protein prescription diets in US

Producer	Product	Form	Protein source	Carbohidrate source	Fat source
Royal Canin	Hypoallergenic hydrolyzed adult HP	Dry	Hydrolyzed soy protein	Brewers rice	Chicken fat / vegetable oil / fish oil
Royal Canin	Hypoallergenic hydrolyzed adult HP small breed	Dry	Hydrolyzed soy protein	Brewers rice	Chicken fat / vegetable oil / fish oil
Royal Canin	Hypoallergenic hydrolyzed adult HP moderate calorie	Dry	Hydrolyzed soy protein	Brewers rice	Chicken fat / vegetable oil / fish oil
Hill's	z/d low allergen	Dry	Hydrolyzed chicken liver / hydrolyzed chicken	Dried potato product / potato starch	Soybean oil
Hill's	z/d ultra allergen free	Dry	Hydrolyzed chicken liver / hydrolyzed chicken	Starch	Soybean oil
Hill's	z/d ultra allergen free	Canned	Hydrolyzed chicken liver	Corn starch	Soybean oil
Purina	HA Hypoallergenic	Dry	Hydrolyzed soy protein isolate	Starch	Vegetable oil / canola oil / corn oil

Table 14.3 (*Continued*)

Uncommon ingredients feline prescription diets in US

Producer	Product	Form	Protein source	Carbohydrate source	Fat source
Royal Canin	Hypoallergenic selected protein PD	Dry	Duck by-product meal/ pea protein	Peas	Coconut oil / vegetable oil / fish oil
Royal Canin	Hypoallergenic selected protein PD	Canned	Duck/ duck by-product meal/ pea protein	Pea flour	Fish oil
Royal Canin	Hypoallergenic selected protein PR	Dry	Rabbit meal/ pea protein	Peas	Coconut oil / vegetable oil / fish oil
Royal Canin	Hypoallergenic selected protein PR	Canned	Rabbit/ pea protein	Pea flour	Vegetable oil / fish oil
Royal Canin	Hypoallergenic selected protein PV	Dry	Venison meal/ pea protein	Peas	Coconut oil / vegetable oil / fish oil
Royal Canin	Hypoallergenic selected protein PV	Canned	Venison/ venison by-products / pea protein	Pea flour	Vegetable oil / fish oil
Hill's	d/d skin support duck formula	Canned	Duck / pea protein concentrate	Ground green pea	Soybean oil / fish oil
Hill's	d/d skin support venison formula	Canned	Venison / pea protein concentrate	Ground green pea	Soybean oil / fish oil
Hill's	d/d skin support duck & green pea formula	Dry	Pea protein concentrate / duck	Ground yellow pea / ground green pea	Pork fat / fish oil
Hill's	d/d skin support rabbit & green pea formula	Dry	Pea protein concentrate / rabbit	Ground yellow pea / ground green pea	Pork fat / fish oil
Hill's	d/d skin support venison & green pea formula	Dry	Pea protein concentrate / venison	Ground yellow pea / ground green pea	Pork fat / fish oil
Eukanuba	Iams veterinary formula skin & coat response LB	Canned	Lamb / lamb meal	Ground pearled barley	Corn oil

Feline Hydrolyzed protein prescription diets in US

Producer	Product	Form	Protein source	Carbohydrate source	Fat source
Royal canin	Hypoallergenic hydrolyzed adult HP	Dry	Hydrolyzed soy protein	Brewers rice	Chicken fat / vegetable oil / fish oil

(*Continued*)

Table 14.3 (*Continued*)

Feline Hydrolyzed protein prescription diets in US

Producer	Product	Form	Protein source	Carbohydrate source	Fat source
Hill's	z/d low allergen	Dry	Hydrolyzed chicken liver / hydrolyzed chicken	Brewers rice	Soybean oil
Hill's	z/d ultra allergen free	Canned	Hydrolyzed chicken liver	Corn starch	Soybean oil
Purina	HA Hypoallergenic	Dry	Hydrolyzed soy protein isolate / hydrolyzed chicken liver / hydrolyzed chicken	Rice starch	Corn oil

Uncommon ingredients canine prescription diets in Europe

Producer	Product	Form	Protein source	Carbohydrate source	Fat source
Royal Canin	Sensitivity control	Dry	Dehydrated fish / hydrolyzed poultry liver	Tapioca	Animal fats / fish oil / soy oil
Royal Canin	Sensitivity control chicken with rice	Canned	Chicken	Rice	Fish oil / sunflower oil
Royal Canin	Sensitivity control duck with rice	Canned	Duck	Rice	Fish oil / sunflower oil
Purina	DRM dermatologic management	Dry	Salmon meal / trout	Brewers rice	Animal fat
Hill's	d/d duck formula	Canned	Duck	Potato / potato starch	Vegetable oil / fish oil
Hill's	d/d lamb formula	Canned	Lamb	Rice flour	Vegetable oil / fish oil
Hill's	d/d venison formula	Canned	Salmon	Potato / potato starch	Vegetable oil / fish oil
Hill's	d/d salmon formula	Canned	Salmon	Potato / potato starch	Vegetable oil / fish oil
Hill's	d/d venison formula	Canned	Venison / potato protein	Potato / potato starch	Vegetable oil / fish oil
Hill's	d/d duck & rice formula	Dry	Duck meal / hydrolyzed chicken	Ground rice	Animal fat / vegetable oil / fish oil
Hill's	d/d salmon & rice formula	Dry	Dried whole egg / hydrolyzed chicken	Ground rice	Animal fat / vegetable oil / fish oil

Table 14.3 (*Continued*)

Uncommon ingredients canine prescription diets in Europe

Producer	Product	Form	Protein source	Carbohydrate source	Fat source
Hill's	d/d egg & rice formula	Dry	Salmon meal / hydrolyzed chicken	Ground rice	Animal fat / vegetable oil / fish oil
Eukanuba	Veterinary diets dermatosis FP	Dry	Fish meal / catfish / hydrolyzed fish protein	Potato	Animal fat
Eukanuba	Veterinary diets dermatosis FP	Canned	Catfish / kipper meal	Modified potato starch	Corn oil
Affinity	Advance dermatosis limited antigen	Dry	Trout / dehydrated salmon protein	Rice	Animal fat /fish oil
Specific	CDD food allergy management	Dry	Egg	Rice	Animal fat / sunflower oil
Specific	CDW food allergy management	Canned	Lamb	Rice	Soybean oil

Canine Hydrolyzed protein prescription diets in Europe

Producer	Product	Form	Protein source	Carbohydrate source	Fat source
Royal Canin	Hypoallergenic	Dry	Hydrolyzed soy protein / hydrolyzed poultry liver	Rice	Animal fat / soybean oil / fish oil
Royal Canin	Hypoallergenic moderate energy	Dry	Hydrolyzed soy protein / hydrolyzed poultry liver	Rice	Animal fat / soybean oil / fish oil
Royal Canin	Hypoallergenic small dog	Dry	Hydrolyzed soy protein / hydrolyzed poultry liver	Rice	Animal fat / soybean oil / fish oil
Purina	HA hypoallergenic	Dry	Hydrolyzed soy protein isolate	Starch	Vegetable oil / canola oil / corn oil
Hill's	z/d low allergen	Dry	Hydrolyzed chicken liver / hydrolyzed chicken	Dried potato product / potato starch	Vegetable oil

(*Continued*)

Table 14.3 (*Continued*)

Canine Hydrolyzed protein prescription diets in Europe

Producer	Product	Form	Protein source	Carbohydrate source	Fat source
Hill's	z/d ultra allergen free	Dry	Hydrolyzed chicken liver	Starch	Vegetable oil
Hill's	z/d ultra allergen free	Canned	Hydrolyzed chicken liver	Corn starch	Vegetable oil
Affinity	Advance Hypo Allergenic	Dry	Hydrolyzed soy protein	Corn starch	Coconut oil / corn oil
Specific	CωD-hy Allergy management plus	Dry	Hydrolyzed salmon protein / rice protein	Rice	Fish oil / pork fat / sunflower oil
Specific	CYD-HY Food allergy management	Dry	Hydrolyzed salmon protein / rice protein	Rice	Pork fat / sunflower oil

Uncommon ingredients feline prescription diets in Europe

Producer	Product	Form	Protein source	Carbohydrate source	Fat source
Royal Canin	Sensitivity control	Dry	Dehydrated duck meat / hydrolysed poultry proteins / rice gluten	Rice	Animal fats / fish oil / soybean oil
Royal Canin	Sensitivity control duck & rice	Canned	Duk /rice protein	Rice	Fish oil
Royal Canin	Sensitivity control chicken & rice	Canned	Chicken	Rice	Fish oil
Eukanuba	Veterinary diets dermatosis lb	Canned	Lamb	Barley	Corn oil
Hill's	d/d skin support duck formula	Canned	Duck / pea protein concentrate	Ground green pea	Soybean oil / fish oil
Hill's	d/d venison formula	Dry	Pea protein extract / venison meal / hydrolyzed poultry liver	Dehydrated peas	Animal fat / vegetable oil / fish oil
Specific	CDW food allergy management	Canned	Lamb	Rice	Soybean oil

Table 14.3 (*Continued*)

Feline Hydrolyzed protein prescription diets in Europe					
Producer	**Product**	**Form**	**Protein source**	**Carbohidrate source**	**Fat source**
Royal Canin	Hypoallergenic	Dry	Hydrolyzed soy protein / hydrolyzed poultry liver	Rice	Animal fat / soybean oil / fish oil
Purina	HA Hypoallergenic	Dry	Hydrolyzed soy protein isolate / hydrolyzed chicken liver / hydrolyzed chicken	Rice starch	Corn oil
Hill's	z/d low allergen	Dry	Hydrolyzed chicken liver / hydrolyzed chicken	Brewers rice	Soybean oil
Hill's	z/d ultra allergen free	Canned	Hydrolyzed chicken liver	Corn starch	Soybean oil
Affinity	Advance Hypo Allergenic	Dry	Hydrolyzed soy protein / hydrolyzed animal protein	Corn starch	Coconut oil / corn oil
Specific	FωD-HY allergy management plus	Dry	Hydrolyzed salmon protein	Rice	Fish oil / pork fat / sunflower oil
Specific	FDD-HY food allergy management	Dry	Hydrolyzed salmon protein / rice protein	Rice	Pork fat / sunflower oil

patients (Table 14.3). However, not all have been tested in dogs and cats with known AFR (Leistra, Markwell and Willemse, 2001; Leistra and Willemse, 2002; Guilford et al., 2001; Sauter et al., 2006). Over the counter foods with uncommon ingredients should be avoided, since some of them may contain multiple protein sources and include traces of common pet food proteins not mentioned on the label, as shown in a recent study (Raditic, Remillard and Tater, 2011).

Diets with hydrolyzed proteins

The aim of hydrolyzing proteins is to sufficiently disrupt the protein structure to a size that does not trigger an immune response, both in patients already sensitized to the intact protein and in naive individuals. Many dry therapeutic commercial diets exist in the market. These diets use either uncommon carbohydrate sources or purified starch.

These diets are good options when the patient has been exposed to multiple protein sources or the diet history is incomplete. They have been reported to be effective in a high percentage of dogs (Loeffler et al., 2006; Biourge, Fontaine and Vroom, 2004; Mandigers et al., 2010a). However, it seems that a small percentage of animals sensitive to the intact protein can react to the hydrolysate (Jackson et al., 2003; Olivry and Bizikova, 2010) or other ingredients of these diets (starch, oils, additives, or new antigens).

Specific considerations
Hospitalized patients
Hospitalized patients diagnosed with AFR
Patients with AFR hospitalized for any reason should have detailed feeding instructions in their hospitalization chart. Owners of those patients should be asked to clearly specify the regular food currently consumed (and tolerated) by the patient and provide some if the hospital does not carry it.

Hospitalized patients with chronic enteropathies
Patients suffering from enteritis (including IBD) might be susceptible to temporary loss of oral tolerance, which may worsen clinical signs. This concern has led to the recommendation of feeding a "sacrificial protein" during recovery in these patients during the initial treatment phase (Cave, 2006). After a few weeks, the diet can be switched to a commercial diet with novel ingredients or hydrolyzed. Another option would be to feed a hydrolyzed protein diet and thus avoid the formation of new AFR during recovery and minimize clinical signs and complications (Cave, 2006).

Thus, in patients with chronic enteropathies or suspected of AFR that are hospitalized (e.g. to obtain biopsies) there are several options: use a highly digestible, energy dense diet ("intestinal" type diet) or use a hydrolyzed diet, which is also highly digestible and may potentially help with recovery. If an elimination trial needs to be instituted at home, the food used while hospitalized should be avoided since the patient may have become sensitized to those ingredients.

Hydrolyzed and uncommon ingredient diets can also be used long term for chronic enteritis, including IBD patients, since there have been reports of improvement using diet, sometimes without the need for immunosuppression (Nelson, Stookey and Kazacos, 1998; Guilford et al., 2001; Fogle and Bissett, 2007; Mandigers et al., 2010b). One study compared the use of a hydrolyzed diet with an intestinal-type diet in the management of chronic small bowel enteropathy in dogs and, while both treatments resulted in clinical improvement, the dogs on the hydrolyzed diets remained free of signs for a longer period of time (Mandigers et al., 2010a).

Diet history
The diet history is key in diagnosis and treatments and should include an exhaustive list of the products regularly supplied to the patients during their lifetime, including commercial and human foods, snacks, treats, supplements, chewable medications, human foods and any other available food

source. This will allow us to choose adequate elimination diets in animals suspected of AFR and know what to avoid in hospitalized patients already diagnosed with AFR.

The objective of the diet history is to make a list of ingredients the pet has been exposed. In the US the majority of pet foods follow AAFCO (Association of American Feed Control Officials) regulations and list all their ingredients in the label, thus, it is relatively easy to identify them. Diets are subject to reformulation which will induce error, but unfortunately this is out of our control.

In Europe, current legislation permits to list ingredients as categories (e.g. "cereal" and "meat"). In some cases, this makes it close to impossible to make a proper list of ingredients the patient has eaten and a hydrolyzed diet or a really exotic ingredient might be the best option.

Monitoring and complications

The most common complication is recurrence of clinical signs. Adequate management of animals with AFR requires avoiding the offending ingredient(s) for life using a complete and balanced diet, be it commercial or home cooked. Given this life-long commitment to a single diet, compliance can be an issue, and it can be involuntary (animal eating a food meant for another animal, scavenging food, unmonitored food source and even changes in formulation of the usual diet) or voluntary (owners giving treats and other food items). Client education both during the elimination trial and after is key to success (Chesney, 2002, Gaschen and Merchant, 2011). Regular visits after diagnosis (every 6–12 months) should include a thorough diet history (to check compliance).

Some pets with diagnosed AFR might conceivably develop eventually another AFR to ingredients in the new diet. In these cases an alternative diet must be found. The other way around could also be possible: in human adults, dietary avoidance of the offending foods for 1 to 2 years resulted in the reestablishment of antigen tolerance in more than 30% of patients with FA (Pastorello et al., 1989). We do not yet have data in animals in this regard.

Concurrent allergies have been reported (Paterson, 1995; Loeffler et al., 2004) and may influence the threshold level of clinical signs. It is important to keep a strict control of atopic and flea allergic dogs that also have AFR.

Summary

Adverse reactions to food result in chronic non-specific skin and gastrointestinal clinical signs that adversely influence the quality of life of dogs and cats. The main treatment consists in avoiding the ingredients responsible for the reaction, and for this a complete and detailed diet history is essential. There are several diet options available, both commercial and homemade, that either include uncommon food ingredients or hydrolyzed protein sources. Care should be taken to avoid other sources of potentially damaging substances (e.g., treats, human foods, flavoured medication) and regular monitoring is important to ensure compliance and avoid recurrence.

KEY POINTS

- In most cases, AFR manifests as dermatological problems (mainly non-seasonal pruritus) and non-specific gastrointestinal problems (such as vomiting and diarrhea).
- The gold standard to diagnose AFR is with an elimination–challenge food trial. A complete and exhaustive diet history is crucial to the success of this trial.
- The main nutritional treatment of animals with AFR is to avoid the offending ingredients. Again, a complete diet history is necessary to ensure the success of the treatment.
- Homemade or commercial diets can be used for diagnosis and treatment of AFR. A specific diet has to be chosen for the particular patient after careful consideration of pros and cons of each option.
- If homemade diets are used long-term (longer than the food trial protocol) they must be formulated by a veterinary nutritionist to ensure nutritional adequacy.
- In hospitalized patients with diagnosed AFR feeding orders must be accurately detailed and followed to avoid recurrence of clinical signs while under our care.

References

Biourge, V. C., Fontaine, J. and Vroom, M. W. (2004) Diagnosis of adverse reactions to food in dogs: efficacy of a soy-isolate hydrolyzate-based diet. *Journal of Nutrition*, **134**, 2062S–2064S.

Bryan, J. and Frank, L. A. (2010) Food allergy in the cat: a diagnosis by elimination. *Journal of Feline Medicine and Surgery*, **12**, 861–866.

Cave, N. J. (2006) Hydrolyzed protein diets for dogs and cats. *Veterinary Clinics of North America: Small Animal Practice*, **36**, 1251–1268.

Cave, N. J. and Marks, S. L. (2004) Evaluation of the immunogenicity of dietary proteins in cats and the influence of the canning process. *American Journal of Veterinary Research*, **65**(10), 1427–1433.

Chesney, C. J. (2002) Food sensitivity in the dog: a quantitative study. *Journal of Small Animal Practice*, **43**, 203–207.

Fogle, J. E. and Bissett, S. A. (2007) Mucosal immunity and chronic idiopathic enteropathies in dogs. *Compendium on Continual Education for the Practicing Veterinarian*, **29**, 290–302.

Garcia, B. E. and Lizaso, M. T. (2011) Cross-reactivity syndromes in food allergy. *Journal of Investigational Allergology and Clinical Immunology*, **21**, 162–170.

Gaschen, F. P. and Merchant, S. R. (2011) Adverse food reactions in dogs and cats. *Veterinary Clinics of North America: Small Animal Practice*, **41**, 361–379.

Guilford, W. G., Jones, B. R., Markwell, P. J. et al. (2001) Food sensitivity in cats with chronic idiopathic gastrointestinal problems. *Journal of Veterinary Internal Medicine*, **15**, 7–13.

Guilford, W. G., Markwell, P. J., Jones et al. (1998) Prevalence and causes of food sensitivity in cats with chronic pruritus, vomiting or diarrhea. *Journal of Nutrition*, **128**, 2790S–2791S.

Harvey, R. G. (1993) Food allergy and dietary intolerance in dogs - a report of 25 cases. *Journal of Small Animal Practice*, **34**, 175–179.

Hensel, P. (2010) Nutrition and skin diseases in veterinary medicine. *Clinics in Dermatology*, **28**, 686–693.

Hobi, S., Linek, M., Marignac, G. et al. (2011) Clinical characteristics and causes of pruritus in cats: a multicentre study on feline hypersensitivity-associated dermatoses. *Veterinary Dermatology*, **22**, 406–413.

Jackson, H. A., Jackson, M. W., Coblentz, L. et al. (2003) Evaluation of the clinical and allergen specific serum immunoglobulin E responses to oral challenge with cornstarch, corn, soy and a soy hydrolysate diet in dogs with spontaneous food allergy. *Veterinary Dermatology*, **14**, 181–187.

Jeffers, J. G., Shanley, K. J. and Meyer, E. K. (1991) Diagnostic testing of dogs for food hypersensitivity. *Journal of the American Veterinary Medical Association*, **198**, 245–250.

Leistra, M. and Willemse, T. (2002) Double-blind evaluation of two commercial hypoallergenic diets in cats with adverse food reactions. *Journal of Feline Medicine and Surgery*, **4**, 185–188.

Leistra, M. H., Markwell, P. J. and Willemse, T. (2001) Evaluation of selected-protein-source diets for management of dogs with adverse reactions to foods. *Journal of the American Veterinary Medical Association*, **219**, 1411–1414.

Loeffler, A., Lloyd, D. H., Bond et al. (2004) Dietary trials with a commercial chicken hydrolysate diet in 63 pruritic dogs. *The Veterinary Record*, **154**, 519–522.

Loeffler, A., Soares-Magalhaes, R., Bond, R. et al., (2006) A retrospective analysis of case series using home-prepared and chicken hydrolysate diets in the diagnosis of adverse food reactions in 181 pruritic dogs. *Veterinary Dermatology*, **17**, 273–279.

Mandigers, P. & German, A. J. (2010) Dietary hypersensitivity in cats and dogs. *Tijdschrift voor Diergeneeskunde*, **135**, 706–710.

Mandigers P. J. J., Biourge, V., van den Ingh, T. S. G. A. M. et al. (2010a) A randomized, open-label, positively-controlled field trial of a hydrolyzed protein diet in dogs with chronic small bowel enteropathy. *Journal of Veterinary Internal Medicine*, **24**, 1350–1357.

Mandigers, P. J., Biourge, V. and German, A. J. (2010b) Efficacy of a commercial hydrolysate diet in eight cats suffering from inflammatory bowel disease or adverse reaction to food. *Tijdschrift voor Diergeneeskunde*, **135**, 668–672.

Nelson, R. W., Stookey, L. J. & Kazacos, E. (1988) Nutritional management of idiopathic chronic colitis in the dog. *Journal of Veterinary Internal Medicine*, **2**, 133–137.

Olivry, T. and Bizikova, P. (2010) A systematic review of the evidence of reduced allergenicity and clinical benefit of food hydrolysates in dogs with cutaneous adverse food reactions. *Veterinary Dermatology*, **21**, 32–41.

Pastorello, E. A., Stocchi, L., Pravettoni, V. et al. (1989) Role of the elimination diet in adults with food allergy. *The Journal of Allergy and Clinical Immunology*, **84**, 475–483.

Paterson, S. (1995) Food hypersensitivity in 20 dogs with skin and gastrointestinal signs. *Journal of Small Animal Practice*, **36**, 529–534.

Philpott, D. J., McKay, D. M., Mak, W. et al. (1998) Signal transduction pathways involved in enterohemorrhagic Escherichia coli-induced alterations in T84 epithelial permeability. *Infection and Immunity*, **66**, 1680–1687.

Raditic, D. M., Remillard, R. L. and Tater, K. C. (2011) ELISA testing for common food antigens in four dry dog foods used in dietary elimination trials. *Journal of Animal Physiology and Animal Nutrition*, **95**, 90–97.

Roudebush, P. and Cowell, C. S. (1992) Results of a hypoallergenic diets survey of veterinarians in North America with a nutritional evaluation of homemade diet prescriptions. *Veterinary Dermatology*, **3**, 23–28.

Sauter, S. N., Benyacoub, J., Allenspach, K. et al. (2006) Effects of probiotic bacteria in dogs with food responsive diarrhoea treated with an elimination diet. *Journal of Animal Physiology and Animal Nutrition*, **90**, 269–277.

Verlinden, A., Hesta, M., Millet, S. et al. (2006) Food allergy in dogs and cats: a review. *Critical Reviews in Food Science and Nutrition*, **46**, 259–273.

Watson, T. D. (1998) Diet and skin disease in dogs and cats. *Journal of Nutrition*, **128**, 2783S–2789S.

CHAPTER 15

Nutritional management of short bowel syndrome in dogs and cats

Daniel L. Chan

Department of Veterinary Clinical Sciences and Services, The Royal Veterinary College, University of London, UK

Introduction

Short bowel syndrome (SBS) refers to a constellation of clinical signs resulting from intestinal malabsorption that develops following extensive resection of the small intestines (Yanoff and Willard, 1989). Affected individuals can develop a number of nutritional and metabolic disturbances typified by weight loss, chronic diarrhea, fluid and electrolyte imbalances. Long-term survival of patients with SBS is dependent on adaptation of the remaining small intestine and response to pharmacological and nutritional management (Wall, 2013). In people, this syndrome is encountered when there is extensive or repeated resection of small bowel for management of chronic inflammatory (e.g., Crohn's disease), ischaemic or neoplastic processes. Disease processes in dogs and cats that may require extensive resection include linear foreign bodies, intussusception, mesenteric volvulus or entrapment/ischaemia. While there is no defined amount of small intestine that is removed for SBS to develop, patients that have > 50% of small intestine resected are believed to be at high risk for developing SBS (Urban and Weser, 1980; Wilmore et al., 1997; Wall, 2013). Although intestinal resection/anastomosis is a relatively common procedure in dogs and cats, resection of > 50% of the small intestine appears to be uncommon (Figure 15.1). Moreover, the development of SBS has mostly been reported in experimental reports that have used canine models of the disease and in sporadic case reports and case series (Wilmore et al., 1971; Joy and Patterson, 1978; Williams and Burrows, 1981; Pawlusiow and McCarthy, 1994; Uchiyama et al., 1996; Yanoff et al., 1992; Gorman et al., 2006). Dogs affected by SBS have been reported to have watery diarrhea, fluid and electrolyte imbalances and significant weight loss (Pawlusiow and McCarthy, 1994; Williams and Burrows, 1981). In the largest retrospective study in dogs and cats published thus far, no relationship between the percentage of resected intestines and the development of SBS has been identified (Gorman et al., 1996). Although data on this syndrome and response rate to treatment in dogs and cats is scarce, there are some general considerations in respect to drug and nutritional therapy that can be used in animals at high risk for developing SBS and these will be discussed in this chapter.

Nutritional Management of Hospitalized Small Animals, First Edition. Edited by Daniel L. Chan.

© 2015 John Wiley & Sons, Ltd. Published 2015 by John Wiley & Sons, Ltd.

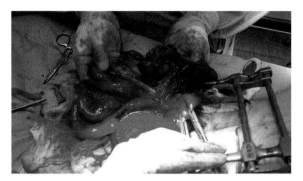

Figure 15.1 Extensive resection of bowel in dogs and cats is not performed commonly but may be required in cases with extreme devitalization of intestines, as depicted in this picture of a dog with intestinal volvulus. Source: Elvin Kulendra. Reproduced with permission of Elvin Kulendra.

Pathophysiology

Following extensive resection of the small intestines, postprandial motility is altered, leading to delayed gastric emptying and increased intestinal transit times in other segments of small intestines (Johnson et al., 1996). Loss of absorptive surface compromises adequate absorption of water, electrolytes and other nutrients. Incomplete digestion and absorption of nutrients may result in osmotic diarrhea. In addition, unabsorbed bile acids and fatty acids may lead to secretory diarrhea in the large bowel. Clinical manifestations of SBS include dehydration, vomiting, diarrhea, cramping and weight loss. Diarrhea may be intermittent or persistent. In chronic cases, animals may become catabolic with significant muscle wasting despite being polyphagic. In cases where the ileum is removed, there is also bile acid and vitamin B_{12} (i.e., cobalamin) malabsorption. Findings on hematology and serum biochemistry are not specific although findings of hypoalbuminemia, mild, normocytic, normochromic non-regenerative anemia may be present. The presence of microcytic anemia may be suggestive of cobalamin deficiency.

Through a process of intestinal recovery and adaptation, the presence of luminal nutrients stimulates the remaining small intestine to undergo a period of hypertrophy and hyperplasia, which may continue for several weeks to months. Exposure to luminal contents, endogenous GI secretions, trophic effects of gut hormones (especially epidermal growth factor, enteroglucagon and gastrin), intraluminal polyamines, and neural factors all contribute to adaptation of the remaining bowel (Cisler and Buchman, 2005). Dilatation, lengthening and thickening of the intestine are observed, along with epithelial cell proliferation in intestinal crypts and migration of cells into intestinal villi (Thompson, Quigley and Adrian, 1999; Cisler and Buchman, 2005). The colon also becomes an important digestive organ in patients with SBS (Jeppensen and Mortensen, 1998). Sodium, water and some amino acids are absorbed in the colon, as well as energy from absorbed short-chain fatty acids (Jeppensen and Mortensen, 1998). Thus, a source of readily available fermentable fiber should be included in all diets, while insoluble fiber should be kept to a minimum to maximize nutrient digestibility (Roth et al., 1995). Short-chain fatty acids promote mucosal hyperplasia and thus support further bowel adaptation. Intestinal adaptation is typified by enterocyte hyperplasia, increases in bowel diameter, villous height, crypt depth and enterocyte density. Ideally, these physical changes will increase the bowel's absorptive capacity. Mucosal changes may start to occur within a few days and can result in a fourfold increase in mucosal surface area within 14 days, if intraluminal contents are provided (Vanderhoof et al., 1992).

Nutritional management strategies

In the initial post-operative period following extensive bowel resection (e.g., >50% of bowel removed), there should be consideration for parenteral nutritional support initially, with introduction of a small amount of enteral nutrition within days following surgery (Figure 15.2). Long-term dietary management is complex and needs to be individualized for each patient depending on residual intestinal function and nutritional status. In addition to nutrient intake, management of SBS also requires appropriate oral rehydration, vitamin and mineral supplementation and pharmacotherapy. Several medications provide a useful adjunctive function to dietary intervention, including antidiarrheal agents (e.g., loperamide), H_2 antagonists (e.g., famotidine) and proton pump inhibitors (e.g., omeprazole) and antimicrobials. Future therapy will likely involve direct stimulation of intestinal adaptation through the administration of trophic factors such as glucagon-like protein 2 (GLP-2) (Bechtold et al., 2014) and is discussed in a later section.

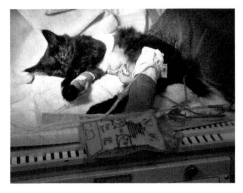

Figure 15.2 Patients with extensive small bowel resection, such as the cat depicted in this picture, may require initial nutritional management consisting of parenteral nutrition (as has been done in this case) with gradual introduction of enteral nutrition.

Specific recommendations based on resultant GI integrity

If only the jejunum is resected, long-term management will require feeding multiple small meals throughout the day as this may help with improving absorption and decrease episodes of vomiting. Diets should have very high digestibility, as is typical in super-premium and prescription diets. Fat content should be limited to a maximum of 25% of metabolized energy as excessive fat will exacerbate diarrhea and vomiting. Dietary fiber is important to stimulate intestinal adaptation, maximize colonic absorption and bind unabsorbed bile acids. However, excessive fiber will decrease digestibility, impair nutrient absorption, and may exacerbate diarrhea. Supplementing the diet with psyllium or wheat bran may be helpful. Diets with high non-fermentable fiber (e.g., cellulose), although low in fat, are not recommended.

If there is greater than 50% of small intestines removed including partial resection of the ilium bile salt-induced diarrhea may develop that may not be controlled with increased dietary fiber. The addition of cholestyramine (100–300 mg/kg PO q 12 h) may help bind bile salts. Supplemental taurine is advised in dogs and cats with long-term cholestyramine treatment as obligate losses of taurine will be increased with binding of bile salts. Vitamin B_{12} supplementation 250 µg (cats) or 500 µg (dogs) subcutaneously or intramuscularly, weekly for 4 weeks then every 1–4 weeks as indicated, may also be advised.

If there is complete resection of the ilium fat restriction is absolutely required and diets may have to be formulated to contain less than 20% calories from fat. With massive (>70% resection of jejunum and ileum), PN may be initially required for several days. Enteral feeding should be initiated as soon as feasible as introduction of enteral feeding will help with bowel adaptation, however, the amount of enteral feeding tolerated may be small. The introduction of enteral feeding can be very gradual within a couple of days postoperatively, supplying as little as 25% of resting energy requirements. This amount of enteral feeding may be sufficient to provide luminal benefits and stimulate trophic factors. These patients will also require medical management including cholestyramine therapy, taurine and parenteral vitamin B_{12} supplementation, as described above.

Special considerations

Removal of the ileocolic valve removes the physical barrier that separates the profuse bacterial flora of the colon and this could lead to small intestinal bacterial overgrowth. Using diets with prebiotic fructooligosaccharides (FOS) have been proposed to help with small intestinal bacterial overgrowth so it may be helpful in cases with SBS. As there are commercial diets designed with low fat, high fermentable fiber content with added FOS, such diets may be ideal for patients with SBS.

As glutamine is a primary energy source for enterocytes, it has been extensively studied in the context of intestinal adaptation (Lund et al., 1990; Rhoads et al., 1991; Tamada et al., 1993). In animal models, the use of glutamine induces intestinal adaptation by increasing the length of intestinal villi and thereby increases absorption capacity (Lund et al., 1990; Rhoads et al., 1991; Tamada et al., 1993).

Growth hormone (in the form of recombinant human growth hormone) has similarly been evaluated for its capacity to increase body weight, lean body mass in human patients with SBS (Ellegard et al., 1997; Seguy et al., 2003). A series of studies combining glutamine and growth hormone in patients with SBS have yielded mixed results and, unfortunately, the effects appear to require continual use, the therapy is expensive and does not affect overall clinical outcome (Bechtold et al., 2014).

Teduglutide, an analogue of glucagon-like peptide 2 (GLP-2) has been shown to be a promising and key agent in stimulating intestinal adaptation and a series of studies have demonstrated reduction of diarrhea, improvement in intestinal structure, reduction of PN-dependence and some resolution in some patients with SBS (Jeppesen et al., 2001; Haderslev et al., 2002; Jeppesen et al., 2011; O'Keefe et al., 2013). However, this drug is not without serious side-effects and is associated with prolific trophic effect on intestinal mucosa to the point of causing partial or complete intestinal obstruction in some patients with SBS (Jeppesen et al., 2011; O'Keefe et al., 2013). As a potent growth factor, teduglutide could also promote growth of intestinal neoplasms (Bechtold et al., 2014). Currently, there are no reports on the use of tediglutide in animals with SBS.

Monitoring and complications

Animals that have undergone extensive bowel resection should be assessed on a weekly to biweekly basis for tolerance to enteral feeding, stool quality and body condition. Additionally, assessing for the presence of anemia is advised as this may require vitamin B_{12} supplementation. Prognosis for patients with SBS can be variable, with some cases stabilizing with appropriate medical and nutritional management. Response to treatment does not appear to be predictable based on length of intestine removed (Gorman et al., 2006).

Summary

Short bowel syndrome may be a serious sequelae to extensive bowel resection comprising at least > 50% of length of the bowel, although the precise percentage of bowel removed that is required to trigger SBS has not been demonstrated in dogs or cats. In animals that undergo extensive bowel resection, there should be consideration for providing parenteral nutrition initially with gradual introduction of enteral feeding within a couple of days following surgery. Patients displaying clinical signs of SBS should be managed with anti-diarrheal agents, antacids, parenteral vitamin injections and nutritional support. The recommended dietary strategy includes frequent and small meals, and use of a diet that is restricted in fat and high in fermentable fiber. There is insufficient evidence to recommend glutamine or growth hormone in dogs at risk for developing SBS, but some human patients with SBS may respond to such therapy. Newer pharmacological agents that have been identified to be potent trophic factors could be used in the future in animals with SBS but as yet are untried in veterinary patients.

> **KEY POINTS**
>
> - Short bowel syndrome results from severe intestinal malabsorption that develops following extensive resection of the small intestines.
>
> - Affected individuals can develop a number of nutritional and metabolic disturbances typified by weight loss, chronic diarrhea, fluid and electrolyte imbalances.
>
> - A definitive percentage of bowel that needs to be resected to trigger short bowel syndrome in dogs has not been established, although those with >50% of bowel resected are believed to be at high risk.
>
> - Survival of affected patients depends on the ability of the remaining intestines and colon to adapt and cope with digestion and assimilation.
>
> - Main nutritional strategy includes feeding small and frequent meals using a diet restricted in fat and high in fermentable fibre.
>
> - Some affected patients also require long-term therapy with anti-diarrheal agents, antacids and antimicrobial agents.
>
> - Goals for management include improvement in fecal quality, decreased fecal output, improved body weight and body condition score.

References

Bechtold, M.L., McClave, S.A., Palmer, L.B. et al. (2014) The pharmacologic treatment of short bowel syndrome: New Tricks and Novel Agents. *Current Gastroenterology Reports,* **16**:392, doi: 10.1007/s11894-014-0392-2.

Cisler, J.J. and Buchman, A.L. (2005) Intestinal adaptation in short bowel syndrome. *Journal of Investigative Medicine,* **53**, 402–413.

Ellegard, L., Bosaeus, I., Nordgren, S. et al. (1997) Low-dose recombinant human growth hormone increases body weight and lean body mass in patients with short bowel syndrome. *Annals of Surgery,* **225**, 88–96.

Gorman, S.C., Freeman, L.M., Mitchell, S.L. et al. (2006) Extensive small bowel resection in dogs and cats: 20 cases (1998–2004). *Journal of the American Veterinary Medicine Association,* **228**, 403–407.

Jeppensen, P.B. and Mortensen, P.B. (1998) The influence of a preserved colon on the absorption of medium chain fat in patients with small bowel resection. *Gut,* **43**, 478–83.

Jeppesen, P.B., Hartmann, B., Thulesen, J. et al. (2001) Glucagon-like peptide 2 improves nutrient absorption and nutritional status in short-bowel patients with no colon. *Gastroenterology,* **120**, 806–815.

Jeppesen, P.B., Gilroy, R., Perkiewicz, M. et al. (2011) Randomized placebo-controlled trial of teduglutide in reducing parenteral nutrition and/or intravenous fluid requirements in patients with short bowel syndrome. *Gut,* **60**, 902–914.

Johnson, C.P., Sarna, S.K., Zhu, Y.R. et al. (1996) Delayed gastroduodenal emptying is an important mechanism for control of intestinal transit in short-gut syndrome. *American Journal of Surgery,* **171**, 90–95.

Joy, C.L. and Patterson, J.M. (1978) Short bowel syndrome following surgical correction of a double intussusception in a dog. *Canadian Veterinary Journal,* **19**, 254–259.

Haderslev, K.V., Jeppesen, P.B., Hartmenn, B. et al. (2002) Short-term administration of glucagon-like peptide-2. Effects on bone mineral density and markers of bone turnover in short bowel syndrome patients with no colon. *Scandinavian Journal of Gastroenterology,* **37**, 392–398.

Lund, P.K., Ulshen M.H., Rountree, D.B. et al. (1990) Molecular biology of gastrointestinal peptides and growth factors: relevance to intestinal adaptation. *Digestion,* **46**, Suppl 2, 66–73.

O'Keefe, S.J., Jeppesen, P.B., Gilroy, R. et al. (2013) Safety and efficacy of teduglutide after 52 weeks of treatment in patients with short bowel intestinal failure. *Clinical Gastroenterology Hepatology*, **11**, 815–823.

Pawlusiow, J.I. and McCarthy, R.J. (1994). Dietary management of short bowel syndrome in a dog. *Veterinary Clinical Nutrition*, **1**, 163–170.

Rhoads, J.M., Keku, E.O., Quinn, J. et al. (1991) L-glutamine stimulates jejunal sodium and chloride absorption in pig rotavirus enteritis. *Gastroenterology*, **100**, 683–691.

Roth, J.A., Frankel, W.L., Zhang, W. et al (1995) Pectin improves colonic function in rat short bowel syndrome. *Journal of Surgical Research*, **58**, 240–246.

Seguy, D., Vahedi, K., Kapel, N. et al. (2003) Low-dose growth hormone in adult home parenteral nutrition-dependent short bowel syndrome patients: a positive study. *Gastroenterology*, **124**, 293–302.

Tamada, H., Nezu, E.O., Quinn, J. et al. (1993) Alanyl-glutamine-enriched total parenteral nutrition restores intestinal adaptation. *Journal of Parenteral and Enteral Nutrition*, **17**, 236–242.

Thompson, J.S., Quigley, E.M. and Adrian, T.E. (1999) Factors affecting outcome following proximal and distal intestinal resection in the dog: an examination of the relative roles of mucosal adaptation, motility, luminal factors, and enteric peptides. *Digestive Disease Science*, **44**, 63–74.

Uchiyama, M., Iwafuchi, M., Matsuda, Y. et al. (1996) Intestinal motility after massive small bowel resection in conscious canines: comparison of acute and chronic phases. *Journal of Pediatric Gastroenterology and Nutrition*, **23**, 217–223.

Urban, E. and Weser, E. (1980) Intestinal adaptation to bowel resection. *Advances in Internal Medicine*, **26**, 265–291.

Vanderhoof, J.A., Lagnas, A.N., Pinch, L.W. et al. (1992) Short Bowel Syndrome. *Journal of Pediatric Gastroenterology and Nutrition*, **14**, 559–570.

Wall, E.A. (2013) An overview of short bowel syndrome management: adherence, adaptation, and practical recommendations. *Journal of the Academy of Nutrition and Dietetics*, **113**, 1200–1208.

Wilmore, D.W., Byren, T.A., Persinger R.L. et al. (1997) Short bowel syndrome: new therapeutic approaches. *Current Problems in Surgery*, **34**, 389–444.

Williams D.A. and Burrows C.F. (1981) Short bowel syndrome—a case report in a dog and discussion of the pathophysiology of bowel resection. *Journal of Small Animal Practice*, **22**, 263–265.

Yanoff S.R., Willard M.D., Boothe H.W. et al. (1992) Short-bowel syndrome in four dogs. *Veterinary Surgery*, **21**, 217–222.

Yanoff S.R. and Willard, M.D. (1989) Short bowel syndrome in dogs and cats. *Seminars in Veterinary Medicine and Surgery*, **4**, 226–231.

CHAPTER 16

Refeeding syndrome in small animals

Daniel L. Chan

Department of Veterinary Clinical Sciences and Services, The Royal Veterinary College, University of London, UK

Introduction

Refeeding syndrome refers to a potentially fatal constellation of metabolic derangements that occur upon refeeding a patient with an extended period of complete anorexia or severe malnutrition (Crook, Hally and Panteli, 2001; Kraft, Btaiche and Sacks, 2005). These metabolic derangements include severe hypophosphatemia, hypomagnesemia, hypokalemia, hyponatremia, hypocalcemia, hyperglycemia and vitamin deficiencies (Skipper, 2012). Clinical manifestations of these abnormalities include peripheral edema, hemolytic anemia, cardiac failure, neurological dysfunction and respiratory failure. Many of these metabolic changes are believed to result from sudden release of insulin (stimulated by carbohydrate intake) in the presence of total body nutrient depletion. The successful management and refeeding of a patient with a history of prolonged starvation, therefore, involves careful use of fluid therapy, frequent monitoring of electrolytes, conservative nutritional therapy, and support of cardiac and respiratory function.

Pathophysiology

Refeeding syndrome is believed to result when enteral or parenteral nutrition is fed to starved or severely malnourished patients (Figure 16.1) leading to changes and redistribution of fluid and electrolytes that cannot be accommodated by the weakened cardiovascular system. (Skipper, 2012). These patients often have an intracellular depletion of electrolytes that may not be identified on evaluation of serum electrolytes. Upon refeeding, there is increased utilization of phosphorus and magnesium to drive metabolic pathways of substrates (e.g., glycolysis) and to act as co-factors for adenosine triphosphate (ATP) synthesis. This increased intracellular need, in conjunction with cotransport of potassium into the cell with insulin-driven glucose uptake, results in the further depletion of these electrolytes. Hypophosphatemia is the most common and consistent abnormality seen

Nutritional Management of Hospitalized Small Animals, First Edition. Edited by Daniel L. Chan.
© 2015 John Wiley & Sons, Ltd. Published 2015 by John Wiley & Sons, Ltd.

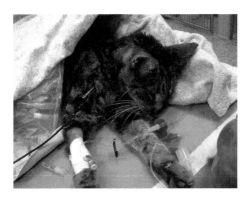

Figure 16.1 Severely malnourished animals (weight loss > 20%) such as the cat depicted above that had been missing for 6 weeks, should be considered at high risk of developing refeeding syndrome and require special nutritional management strategies to ensure safe nutritional recovery.

in refeeding syndrome and also results in many of the complications seen. Moreover, depletion of magnesium and potassium contribute to the clinical manifestation of this syndrome. The ensuing depletion in phosphate results in neuromuscular, cardiovascular and respiratory compromise (e.g., diaphragmatic muscle fatigue, respiratory failure). Arrhythmias could be induced by hypokakemia in combination with hypocalcemia and hypomagnesemia. Upregulation of carbohydrate metabolism may also explain the increased demand for magnesium and thiamine, which then leads to neurological and neuromuscular complications (Crook et al., 2001; Kraft et al., 2005; Skipper, 2012). Typically, refeeding syndrome occurs within the first 2 to 5 days after initiation of feeding (Skipper, 2012), but signs can be detected within hours of refeeding or delayed up to 10 days (Armitage-Chan, O'Toole and Chan, 2006; Hofer et al., 2014).

Systemic responses to prolonged starvation reported in people with severe weight loss secondary to anorexia nervosa include severe bradycardia, hypothermia and hypoventilation. These changes reflect a decrease in resting metabolic rate that occurs within a few days of anorexia. Decreased energy expenditure stems from decreased insulin activity, reduction of glucose utilization, and loss of metabolically active lean body mass (Crook et al., 2001). Skeletal muscle wasting and reduction in respiratory muscle function leads to poor shivering ability and further compromises ventilatory function and body temperature regulation. Eventually, decreased myocardial mass and ventricular contractility occur, leading to decreased cardiac output. The reported incidence of cardiovascular related complications in anorexia nervosa is high (up to 95%), and these include bradycardia, postural hypotension, fluid overload and cardiac arrhythmias, and result in a high incidence of cardiovascular-related mortality (Crook et al., 2001; Mehler et al., 2010).

During starvation, depletion of electrolytes, such as potassium and magnesium, occurs because of decreased dietary intake. Catabolism of fat and muscle also contributes to further electrolyte losses. Adjustments in renal electrolyte excretion maintain serum concentrations and clinical signs of electrolyte depletion may not be seen initially. During refeeding, intake of carbohydrate stimulates insulin release, resulting in conversion from a catabolic to an anabolic state, which increases cellular demand for phosphorus, potassium and water. Newly synthesized cells require potassium for maintenance of electrical gradients and translocate serum potassium and phosphorus intracellularly.

Stimulated processes, such as glycolysis and protein synthesis, also require cellular uptake of phosphate and magnesium. The increase in cellular activity resulting from insulin release therefore rapidly increases the cellular requirement for magnesium, depleting serum magnesium concentration. As starvation leads to whole-body depletion of these electrolytes, cellular translocation can cause severe serum depletion and life-threatening complications. Inorganic phosphate is required for generation of ATP and 2,3-diphosphoglycerate (2,3-DPG). Protein phosphorylation is also required for many intracellular enzymatic processes. Hypophosphatemia decreases ATP synthesis causing an energy deficit that is responsible for many of the clinical signs associated with refeeding syndrome. Refeeding-associated hypophosphatemia has been reported previously in cats when it resulted in hemolytic anemia (Justin and Honenhaus, 1995). Thiamine deficiency is an important component of refeeding syndrome in people and has also been reported in cats (Justin and Hohenhaus, 1995; Armitage-Chan et al., 2006; Brenner, KuKanich and Smee, 2011). Signs of thiamine deficiency include ataxia, vestibular dysfunction and visual disturbances. Thiamine is a cofactor in many enzymatic reactions involved in carbohydrate metabolism and clinical deficiencies may develop as refeeding of carbohydrates dramatically increases cellular thiamine utilization.

There is a single report of apparent refeeding syndrome in dogs that were starved then fed with enteral hyperalimentation resulting in hypophosphatemia, hemolytic anemia and neurological signs (Silvis, DiBartolomeo and Aaker, 1980). However, given the lack of any other information, it is unknown whether dogs with severe malnutrition are at increased risk for developing refeeding syndrome.

Nutritional management strategies

The risk of developing refeeding syndrome may be related to the degree of prior malnutrition, although it has been reported to occur in critically ill patients after a brief period of starvation (48 hours). (Marik and Bedigian, 1996; Ornstein et al., 2003). Proposed guidelines for identification of patients at high risk for developing refeeding syndrome in people include decreased body mass index (BMI), unintentional weight loss >10% in previous 3 to 6 months, complete lack of food intake, decreased serum concentrations of potassium, phosphorus or magnesium before initiation of feeding (Mehler et al., 2010). General guidelines for the prevention of refeeding syndrome state that nutritional support should not be initiated prior to correction of fluid and electrolyte imbalances. Once stabilization is achieved, nutrition should be administered gradually and only increased incrementally. Recommendations for prevention of refeeding complications in people suggest that initial refeeding should not exceed 20 kcal/kg/day (Crook et al., 2001). Refeeding syndrome has been reported to occur in cats fed only approximately 6 kcal/kg/day; it is therefore possible that refeeding complications in cats may be triggered at a lower level of caloric intake than is typically seen with people (Justin and Hohenhaus, 1995;Armitage-Chan et al., 2006). A loading dose of thiamine administered before initiation of feeding, followed by daily injections until day 3 of nutritional therapy is recommended (Solomon and Kirby, 1990; Stanga et al., 2008; Boateng et al., 2010; Sriram, Manzanares and Joseph, 2012).

Although there is insufficient information available from dogs and cats at risk for developing refeeding syndrome, protocols for reducing the risk for this disorder are available in people. In a protocol proposed by Hofer et al., (2014), which has been adopted by the European Society of Clinical Nutrition and Metabolism (ESPEN), there should be careful patient assessment of patients at risk for developing refeeding syndrome, restoration of fluid balance without overloading the cardiovascular system, initiation empirical supplementation of phosphate, potassium and magnesium (unless serum concentrations of these electrolytes are increased), initiation of thiamine and other B vitamins and trace minerals with the exception of iron (Hofer et al., 2014). The caloric intake is gradually increased from 10 kcal/kg to 30 kcal/kg over the course of 10 days with daily monitoring of potassium, phosphate, magnesium and glucose (Hofer et al., 2014).

Extrapolating from recommendations in people and recommended supplementation regimens in animals, a sensible approach would be to empirically supplement high risk patients with phosphate at 0.01–0.03 mmol/kg/h, potassium at 0.05 mEq/kg/h, and magnesium at 0.01 to 0.02 mEq/kg/h for the first 24 hours of therapy, provided the patient does not have any of these electrolytes above the reference interval for the first 3 days. Thiamine should be administered prior to feeding at 25 mg total dose (cats) or 100 mg total dose (dogs) either subcutaneously or intramuscularly daily until signs resolve. When nutritional support is instituted, no greater than 20% of RER should be provided on the first day and nutritional support should be increased gradually over 4–10 days.

Monitoring

Patients considered at risk for developing refeeding syndrome should be monitored daily as successful treatment may be dependent on identifying this condition in the early stages. Body weight, urine output, serum electrolytes (i.e., phosphorus, potassium, magnesium, calcium) electrocardiography, haematocrit, presence of hemolysis, serum glucose, cardiovascular and respiratory function should be monitored closely. Detection of metabolic abnormalities should prompt adjustments of nutritional therapy along with further correction of serum electrolyte concentrations.

Summary

Refeeding syndrome is an uncommon but potentially fatal complication associated with the initiation of nutritional support in severely malnourished animals, particularly cats. Typical metabolic derangements include severe hypophosphatemia, hypomagnesemia, hypokalemia, hyponatremia, hypocalcemia, hyperglycemia and vitamin deficiencies. Clinical manifestations of these abnormalities include peripheral edema, hemolytic anemia, cardiac failure, neurological dysfunction and respiratory failure. The successful management and refeeding of a patient with a history of prolonged starvation involves careful use of fluid therapy, nutritional replacement, and support of cardiac and respiratory function. Before initiation of feeding, patients should be supplemented with thiamine as well as phosphorus, potassium and magnesium. Energy targets should be very conservative (e.g., 20% of RER on the first day) and only gradually increasing over the next several days. With careful management of cases at risk for developing refeeding syndrome, nutritional support can play a key role in the recovery of these patients.

KEY POINTS

- Metabolic derangements associated with refeeding syndrome include severe hypophosphatemia, hypomagnesemia, hypokalemia, hyponatremia, hypocalcemia, hyperglycemia and thiamine deficiency.

- Clinical manifestations of these abnormalities include peripheral edema, hemolytic anemia, cardiac failure, neurological dysfunction and respiratory failure.

- Many of these metabolic changes are believed to result from sudden release of insulin (stimulated by carbohydrate intake) in the presence of total body nutrient depletion.

- Proposed recommendations for reducing risk of refeeding syndrome include empirically supplementing phosphate, potassium, and magnesium for the first 24 hours of therapy, provided the patient does not have any of these electrolytes above the reference interval for the first 3 days.

- Thiamine should be administered prior to feeding at 25 mg total dose (cats) or 100 mg total dose (dogs) either subcutaneously or intramuscularly daily until signs resolve.

- When nutritional support is instituted, no greater than 20% of RER should be provided on the first day and this target is gradually increased to 100% RER over the next several days

References

Armitage-Chan, E.A., O'Toole, T. and Chan, D.L. (2006) Management of prolonged food deprivation, hypothermia, and refeeding syndrome in a cat. *Journal of Veterinary Emergency and Critical Care*, **16**, S34–S41.

Boateng, A.A., Sriram, K., Meguid, M.M. et al. (2010) Refeeding syndrome: treatment considerations based on collective analysis of literature case reports. *Journal of Nutrition*, **26**,156–67.

Brenner, K., KuKanich, K.S. and Smee, N.M. (2011) Refeeding syndrome in a cat with hepatic lipidosis. *Journal of Feline Medicine and Surgery*, **13**, 614–617.

Crook, M.A., Hally, V. and Panteli, J.V. (2001) The importance of the refeeding syndrome Nutrition. **17**, 632–637.

Hofer, M., Pozzi, A., Joray, M. et al. (2014) Safe refeeding management of anorexia nervosa inpatients: an evidence-based protocol. *Journal of Nutrition*, **30**, 524–530.

Justin, R.B. and Hohenhaus, A.E. (1995) Hypophosphatemia associated with enteral alimentation in cats. *Journal of Veterinary Internal Medicine*, **9**, 228–233.

Kraft, M.D., Btaiche, I.F. and Sacks, G.S. (2005) Review of the refeeding syndrome. *Nutrition in Clinical Practice*, **20**, 625–633.

Marik, P.E. and Bedigian, M.K. (1996) Refeeding hypophosphatemia in critically ill patients in an intensive care unit A prospective study. *Archives of Surgery*, **131**,1043–1047.

Mehler, P.S., Winkelman, A.B., Andersen, D.M. et al. (2010) Nutritional rehabilitation: Practical guidelines for refeeding the anorectic patient. *Journal of Nutrition and Metabolism*, **pii**: 625782. doi: 10.1155/2010/625782

Ornstein, R.M., Golden, N.H., Jacobson, M.S. et al. (2003) Hypophosphatemia during nutritional rehabilitation in anorexia nervosa: implications for refeeding and monitoring. *Journal of Adolescent Health*, **32**, 83–88.

Skipper, A. (2012) Refeeding syndrome or refeeding hypophosphatemia: a systematic review of cases. *Nutrition in Clinical Practice*, **27**, 34–40.

Silvis, S.E., DiBartolomeo, A.G. and Aaker, H.M. (1980) Hypophosphatemia and neurological changes secondary to oral caloric intake: a variant of hyperalimentation syndrome. *American Journal of Gastroenterology*, **73**, 215–222.

Solomon, S. and Kirby, D. (1990) The refeeding syndrome: a review. *Journal of Parenteral and Enteral Nutrition*, **14**, 90–97.

Sriram, K., Manzanares, W. and Joseph, K. (2012) Thiamine in nutrition therapy. *Nutrition in Clinical Practice*, **27**, 41–50.

Stanga, Z., Brunner, A., Leuenberger, M. et al. (2008) Nutrition in clinical practice – the refeeding syndrome: illustrative cases and guidelines for prevention and treatment. *European Journal of Clinical Nutrition*, **2**, 687–694.

CHAPTER 17

Feeding small animal patients with gastrointestinal motility disorders

Karin Allenspach[1] and Daniel L. Chan[2]

[1] Department of Clinical Science and Services, The Royal Veterinary College, University of London, UK
[2] Department of Veterinary Clinical Sciences and Services, The Royal Veterinary College, University of London, UK

Introduction

For normal gastrointestinal(GI) function and digestion, maintenance of GI motility is essential. As the GI tract is frequently affected by disease and pharmacological agents for treatment of various conditions, GI dysmotility disorders are commonly encountered complications in critically ill people (Adam and Baston, 1997; Fruhwald, Holzer and Metzler, 2007). In animals the most commonly recognized GI dysmotility disorders include esophageal dysmotility, delayed gastric emptying, functional intestinal obstruction (ileus) and colonic motility abnormalities (Washabau, 2003; Boillat et al., 2010).

Most GI dysmotility disorders in small animals occur secondary to an underlying disease process or following surgery and are therefore very common in hospitalized patients. It is important to recognize GI motility disorders early in these patients in order to initiate appropriate treatment, which usually consists of changes in nutritional therapy and may require GI motility modifying therapies. In this chapter, common GI motility disorders in hospitalized patients and their management will be discussed.

Pathophysiology of GI dysmotility disorders

Esophageal motility disturbances are frequently encountered in hospitalized patients. For example, in patients requiring mechanical ventilation, the frequency, amplitude, and percentage of propulsive contractions of the esophagus are reduced (Kölbel et al., 2000). The most pressing clinical concern with oesophageal dysmotility disorders is the development of gastroesophageal reflux, esophagitis, and subsequent aspiration (Nind et al., 2005).

Delayed gastric emptying, or gastric stasis, has been associated with many diseases in veterinary patients, including both primary and secondary disorders. Delayed gastric emptying is a functional disorder caused by defects in myenteric neuronal and gastric smooth-muscle function, leading to impaired emptying of

Nutritional Management of Hospitalized Small Animals, First Edition. Edited by Daniel L. Chan.
© 2015 John Wiley & Sons, Ltd. Published 2015 by John Wiley & Sons, Ltd.

digesta from the stomach. The pathophysiology of delayed gastric emptying in critically ill human and small animal patients is not fully understood. Normally, the gastric antrum in the stomach acts as a pump for peristaltic waves passing through the rest of the GI tract. This so-called 'antral pump' is stimulated by distension of the gastric body, which excites mechano- and chemo-receptors to produce acetylcholine, which in turn leads to excitation of afferent nerves and, finally, to antral contractions. One theory suggests that delayed gastric emptying is the result of a primary motor dysfunction ("pump failure"), resulting in decreased antral motility and the presence of the fasting motility pattern during feeding (Dive et al., 1994).

Another theory for delayed gastric emptying relates to neuroendocrine feedback mechanisms. Normally, the release of choleocystokinin (CCK) by the intestinal epithelium after sensing luminal hydrochloric acid, amino acids and fatty acids provides feedback to the antrum that contractions should diminish, which leads to relaxation of the gastric body. Once the chyme arrives in the distal small intestine, glucagon-like peptide 1 (GLP-1) is released from the intestinal epithelium which again provides negative feedback on gastric emptying (Hall and Washabau, 1999). This phenomenon is called 'ileal brake' (Lin et al., 1996). The rate of gastric emptying in dogs is regulated to a large degree by the composition of the diet, with the amount of moisture, fat, protein and carbohydrates all playing a role. During some disease states there appears to be a disproportionate activation of an inhibitory feedback pathway originating in the proximal small intestine or duodenum ("excessive feedback") leading to inhibitioning and vagal and spinal afferent neurons and delayed gastric emptying. (Chapman, Nguyen and Fraser, 2005).

In the small intestine, three types of motility patterns occur: peristaltic waves, which move chyme aborally over long intestinal segments, stationary contractions which segment the chyme for better absorption, and clusters of contraction which mix the chyme over short segments in aboral movements. Diarrhea is associated with the occurrence of pathologic giant aboral contractions in the small intestine. Colonic motor complexes occur in the colon and mix the content and slowly move it aborally.

Ileus is characterized by lack of borborygmi, accumulation of gas and fluid in the bowel with subsequent abdominal distension, patient discomfort and decreased advancement of GI contents (Washabau, 2003). A functional ileus appears to occur more commonly in critically ill patients (Madl, 2003). There is also some recent suggestion that ileus in the critically ill patient results from a loss of synchronized coordination of peristalsis (Chapman et al., 2007).

This is in contrast to previous suggestions that GI paralysis and decreased motor activity was the cause of ileus. Inflammatory mediators have also been implicated in the pathophysiology of ileus.

Clinical manifestations of GI dysmotility

The clinical signs of gastric emptying disorders are mainly vomiting, which occurs approximately 10–12 hours after food intake. In addition, bloating, regurgitation, abdominal pain and colic can be seen. Some clinical signs are relatively subtle and include decreased appetite, nausea, belching and pica. These signs are commonly seen in hospitalized patients and it is therefore helpful to keep a list of diseases in mind that can result in the development of secondary gastric emptying disorders so that appropriate action can be initiated early in the hospitalized patient.

Diagnosis of GI dysmotility disorders

Definitive identification of GI motility in small animals is challenging because we are lacking sufficiently sensitive and specific diagnostics modalities to fully characterize these disorders. A number of diagnostic modalities have been evaluated to investigate GI function in animals (Wyse et al., 2003) Contrast radiography can be used qualitatively to assess gastrointestinal motility disturbances in critically ill dogs and cats. Although widely available, radiographic assessment has limited use for the evaluation of subtle gastrointestinal dysmotility disorders in animals (Guilford, 2000; Lester et al., 1999). Ultrasonography may be more useful for qualitative and semi-quantitative assessment of delayed gastric emptying and ileus compared with radiography, however, the main disadvantages relates to its inherent subjectivity.

As many hospitalized animals with GI disorders have gastric feeding tubes in place, the measurement of gastric residual volume (GRV), defined as the volume of fluid aspirated from the stomach after a given time and before each new feeding, can be used to quantify and evaluate gastric tolerance of enteral feeding and can be used to infer the presence of delayed gastric emptying. In human adults, GRV exceeding 150 mL in a 4-hour period is indicative of intolerance of enteral feeding (MacLeod et al., 2007). In infants, GRVs in excess of 5 mL/kg in a 4-hour period were considered a marker for delayed gastric emptying in one study (Horn, Chaboyer and Schluter, 2004). Unfortunately, veterinary guidelines as to acceptable GRV have not been defined but in a recent study, Holahan et al., (2010) reported a median GRV of 4.5 mL/kg in a group of dogs prospectively being evaluated for complications associated with bolus versus continuous nasogastric tubes. The range of GRV in that same population ranged from 0 to 213 mL/kg and the volume of GRV was not associated with increased incidence of vomiting or regurgitation. Therefore it is still unclear what level of GRV should be considered as acceptable or indicative of gastric emptying problems in animals.

Therapeutic and nutritional management strategies

The mainstay approach for animals with GI dysmotility includes identification and treatment of the underlying condition, institution of early nutritional interventions, early ambulation, correction of metabolic derangements, multimodal pain management and pharmacological interventions that are aimed to restore normal GI motility. The use of pharmacological agents for management of GI dysmotility is a major area of investigation and the reader is referred elsewhere (Washbau, 2005; Chapman et al., 2007; Fraser and Bryant, 2010). Table 17.1 lists commonly used prokinetic agents and dosages that are

Table 17.1 Prokinetic agents used in small animals for management of gastrointestinal dysmotility disorders.

Agent	Dosage	Mode of action
cisapride	Dogs: 0.2–1.0 mg/kg PO q8h	Serotonergic agonist (5HT$_4$)
	Cats: 2.5–5 mg/cat, PO q8h	Serotonergic antagonist (5HT$_{1,3}$)
domperidone	0.05–0.1 mg/kg PO q12h	Dopaminergic (D$_2$) antagonist
erythromycin	0.5–1.0 mg/kg, IV, PO q8h	Motilin agonist
	– q12h	Serotonergic antagonist (5HT$_3$)
metoclopramide	Constant rate infusion:	Dopaminergic (D$_2$) antagonist
	1–2 mg/kg/day IV	Serotonergic agonist (5HT$_4$)
	0.2–0.5 mg/kg PO, IV, SQ q8h	
nizatidine	2.5–5.0 mg/kg PO q24h	H$_2$- histaminergic antagonist
ranitidine	1.0–2.0 mg/kg PO q8h - q12h	H$_2$- histaminergic antagonist

recommended in small animals. The focus of this chapter will cover nutritional modulation of GI motility dysfunction.

Nutritional management

Although animals with GI dysmotility disorders may manifest regurgitation, vomiting and diarrhea, institution of early enteral nutrition can help normalize GI motility and therefore should be considered a key treatment strategy (Stupak, Abdelsayed and Soloway, 2012). Proposed mechanisms for the positive effects of enteral nutrition on GI function include improving gut perfusion, promoting secretion of bicarbonate and various gut hormones and growth factors and stimulating motility (Stupak et al., 2012, Marik and Zaloga, 2001).

The actual composition of the food can impact GI motility and is worthy of consideration in selecting diets for affected patients. Formulations that are highly digestible (>95% digestibility), have high moisture content, with a low to medium content of fat (15% dry matter in cats and 6–15% of dry matter in dogs) may be desirable. However, specific formulations for use in animals with GI dysfunction have not been evaluated. Whereas protein content in the diet increases gastric emptying and intestinal transit time, dietary fat slows gastric emptying in dogs and humans but not in cats (Lin et al., 1996; Zhao, Wang and Lin, 2000). Furthermore, fat content lowers the tone of the lower esophageal sphincter and may therefore lead to gastro-esophageal reflux and vomiting. Interestingly, in a recent study evaluating bolus feeding versus intermittent feeding in dogs with nasoenteric tubes, investigators used a liquid diet with moderate to high fat contents and this was not associated with increased complication rates. Although fat is in general more digestible for small animals than protein or carbohydrates, the digestion and absorption of fat is a complex process involving various enzymes and bicarbonate secreted from the pancreas and the intestinal epithelial cells. Malassimilation of fat is

Table 17.2 Recommended dosages of cobalamin supplementation subcutaneously once weekly for at least 6 weeks in dogs with chronic enteropathies.

Body weight (kg)	<5	5–10	10–20	20–30	30–40	40–50
Dosage of cobalamin (µg)	250	400	600	800	1000	1200

therefore a common concern in hospitalized animals, and could lead to bacterial fermentation of the fat in the distal small intestine and colon. This reinforces the recommendation made above that diets for these patients should contain reduced amounts of fat.

Soluble fibers in the diet form gels in solution and delay gastric emptying and slow the intestinal transit time (Papasouliotis et al., 1993), so these should be avoided in patients with GI motility disorders. Insoluble fibers on the other hand do not form gels in solution and have no effect on gastric emptying. They can increase the intestinal transit time, are good bulking agents and have no effect on nutrient absorption. These fibres can promote colonic health, however, they can also decrease digestibility of the diet. Fructo-oligosaccharides (FOS) are fibres that have been shown to decrease intestinal inflammation in human patients and may therefore also have an anti-inflammatory effect in small animals with GI inflammation (Rose et al., 2010).

Liquid formulations may be delivered via continuous or intermittent bolus feedings. Critically ill animals with GI dysmotility have been suggested to tolerate continuous infusion feedings better than intermittent bolus feeding. A recent veterinary study defined 'feeding intolerance' as vomiting or regurgitation twice within a 24-hour period (Holahan et al., 2010). Although continuous feeding may be helpful in animals in which high feeding volumes may not be tolerated, a recent study demonstrated that GRVs and clinical outcome did not differ between the two feeding methods (Holahan et al., 2010). Furthermore, Holahan et al. (2010) suggested that terminating of enteral feeding when GRVs are high may be unwarranted in dogs as they found no relationship between GRVs and incidence of complications.

In addition, it should be kept in mind that many patients with GI diseases or GI motility disorders in the ICU have cobalamin malabsorption, leading to severe whole-body cobalamin deficiency. This cobalamin deficiency can by itself lead to clinical GI disease. Therefore it is never contraindicated to supplement any hospitalized patient with chronic GI disease with cobalamin parenterally, even if there are no serum concentrations available for that particular patient. This is especially true for cats, where it has been shown that GI diseases will not be treatable unless cobalamin supplementation is initiated (Ruaux et al., 2005). The recommended dosages for cobalamin supplementation can be found in Table 17.2.

Summary

GI motility disorders are common in the small animal critical care setting and can occur secondary to GI as well as many systemic diseases. Manifestations of GI motility dysfunction include regurgitation, vomiting, diarrhea, abdominal pain, nausea and anorexia. In addition to pharmacological therapy, nutritional management of these animals may help restore normal GI motility and alleviate clinical signs. Although not formally evaluated, the use of highly digestible, high moisture, low-fat diets fed in frequent small feedings throughout the day may help improve tolerance to enteral feeding in these patients.

KEY POINTS

- In animals the most commonly recognized GI dysmotility disorders include esophageal dysmotility, delayed gastric emptying, and functional intestinal obstruction (ileus).
- Most GI dysmotility disorders in small animals occur secondary to an underlying disease process or following surgery.
- Management of GI dysmotility disorders include addressing the underlying cause, use of prokinetic therapy, analgesia and nutritional management.
- Early enteral nutrition may be useful in mitigating dysmotility disorders and should be encouraged.
- The optimal composition of diets suitable for animals with GI dysmotility disorders is unknown, but diets with high moisture content, high digestibility with reduced or moderate fat content are commonly recommended.

References

Adam, S. and Baston, S. (1997) A study of problems associated with the delivery of enteral feed in critically ill patients in five ICUs in the UK. *Intensive Care Medicine*, **3**, 261–266.

Boillat, C.S., Gaschen, F.P., Gaschen, L. et al. (2010) Variability associated with repeated measurements of gastrointestinal tract motility in dogs obtained by use of a wireless motility capsule system and scintigraphy. *American Journal of Veterinary Research*, **71**, 903–907.

Chapman, M., Fraser, R., Vozzo, R. et al. (2005) Antro-pyloro-duodenal motor responses to gastric and duodenal nutrient in critically ill patients. *Gut*, **54**, 1384–1390.

Chapman M.J., Nguyen N.Q. and Fraser R.J. (2007) Gastrointestinal motility and prokinetics in the critically ill. *Current Opinion in Critical Care*, **13**, 187–194.

Dive, A., Miesse, C., Jamart, J. et al. (1994) Duodenal motor response to continuous enteral feeding is impaired in mechanically ventilated critically ill patients. *Clinical Nutrition*, **13**, 302–306.

Fraser, R.J. and Bryant, L. (2010) Current and future therapeutic prokinetic therapy to improve enteral feed intolerance in the ICU patient. *Nutrition Clinical Practice*, **25**, 26–31.

Fruhwald, S., Holzer, P. and Metzler, H. (2007) Intestinal motility disturbances in intensive care patients pathogenesis and clinical impact. *Intensive Care Medicine*, **33**, 36–44.

Guilford, G. (2000) Gastric emptying of BIPS in normal dogs with simultaneous solid-phase gastric emptying of a test meal measured by nuclear scintigraphy. *Veterinary Radiology and Ultrasound*, **41**, 381–383.

Hall, J. A. and Washabau, R. J. (1999) Diagnosis and treatment of gastric motility disorders. *Veterinary Clinics of North America Small Animal Practice*, **29**, 377–395.

Holahan, M., Abood, S., Hautman, J. et al. (2010) Intermittent and continues enteral nutrition in critically ill dogs: A prospective randomized trial. *Journal of Veterinary Internal Medicine*, **24**, 520–536.

Horn, D.,Chaboyer, W. and Schluter, P. (2004) Gastric residual volumes in critically ill paediatric patients: a comparison of feeding regimens. *Australian Critical Care*, **17**, 98–103.

Kölbel, C.B., Rippel, K., Klar, H. et al. (2000) Esophageal motility disorders in critically ill patients: a 24-hour manometric study. *Intensive Care Medicine*, **26**, 1421–1427.

Lester, N. V., Roberts, G. D., Newell, S. M. et al. (1999) Assessment of barium impregnated poly-ethylene spheres (BIPS) as a measure of solid-phase gastric emptying in normal dogs–comparison to scintigraphy. *Veterinary Radiology and Ultrasound*, **40**, 465–471.

Lin, H. C., Zhao, X. T., Wang, L. et al., (1996) Fat-induced ileal brake in the dog depends on peptide YY. *Gastroenterology*, **110**, 1491–1495.

MacLeod, J.B.A., Lefton, J., Houghton, D. et al. (2007) Prospective randomized control trial of intermittent versus continuous gastric feeds for critically ill trauma patients. *Journal of Trauma*, **63**, 57–61.

Madl C.D.W. (2003) Systemic consequences of ileus. *Best Practice and Research: Clinical Gastroenterology*, **17**(3), 445–456.

Marik, P.E. and Zaloga, G.P. (2001) Early enteral nutrition in acutely ill patients: A systematic review. *Critical Care Medicine*, **29**, 2264–2270.

Nind, G., Chen, W-H., Protheroe, R. et al. (2005) Mechanisms of gastroesophageal reflux in critically ill mechanically ventilated patients. *Gastroenterology*, **128**, 600–606.

Papasouliotis, K., Muir, P., Gruffydd-Jones, T. J. et al. (1993) The effect of short-term dietary fibre administration on oro-caecal transit time in dogs. *Diabetologia*, **36**, 207–211.

Rose, D. J., Venema, K., Keshavarzian, A. et al. (2010) Starch-entrapped microspheres show a beneficial fermentation profile and decrease in potentially harmful bacteria during in vitro fermentation in faecal microbiota obtained from patients with inflammatory bowel disease. *British Journal of Nutrition*, **103**, 1514–1524.

Ruaux, C. G., Steiner, J. M. and Williams, D. A. (2005) Early biochemical and clinical responses to cobalamin supplementation in cats with signs of gastrointestinal disease and severe hypoc-obalaminemia. *Journal of Veterinary Internal Medicine*, **19**, 155–160.

Stupak, D.P., Abdelsayed, G.G. and Soloway, G.N. (2012) Motility disorders of the upper gastro-intestinal tract in the intensive care unit: pathophysiology and contemporary management. *Journal of Clinical Gastroenterology*, **46**, 449–456.

Washabau, R. J. (2003) Gastrointestinal motility disorders and gastrointestinal prokinetic therapy. *Veterinary Clinics of North America Small Animal Practice*, **33**, 1007–1028.

Wyse C.A., McLellan J., Dickie A.M. et al. (2003) A review of methods for assessment of the rate of gastric emptying in the dog and cat: 1998–2002. *Journal of Veterinary Internal Medicine*, **17**, 609–621.

Zhao, X. T., Wang, L. and Lin, H. C. (2000) Slowing of intestinal transit by fat depends on naloxone-blockable efferent, opioid pathway. *America Journal of Physiology. Gastrointestinal and Liver Physiology*, **278**, G866–G870.

CHAPTER 18

Immune modulating nutrients in small animals

Daniel L. Chan

Department of Veterinary Clinical Sciences and Services, The Royal Veterinary College, University of London, UK

Introduction

In critically ill and hospitalized animals, the role of nutritional support in the overall management of patients is well established. However, nutrition is most often simply regarded as a supportive measure. Recently, further understanding of the underlying mechanisms of various disease processes and the recognition that certain nutrients possess pharmacological properties have led to investigations on how nutritional therapies themselves could modify the behavior of various conditions and improve patient outcomes and this has been dubbed 'therapeutic nutrition'(Wischmeyer and Heyland, 2010). Nutrients, such as certain vitamins, amino acids, and polyunsaturated fatty acids, can modulate inflammation and the immune response (Cahill et al., 2010; Hegazi and Wischmeyer, 2011). A major focus of nutrition in critically ill human patients now involves the development of strategies that target or modulate metabolic pathways, inflammation and the immune system. (Hegazi and Wischmeyer, 2011) Exploiting pharmacological effects of certain nutrients to modulate disease processes and patient outcomes has been the subject of various clinical trials in people, however, a similar focus on clinical veterinary patients has not yet taken place. The use of nutritional strategies in ameliorating animal diseases has been shown to be beneficial in the areas of chronic kidney disease (e.g., protein and phosphorus restriction) (Bauer et al., 1999; Brown et al., 1998) and cardiac disease (e.g., omega-3 fatty acids) (Freeman et al., 1998; Smith et al., 2007). In people, there is mounting evidence that certain nutrients, such as glutamine, omega-3 fatty acids and antioxidants, can positively impact both morbidity and mortality in critically ill populations. It is hoped that a greater understanding of how these nutrients impart such beneficial effects may lead to developments of novel strategies for modulating various diseases in small animals. To this end, a review of how nutritional strategies could be used to modulate disease, especially in critically ill animals, is the focus of this chapter and is discussed in greater detail.

Nutritional Management of Hospitalized Small Animals, First Edition. Edited by Daniel L. Chan.
© 2015 John Wiley & Sons, Ltd. Published 2015 by John Wiley & Sons, Ltd.

Nutritional management strategies

Omega-3 fatty acids

As inflammation plays a crucial role in many diseases, modulation of the inflammatory response has become an important target of therapy. Inflammation yields several lipid mediators that are involved in a complex regulatory array of the inflammatory process. Lipid mediators are synthesized by three main pathways, namely the cyclooxygenase, 5-lipoxygenase and cytochrome P450 pathways and they each use polyunsaturated fatty acids (PUFA) such as arachidonic acid (AA), eicosapentaenoic acid (EPA) and γ-linolenic acid (GLA) as substrates (Mayer, Schaefer andSeeger, 2006). Potent proinflammatory eicosanoids, leukotrienes, and thromboxanes of the 2 and 4 series are produced from AA metabolism. Classically, modulation of inflammation was thought to result from greater substitution of omega-6 fatty acids i.e., AA with EPA and docosahexaenoic acid (DHA) in cell membranes, such that when these PUFAs were cleaved by phospholipases and oxidized by several enzymes it led to less inflammatory eicosanoids of the 3 and 5 series (Mayer et al., 2006).

However, it is now clear that the biological anti-inflammatory activities of omega-3 fatty acids are far beyond the simple regulation of eicosanoid production. Namely, these PUFAs can affect immune cell responses through the regulation of gene expression, subsequent downstream events by acting as ligands for nuclear receptors and through control of some key transcription factors (Singer et al., 2008). EPA can also inhibit the activity of the proinflammatory transcription nuclear factor B (NF- κB) at several levels, which regulates the expression of many proinflammatory mediators (e.g., cytokines, chemokines) and other effectors of the innate immune response system (Singer et al., 2008). In addition, recent research has revealed that free EPA and DHA also inhibit the activation of Toll-like receptor 4 by endotoxin and thereby further inhibit the inflammatory response (Lee and Hwang, 2006). Finally, recent discoveries have identified that EPA and DHA are also substrates of two novel classes of mediators called resolvins and protectins, which are involved in the inhibition and resolution of the inflammatory process, which now appears to be a well orchestrated, complex, active process involving these mediators (Singer et al., 2008; Willoughby et al., 2000). Therefore, in the context of disease modulation, omega-3 fatty acids help reduce the production of inflammatory mediators and are incorporated in the synthesis of anti-inflammatory and "pro-resolution" factors, which serve to attenuate the inflammatory response and the innate immune response.

In regards to the clinical use of omega-3 fatty acids in critically ill populations, the evidence is exclusively from human medicine. Enteral supplementation of EPA/DHA with concurrent antioxidants has been described in ventilated patients with acute lung injury (Pontes-Arruda et al., 2008) and, more recently, it has been shown to improve outcome in patients with early sepsis.(Pontes-Arruda et al., 2011) However, the data are not entirely conclusive, especially when omega-3 fatty acids are administered intravenously via parenteral nutrition. In a recent meta-analysis of studies evaluating supplemental omega-3 fatty acids in parenteral nutrition, no statistically significant benefits were identified in regards to mortality, infection or ICU stay and only weak evidence that such supplementation shortens overall hospitalization. (Palmer et al., 2013) However, the analysis should be considered preliminary as there were fewer than 10 trials included in the analysis and 6 of these trials contained fewer than 50 patients and therefore the conclusions regarding the utility of parenteral omega-3 fatty acids should be reserved until more data are available (Palmer et al., 2013). It is worth noting that the analysis did possibly uncover that timing of supplementation (i.e., early versus late in the disease process) may have a large impact on the results. Many of the trials included in the analysis recruited patients in septic shock and therefore the ability to demonstrate treatment benefit would be extremely difficult (Palmer et al., 2013). The recent results of the INTERSEPT Study (Pontes-Arruda et al., 2011) using enteral EPA/DHA would support this hypothesis as they recruited patients with early sepsis without organ dysfunction and were able to demonstrate various improvements in outcome. Currently, no data are available on the use of omega-3 fatty acids in critically ill veterinary populations. Given the number of potential benefits in modulation of inflammation and patient outcome, further research in this area is warranted.

Antioxidants

Similar to inflammation, oxidative stress is also recognized to be a prominent and common feature of many disease processes, including neoplasia, cardiac disease, trauma, burns, severe pancreatitis, sepsis, and critical illness. During various pathophysiological states, particularly those typified by an inflammatory response, cells of the immune system, such as neutrophils, macrophages and eosinophils, contribute substantially to the production of reactive oxygen species (ROS) and reactive nitrogen species (RNS). With the depletion of normal anti-oxidant defences, the host is more vulnerable to free radical species and prone to cellular and subcellular damage (e.g., DNA, mitochondrial damage) (Manzanares et al., 2012). The degree of antioxidant depletion appears to reflect the severity of illness in human patient populations(Alonso de Vega, Serrano and Carbonell, 2002). Oxidative stress is believed not only to be a promoter of inflammation but also a key factor leading to multiple organ failure (Manzanares et al., 2012).

Replenishment of antioxidant defences attempts to lessen the intensity of the injury caused by ROS and RNS. Antioxidants can be classified in three different systems: (i) Antioxidant proteins such as albumin, haptoglobin and ceruloplasmin, (ii) enzymatic antioxidants such as superoxide dismutase, glutathione peroxidase, and catalase and (iii) non-enzymatic or small molecule antioxidants, such as ascorbate (vitamin C), alpha-tocopherol (vitamin E), glutathione, selenium, lyco-pene and beta-carotene. N-acetylcysteine is a powerful progenitor of glutathione and has been associated with some positive results in several patient populations. Treatment with n-acetylcysteine not only scavenges ROS but also enables continual production of glutathione and even blocks transcription of inflammatory cytokines (Manzanares et al., 2012).

In regards to clinical evidence in critically ill people, a number of meta-analyses have indicated that the administration of antioxidant micronutrients (as mono-therapy or combination therapy or antioxidant cocktails) is associated with a mor-tality risk reduction, reduced mechanical ventilator dependence but only a trend for reduced infectious complications (Manzanares et al., 2012; Heyland et al., 2005; Visse, Labadarios and Blaauw, 2011). It is interesting to note that the effect on mortality reduction was most apparent in populations with the expected highest mortality rates but a difference could not be detected when the mortality rate between the critically ill population and control population was less than 10% (Manzanares et al., 2012). However, not all of the data regarding the use of antioxidants in the critically ill are positive. In a recent Cochrane review (Szakmany, Hauser and Radermacher, 2012) of the use of N-acetylcysteine for sepsis and systemic inflammatory responses syndrome (SIRS) in adult human patients, the authors concluded that their analysis casts "doubt on the safety and utility of intravenous N-acetylcysteine as an adjuvant therapy in SIRS and sepsis. At best, N-acetylcysteine is ineffective in reducing mortality and complications in this patient population" (Szakmany et al., 2012). The analysis also highlighted concern that administration of N-acetylcysteine after 24 hours of onset of symptoms could lead to cardiovascular depression (Szakmany et al., 2012). Typically, Cochrane reviews are very conservative in their analytical methods and seldom support novel interventions in critically ill populations. It is clear that further research is required to identify the most appropriate approach in modulating oxidative stress in the critically ill patients.

Despite the clear importance of oxidative stress in various diseases in veterinary species, investigations evaluating the effect of antioxidants on disease processes are limited. Positive results have been demonstrated in experimental models of oxidative stress including in conditions such as congestive heart failure(Amado et al., 2005), acute pancreatitis (Marks et al., 1998) gastric dilatation-volvulus (Badylak, Lanz and Jeffries, 1990), renal transplantation (Lee, Son and Kim, 2006), gentamicin-induced nephrotoxicity (Varzi et al., 2007), and acetaminophen toxicity (Webb et al., 2003; Hill et al., 2005). Supplementation of vitamin E alone did not prevent oxidative injury (i.e., development of Heinz body anemia) in cats fed onion powder or propylene glycol but the same group of investigators later showed that supplementation of vitamin E with cysteine in cats decreased the production of methemoglobinemia following acetaminophen challenge (Hill et al., 2005).

In naturally-occurring disease such as chronic valvular disease (Freeman et al., 1998) and renal insufficiency (Plevraki et al., 2006) there have also been some positive results that support the need for further evaluation. Unfortunately, the use of antioxidants in the setting of critically ill veterinary patients has not been published.

Immune modulating amino acids

Amino acids fulfill a vast array of functions in the body. They primarily serve as building blocks for protein synthesis and participate in various chemical reactions. Certain amino acids have immune-modulating properties and they help maintain the functional integrity of immune cells and aid in wound healing and tissue repair. They may also serve as an energy source for certain cells; perhaps the most pertinent example being glutamine which is the preferred fuel source for enterocytes and cells of the immune system. During disease states, the body undergoes marked alterations in substrate metabolism that could lead to a deficiency in these amino acids. In the response to stress there may be a dramatic increase in demand by the host for particular amino acids such as arginine and glutamine. In health these amino acids are adequately synthesized by the host. However, during periods following severe trauma, infection or inflammation, the demand for these amino acids cannot be met by the host, and they become "conditionally essential" and must be obtained from the diet. Given the importance of these amino acids, the sudden depletion in these important substrates led to the hypothesis that dietary supplementation of these amino acids during disease would improve outcome. In addition, in times of injury and tissue repair and rapid cellular proliferation, nucleotide availability may become depleted and rate-limiting for the synthesis of nucleotide-derived compounds (Hegazi and Wischmeyer, 2011).

Arginine

Arginine is a conditionally essential amino acid that is required for polyamine synthesis (for cell growth and proliferation), proline synthesis (for wound healing) and is a precursor for nitric oxide (signalling molecule for immune cells). Following extensive injury or surgery, immature cells of myeloid origin produce arginase-1, an enzyme that breaks down arginine. The ensuing arginine deficiency is associated with suppression of T-lymphocyte function (Popovic, Zeh and Ochoa, 2011). When steps are taken to replenish arginine along with omega-3 fatty acids, T cell number and function improves. There are also data that demonstrate a significant treatment benefit following supplementation after major surgery. Clinical benefits included fewer infectious complication rates and decreased overall length of stay when compared with standard nutritional support. (Hegazi and Wischmeyer, 2011)

The one population where arginine therapy is likely to be contraindicated is patients with severe sepsis (Hegazi and Wischmeyer, 2011). Likely causes of this detrimental effect relate to promotion of excessive nitric oxide synthesis, worsening of cardiovascular tone and decreasing organ perfusion (Hegazi and Wischmeyer, 2011).

Glutamine

Glutamine, another conditionally-essential amino acid, is the most abundant free amino acid in circulation, however, stores are rapidly depleted during critical illness in people. A deficiency in glutamine has been documented to impair several important defence mechanisms of the host. Supplementation of glutamine during critical illness is well accepted to confer beneficial effects on patient outcomes. The evidence had been so strong that nutritional guidelines for critically ill people recommended supplemental glutamine to any patient receiving parenteral nutrition. (Wernerman, 2011; McClave et al., 2009; Kreymann et al., 2006) The proposed mechanisms by which glutamine improves outcomes involve: (i) Tissue protection (e.g., heat shock protein expression, maintenance of gut barrier integrity and function, and decreased apoptosis), (ii) anti-inflammatory and immune-modulation (e.g., decreased cytokine production, inhibition of NF-kB), (iii) preservation of metabolic function (e.g., improved insulin sensitivity, ATP synthesis) (iv) Antioxidant effects (i.e., enhance glutathione generation) and (v) Attenuation of inducible nitric oxide synthase activity (Wischmeyer and Heyland, 2010).

The evidence supporting the use of glutamine in critically ill human patients had been overwhelmingly positive, until the publication of the largest randomized placebo-controlled, double-blinded clinical trial evaluating high dose glutamine and antioxidants in severely ill patients (Heyland et al., 2013). In this seminal study, over 1200 critically ill patients, with at least two failing organ systems and requiring mechanical ventilation were randomly allocated to glutamine versus placebo treatment and antioxidants versus placebo treatment. Unexpectedly, there was a trend for increased mortality associated with glutamine use (Heyland et al., 2013). There was no effect of glutamine on rates of organ failure or infectious complications and antioxidants had no discernible effects (Heyland et al., 2013). The exact reasons for the observed trend in increased mortality were not identified, but it is worth noting that the dose of glutamine used in this study was much higher than any previous study to date and also that this study population included patients in shock being treated with nutritional support prior to achieving hemodynamic stability. Most recommendations for nutrition support (both enteral and parenteral) in the critically ill patient stipulate that cardiovascular stability must be achieved before commencing nutritional support (McClave et al., 2009).

Despite ample evidence guiding treatment recommendations in people, there are no equivalent recommendations in the veterinary literature pertaining to glutamine use. This is likely due to the lack of supporting data and limited availability of parenteral glutamine. To date, there are only a few published veterinary trials that have evaluated the use of glutamine (enteral or parenteral) in dogs and cats. In a trial of cats treated with methotrexate, enteral glutamine offered no intestinal protection in terms of reducing intestinal permeability or improving the severity of clinical signs(Marks et al., 1999). Another trial evaluating the effects of enteral glutamine on plasma glutamine concentrations and prostaglandin E_2 concentrations in radiation-induced mucositis showed no measurable benefit (Lana et al., 2003). Possible reasons for the apparent failures in both of these trials could be attributed to inadequate doses used or because the form used, enteral, was not effective in these conditions. In contrast, a recent experimental canine model of post-operative ileus by Ohno et al., (2009) evaluated the effects of glutamine on restoration of interdigestive migrating contraction in the intestines and they were able to demonstrate a statistically significant reduction in the time to restore contractions in the glutamine treated group. The authors hypothesized that the benefit was derived from glutamine's ability to maintain glutathione concentration and thereby counteract the deleterious effects from surgical injury, inflammation and oxidative stress. They concluded that administration of glutamine following gastrectomy could shorten the duration of ileus (a major problem post-operatively in critically ill people) and may protect against surgical stress in general. Given these positive results, further studies should evaluate the possible beneficial effects of glutamine supplementation in treating ileus and other gastrointestinal motility disorders in dogs with natural occurring disease.

Most recently, Kang, Kim and Yang (2011) demonstrated that the immune suppression induced by high-dose methylprednisolone sodium succinate therapy can be ameliorated by parenteral administration of L-alanyl-L-glutamine. The study was designed to address a common concern associated with high dose glucocorticoid therapy, namely, immune-suppression. The model employed did demonstrate that such high doses of glucocorticoid can suppress oxidative burst activity and phagocytic capacity of neutrophils. Although the study used an experimental model, it does suggest that parenteral glutamine does have immu-nomodulatory effects in dogs, and that in the future more clinically applicable uses should be explored. Unfortunately, parenteral glutamine is not routinely available in North America and the majority of studies evaluation parenteral glutamine are performed in Europe and Asia.

Nucleotides

These low molecular weight intracellular compounds (i.e., pyrimidine and purine) are the basic building blocks for the synthesis of DNA, RNA, ATP and key coenzymes involved in essential metabolic reactions. Similarly to amino acids, nucleotides can be synthesized *de novo* or can be salvaged and recycled from other molecules. The reason nucleotides are included in this discussion of therapeutic nutrition is that during disease states and injury, the rapid cell proliferation required for tissue healing leads to nucleotide depletion (Hegazi and Wischmeyer, 2011). Dietary supplementation can compensate for such depletions and support cell proliferation and differentiation. As the cell types most affected by shortfall in nucleotides are cells of the immune systems and of the gastrointestinal tract, nucleotide supplementation is often included in 'immune-enhancing diets'. The evidence for the beneficial effects of dietary nucleotides is mostly from pre-clinical trials and rodent models, therefore further research is still warranted (Hess and Greenberg, 2012). From the pathophysiological point of view, supplementation of dietary nucleotides may be particularly important in animals with prolonged anorexia as supplementa-tion in rodent models enhance intestinal repair, restore brush-border enzyme activity and improve gut barrier function (Hess and Greenberg, 2012). Additional benefits of dietary nucleotides include positive effects on gut flora, gastrointestinal microcirculation, immune function and inflammation (Hess and Greenberg, 2012) Given the plethora of potential beneficial effects with-out clear detrimental effects, it is not surprising that nucleotides have been included in some immune-enhancing diet cocktails despite the lack of defini-tive results. Although results of trials using these immune-enhancing cocktails are encouraging and mostly positive, it is unknown if these effects are syner-gistic or whether they result from the summation of the individual compo-nents. To date, no veterinary studies have evaluated the potential utility of supplementing nucleotides to critically ill patients.

Probiotics

Probiotics are live microorganisms that, when ingested in sufficient amounts, have a positive effect on the health of the host. Some of the benefits purport-edly related to probiotics include reduced production of toxic bacterial metab-olites, increased production of certain vitamins, enhanced resistance to bacterial colonization and reinforcing host natural defences. Probiotics are also believed to shorten the duration of infections or decrease host suscepti-bility to pathogens. (Morrow, Gogineni and Malesker, 2012) The proposed mechanisms underlying the positive effects include restoration of gastrointes-tinal barrier function, modification of the gut flora by inducing host cell antimicrobial peptides (i.e., defensins, cathelicidins) or releasing probiotic antimicrobial factors (e.g., bacteriocins, microsins), competing for epithelial adherence and immunomodulation (Morrow et al., 2012). Probiotics are therefore believed to have a role in balancing gut microflora and increasing host resistance to pathogenic bacteria. It is worth bearing in mind that the effects of probiotics are not only dose-dependent but also both strain and species-specific (Petrof et al., 2012). In people, probiotics used include various species of *Lactobacillus, Bifidobacterium* and *Streptococcus* (Morrow et al., 2012). Microorganisms approved for use in animal feeds include strains belonging to the *Bacillus, Enterococcus* and *Lactobacillus* bacterial groups.

The mechanism by which probiotics enhance gut barrier function may involve how certain bacteria, for example, *Lactobacillus*, stimulate mucin production and thereby inhibit pathogenic bacteria from invading and attaching to the gut epithelium (Morrow et al., 2012). One of the concerns with the use of probiotics is that there is a risk that certain microorganisms, such as *enterococci*, may harbor transmissible antimicrobial resistance determinants (i.e., plasmids), thus contributing to the problem of antimicrobial resistance. The use of probiotics in the critically ill is controversial and guidelines recommend further safety trials before further use in critically ill patients (Petrof et al., 2012).

In human critical care, probiotics have been used to combat antimicrobial-associated diarrhea, *Clostridium difficile* infections, and ventilator-associated pneumonia (Morrow et al., 2012) The probiotic yeast *Saccharomyces boulardii* apparently produces a protease which degrades *C difficile* toxins and may also stimulate IgA secretions against *C difficile* toxins (Petrof et al., 2012). The only meta-analysis evaluating probiotics to prevent ventilator-associated pneumonia demonstrated a significant reduction in the incidence of ventilator-associated pneumonia and length of ICU stay (Siempos, Ntaidou and Falagas, 2010). Thus far, trials evaluating probiotics in critically ill patients have only demonstrated a trend towards reduced ICU mortality (Petrof et al., 2012).

Probiotics have the theoretical risk of transferring the antibiotic resistance gene, translocating from intestine to other areas or developing adverse reactions via interactions with the host's microflora. While bacteremia has not been documented with probiotic use in critically ill people, there are single case reports detailing infections with probiotic strains in patients that are immune-suppressed (Boyle, Robbins-Browne and Tang, 2006).

In veterinary medicine, there are no trials evaluating the use of probiotics in a critically ill patient population. However, there have been trials in dogs with gastrointestinal signs. A prospective placebo-controlled probiotic trial using a canine-specific probiotic cocktail containing three different *Lactobacillus spp* strains in addition to a novel protein diet was able to demonstrate a dramatic improvement in clinical signs after dietary change but no additional benefit attributed to the addition of a probiotic (Sauter et al., 2006). Other studies have documented some positive effects, such as improvements in immunological markers or desirable changes in microbiota, however, these trials have mostly been performed on healthy dogs. It is uncertain whether these benefits would improve clinical signs in dogs with critical illness.

Summary

Despite the many pitfalls discussed, nutritional modulation of diseases appears to be a potentially useful strategy for companion animals. However, until trials can elucidate which specific nutrients and what dosages confer beneficial effects to particular patient populations, a certain degree of caution is advised. Of particular concern is the distinct possibility that significant species differences may reduce the usefulness of some of these approaches in veterinary patients. Before general recommendations for the use of immunomodulating nutrients in veterinary patients can be made, many questions must be answered. Central issues of safety, purity and efficacy must be addressed. However, as our understanding of the interactions between nutrients and disease processes grows, we may yet identify specific nutrients that could modulate serious diseases. Based on the progress being made in the area of clinical nutrition, it is quite evident that there should be a greater appreciation for the role nutrients play in ameliorating diseases, and how treatment strategies for certain conditions in companion animals may one day depend heavily on nutritional therapies.

KEY POINTS

- Recently, it has been recognized that certain nutrients possess pharmacological properties that could modify the behavior of various conditions.
- Using nutrients to modulate disease has been dubbed 'therapeutic nutrition'.
- Nutrients such as certain vitamins, amino acids, polyunsaturated fatty acids can modulate inflammation and the immune response.
- It is hoped that a greater understanding of how these nutrients impart such beneficial effects may lead to developments of novel strategies for modulating various diseases in small animals.

References

Alonso de Vega, J.M., Serrano, E. and Carbonell, L.F. (2002) Oxidative stress in critically ill patients with systemic inflammatory response syndrome. *Critical Care Medicine*, **30**, 1782–1786.

Amado, L.C., Saliaris, A.P., Raju, S.V. et al. (2005) Xanthine oxidase inhibition ameliorates cardiovascular dysfunction in dogs with pacing induced heart failure, *Journal of Molecular Cell Cardiology*, **39**, 531–536.

Badylak, S.F., Lanz, G.C. and Jeffries, M. (1990) Prevention of reperfusion injury in surgical induced gastric dilatation volvulus in dogs. *American Journal of Veterinary Research*, **51**, 294–299.

Bauer, J.E., Markwell, P.J , Rauly, J.M. et al. (1999) Effects of dietary fat and polyunsaturated fatty acids in dogs with naturally developing chronic renal failure. *Journal of the American Veterinary Medical Association*, **215**, 1588–1591.

Boyle, R.J., Robbins-Browne, R.M. and Tang, M.L.K. (2006). Probiotic use in clinical practice: what are the risks? *American Journal of Clinical Nutrition*, **83**, 1256–1264.

Brown, S.A., Brown, C.A., Crowel, W.A. et al. (1998) Beneficial effects of chronic administration of dietary omega-3 polyunsaturated fatty acids in dogs with renal insufficiency. *Journal of Laboratory Clinical Medicine*, **131**, 447–455.

Cahill, N.E., Dhaliwal, R., Day, A.G. et al. (2010) Nutrition therapy in the critical care setting: what is "best achievable" practice? An international multicenter observational study. *Critical Care Medicine*, **38**, 395–401.

Freeman, L.M., Rush, J.E., Khayias, J.J. et al. (1998) Nutritional alterations and effect of fish oil supplementation in dogs with heart failure. *Journal of Veterinary Internal Medicine*, **12**, 440–448.

Hegazi, R.A. and Wischmeyer, P.E. (2011) Clinical review: optimizing enteral nutrition for critically ill patients –a simple data-driven formula. *Critical Care*, **15**, 234–245.

Hess, J.R. and Greenberg, N.A. (2012) The role of nucleotides in the immune and gastrointestinal systems: potential clinical applications. *Nutrition Clinical Practice*, **27**, 281–294.

Heyland, D.K., Dhaliwal, R., Suchner, U. et al. (2005) Antioxidants nutrients: a systematic review of trace elements and vitamins in the critically ill patient. *Intensive Care Medicine*, **31**, 327–337.

Heyland, D., Muscedere, J., Wischmeyer, P.E. et al. (2013) A randomized trial of glutamine and antioxidants in critically ill patients. *New England Journal of Medicine*, **368**, 1489–1497.

Hill, A.S., Rogers, Q.R., O'Neill, S.L. et al. (2005) Effects of dietary antioxidant supplementation before and after oral acetaminophen challenge in cats. *American Journal of Veterinary Research*, **66**, 196–204.

Kang, J.H., Kim, S.S. and Yang, M.P. (2011) Effect of parenteral L-alanyl-L-glutamine administration on phagocytic responses of polymorphonuclear neutrophilic leukocytes in dogs undergoing high-dose methylprednisolone sodium succinate treatment. *American Journal of Veterinary Research*, **73**, 1410–1417.

Kreymann, K.G., Berger, M.M., Deutz, N.E. et al. (2006) ESPEN guidelines on enteral nutrition: intensive care. *Clinical Nutrition*, **25**, 210–223.

Lana, S.E., Hansen, R.A., Kloer, L. et al. (2003) The effects of oral glutamine supplementation on plasma glutamine concentrations and PGE2 concentrations in dogs experiencing radiation-induced mucositis. *Journal of Applied Research in Veterinary Medicine*, **1**, 259–265.

Lee, J.I., Son, H.Y. and Kim, M.C. (2006) Attenuation of ischemia-reperfusion injury by ascorbic acid in the canine renal transplantation. *Journal of Veterinary Science*, **7**, 375–379.

Lee, J.Y. and Hwang, D.H. (2006) The modulation of inflammatory gene expression by lipids: mediation through Toll-like receptors. *Molecular Cell*, **21**, 176–185.

Manzanares ,W., Dhaliwal, R., Jiang, X. et al. (2012) Antioxidant micronutrients in the critically ill: a systemic review and meta-analysis. *Critical Care*, **16**, R66.

Marks, J.M., Dunkin, B.J., Shillingstad, B.L. et al. (1998) Preteratment with allopurinol diminishes pancreatography-induced pancreatitis in a canine model, *Gastrointestinal Endoscopy*, **48**, 180–183.

Marks, S.L., Cook, A.K., Reader, R. et al. (1999) Effects of glutamine supplementation of an amino acid-based purified diet on intestinal mucosal integrity in cats with methotrexate-induced enteritis. *American Journal of Veterinary Research*, **60**, 755–763.

Mayer, K., Schaefer, M.B. and Seeger, W, (2006) Fish oil in the critically ill: from experimental to clinical data. *Current Opinion on Clinical Nutrition Metabolic Care*, **9**, 140–148.

McClave, S.A., Martindale, R.G., Vanek, V.W. et al. (2009) Guidelines for the provision and assessment of nutritional support therapy in adult critically ill patient: Society of Critical Care Medicine (SCCM) and the American Society for Parenteral and Enteral Nutrition (ASPEN). *Journal of Parenteral and Enteral Nutrition*, **33**, 277–316.

Morrow, L.E., Gogineni, V. and Malesker, M,A, (2012) Probiotics in the intensive care unit. *Nutrition Clinical Practice*, **27**, 235–241.

Ohno, T., Mochiki, E., Ando, H. et al. (2009) Glutamine decreases the duration of postoperative ileus after abdominal surgery: an experimental study of conscious dogs, *Digestive Disease Science*, **54**, 1208–1213.

Palmer, A.J., Ho, C.K.M., Ajinola, O. et al. (2013) The role of omega-3 fatty acid supplemented parenteral nutrition in critical illness in adults: a systemic review and meta-analysis, *Critical Care Medicine*, **41**, 307–316.

Petrof, E.O., Dhaliwal, R., Manazanares, W. et al. (2012) Probiotics in the critically ill: a systematic review of the randomized trial evidence. *Critical Care Medicine*, **40**, 3290–3302.

Plevraki, K,, Koutinas, A.F., Kaldrymidou, H. et al. (2006) Effects of allopurinol treatment on the progression of chronic nephritis in canine leishmaniosis (Leishmania infantum), *Journal of Veterinary Internal Medicine*, **20**, 228–233.

Pontes-Arruda, A., Demichele, S., Seth, A. et al. (2008) The use of an inflammation-modulating diet in patients with acute lung injury or acute respirator distress syndrome: a meta-analysis of outcome data. *Journal of Parenteral and Enteral Nutrition*, **32**, 596–605.

Pontes-Arruda, A., Martins, L.F., de Lima, S.M. et al. (2011) Enteral nutrition with eicosapentaenoic acid, gamma-linolenic acid and antioxidants in the early treatment of sepsis: results from a multicenter, prospective, randomized, double-blinded, controlled study: the INTERSEPT Study, *Critical Care*, **15**, R144.

Popovic, P.J., Zeh, H.J. and Ochoa, J.B. (2011) Arginine and immunity. *Journal of Nutrition*, **136**, 1681S–1686S.

Sauter, S.N., Benyacoub, J., Allenspach, K. et al. (2006) Effects of probiotic bacteria in dogs with food responsive diarrhoea treated with an elimination diet. *Journal of Animal Physiology and Animal Nutrition*, **90**, 269–277.

Siempos, I., Ntaidou, T.K. and Falagas, M.E. (2010) Impact of the administration of probiotics on the incidence of ventilator-associated pneumonia: a metaanalysis of randomized, controlled trials. *Critical Care Medicine*, **38**, 954–962.

Singer, P., Shapiro, H., Theilla, M. et al. (2008) Anti-inflammatory properties of omega-3 fatty acids in critical illness: novel mechanisms and an integrative perspective. *Intensive Care Medicine*, **34**, 1580–1592.

Smith, C.E., Freeman, L.M., Rush, J.E. et al. (2007) Omega-3 fatty acids in Boxer dogs with arrhythmogenic right ventricular cardiomyopathy. *Journal of Veterinary Internal Medicine*, **21**, 265–273.

Szakmany, T., Hauser, B., and Radermacher, P. (2012) N-acetylcysteine for sepsis and systemic inflammatory response in adults, *Cochrane Database of Systematic Reviews*. **9**, CD006616.

Varzi, H.N., Esmailzadeh, S., Morovvati, H. et al. (2007) Effect of silymarin and vitamin E on gentamycin-induced nephrotoxicity in dogs. *Journal of Veterinary Pharmacology and Therapeutics*, **30**, 477–481.

Visse, J., Labadarios, D. and Blaauw, R. (2011) Micronutrient supplementation for critically ill adults: a systemic review and meta-analysis. *Nutrition*, **27**, 745–758.

Webb, C.B., Twedt, D.C., Fettman, M.J. et al. (2003) S-adenosylmethionine (SAMe) in a feline acetaminophen model of oxidative injury. *Journal of Feline Medicine and Surgery*, **5**, 69–75.

Wernerman, J. (2011) Glutamine supplementation. *Annals of Intensive Care*, **1**, 25–31.

Willoughby, D.A., Moore, A.R., Colville-Nash, P.R. et al/ (2000) Resolution of inflammation. *International Journal of Immunopharmacology*, **22**, 1131–1135.

Wischmeyer, P.E. and Heyland, D.K. (2010) The future of critical care nutrition therapy. *Critical Care Clinics*, **26**, 433–441.

CHAPTER 19

Nutritional management of superficial necrolytic dermatitis in dogs

Andrea V. Volk and Ross Bond

Department of Clinical Sciences and Services, The Royal Veterinary College, University of London, UK

Introduction

Superficial necrolytic dermatitis (SND) (also known as hepatocutaneous syndrome, metabolic epidermal necrosis, canine diabetic dermatosis, necrolytic migratory erythema and glucagonoma syndrome) is a rare skin disease of dogs, which accounted for 0.3% (10/3387) of cases of various non-neoplastic dermatoses recorded by the pathology service of Cornell University. (Miller et al., 1990). It comprises a characteristic symmetrical cutaneous pathology most commonly associated with a particular hepatopathy (Byrne, 1999; Outerbridge, 2013, pp. 143–145). The first case was described by Ehrlein, Loeffler and Trautwein (1968). This was followed by a series of four cases reported by Walton, Center and Scott (1986). The various names for this disease reflect the incomplete understanding of its etiopathogenesis.

In people, an analogous syndrome with equivalent dermatohistopathological features was first reported by Becker, Kahn and Rothman (1942), and is most commonly seen as a paraneoplastic syndrome involving a glucagon-secreting tumour, mainly originating from the pancreas (Stacpoole, 1981). There have been rare reports correlating typical skin lesions to extra-pancreatic glucagonomas (right kidney, Gleeson et al., 1971; proximal duodenum, Roggli, Judge and McGavran, 1979), to cirrhosis (Doyle, Schroeter and Rogers, 1979; Blackford, Wright and Roberts, 1991; Delaporte, Catteau and Piette, 1997), or small bowel villous atrophy and malabsorptive syndrome (Goodenberger, Lawley and Strober, 1979). By contrast, most canine cases have hepatic rather than pancreatic pathology; in one review of canine SND cases only 5 out of 75 dogs had pancreatic neoplasia (Scott, Miller and Griffin, 2001).

SND has rarely been reported in cats (Patel, Whitbread and McNeil, 1996; Day, 1997; Byrne, 1999; Godfrey and Rest, 2000; Mauldin, Morris and Goldschmidt

2002; Kimmel, Christiansen and Byrne, 2003; Asakawa, Cullen and Linder, 2013). The clinical presentation is quite variable and there is no information available on treatment. There is one report of SND in a red fox in conjunction with hepatic lipidosis (van Poucke and Rest, 2005) and conflicting reports about a similar cutaneous manifestation in captive black rhinoceros (Munson et al., 1998; Dorsey et al., 2010).

Clinical presentation

SND is typically a disease of older dogs, with the mean age at presentation being approximately 10 years (Miller, 1992; Gross, Song and Havel, 1993; Outerbridge, 2013). Further reports suggest an increased prevalence in small breeds and male animals (Byrne, 1999; Outerbridge, Marks and Rogers, 2002). The most striking feature at initial presentation is severe hyperkeratosis with fissuring of the footpads (Figure 19.1), causing lameness or reluctance to walk. Similar hyperkeratosis and fissuring can also affect the nasal planum, muzzle and lips. Other cutaneous lesions include progressive crusts with coalescing erosions and ulcers, interdigital erythema, and circular, well-demarcated areas with peripheral erythema, vesiculation, central alopecia and hyperpigmentation (Outerbridge, 2013). Lesions often affect the facial mucocutaneous junctions (perilabial, periocular), pinnal margins, ventral abdomen, flanks, distal extremities, bony prominences, external genitalia and the ventral aspect of the tail. Stomatitis is common in human cases but very rare in dogs (Gross et al., 1993). Pruritus likely reflects secondary infections with bacteria or fungi.

Systemic signs, such as lethargy, decreased appetite, weight loss, polydipsia / polyuria, muscle wastage, peripheral lymphadenopathy, may precede the cutaneous

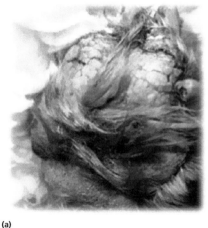 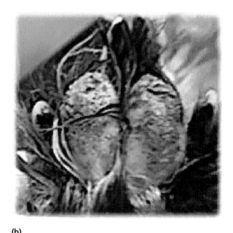

(a)   (b)

Figure 19.1 Images depicting a footpad of a dog with superficial necrolytic dermatitis (SND) before and after treatment. **a**) Characteristic severe hyperkeratosis and deep fissuring in a footpad of a dog with SND. **b**) The same footpad as in **a**) after 3rd intravenous amino acid/ essential fatty acids infusion, showing a marked reduction in hyperkeratosis with new skin visible on pad margins.

signs or become apparent shortly after presentation (Miller, 1992,; Bond et al., 1995; Torres, Johnson and McKeever, 1997b; Cerundolo, McEvoy and McNeil, 1999; Allenspach et al., 2000; Koutinas et al., 2001; Outerbridge et al., 2002; Bexfield and Watson, 2009; Mizuno, Hiraoka and Yoshioka, 2009; Papadogianniakis, Frangia and Matralis, 2009; Brenseke, Belz and Saunders, 2011).

Diagnosis

Diagnosis in dogs is commonly based on history, clinical presentation and dermatohistopathology (Miller, 1992; Gross et al., 1993; Byrne, 1999; Outerbridge, 2013), accompanied by evaluation of routine blood parameters, and imaging of liver and pancreas (Gross et al., 1993; Bond et al., 1995; Cerundolo et al., 1999; Koutinas et al., 2001; Mizuno et al., 2009; Papadogiannakis et al., 2009; Brenseke et al., 2011). Identifying the nature of the underlying pathology (hepatic versus pancreatic pathology) may lead to a different therapeutic approach (Table 19.1).

Pathophysiology

Although the etiopathogenesis is incompletely understood, a common finding in all cases of canine SND is marked hypoaminoacidemia (Outerbridge, 2013). Gross et al., (1993) speculated that reduced plasma amino acid concentrations result in protein depletion in the epidermis with subsequent necrolysis, since amino acids are necessary for maintenance of epidermal stability (Dorsey et al., 2010), growth and keratohyalin granule formation (Byrne, 1999), reflecting some features seen on histopathology in SND lesions.

In glucagonoma-related SND increased plasma glucagon concentrations lead to increased hepatic gluconeogenesis and ureagenesis, which subsequently deplete circulating amino acids (Cellio and Dennis, 2005). Further marked inflammation seen in the epidermis of SND cases could also be glucagon related, as incubation of human keratinocytes *in vitro* with glucagon caused increased concentrations of arachidonic acid (Peterson et al., 1984).

By contrast, dogs with hepatic-related SND have normal plasma glucagon concentrations, at least on current available assays, although it has been suggested that pancreatic and enteric-derived glucagon may influence the liver via the portal route without detection in peripheral blood samples (Gross et al., 1993).

A remarkable difference in canine hepatic-related SND compared to glucagonoma-related ones is the liver appearance. In glucagonoma-related SND the liver is unremarkable (apart from possible discrete metastases of the primary tumour). However, a specific hepatopathy is found in the majority of SND cases in the absence of a glucagonoma, characterized by vacuolar degeneration of hepatocytes and parenchymal collapse. This hepatopathy is, like the glucagonoma cases, associated with hypoaminoacidemia, and diabetes mellitus in 25% of the cases (Outerbridge et al., 2002). Neither the characteristic cutaneous features of SND nor these biochemical changes are seen in primary hepatopathies of dogs, but are more

Table 19.1 Diagnostic approach in dogs possibly affected by superficial necrolytic dermatitis.

Diagnostic procedure	Typical findings
Tests for skin infections and infestations (e.g., scrapings, hair plucks, cytology, bacterial or fungal cultures)	Unremarkable with possible identification of secondary infections
Dermatohistopathology	Parakeratotic hyperkeratosis ('red'), striking pallor of keratinocytes creating a pale middle layer caused by intra-and intercellular edema ('white') and irregular epidermal hyperplasia ('blue') with a mild superficial perivascular dermatitis with mononuclear cells ('French flag'; Gross et al., 2005).
Hematology	Typically unremarkable (early stages) or mild, often non-regenerative anemia
Serum biochemistry	Typically unremarkable (early stages) or increased activity of alkaline phosphatase (ALP) and aminoalanine transferase (ALT), hyperglycemia, hypoalbuminemia, hypocalcemia (Gross et al., 1993; Bond et al., 1995; Cerundolo et al., 1999; Koutinas et al., 2001).
Abdominal ultrasonography	(a) 'Honeycomb' / 'Swiss-cheese' like liver (Jacobson et al., 1995; Nyland et al., 1996; Scott et al., 2001; Outerbridge et al., 2002; ultrasound being a highly sensitive tool) followed by liver biopsy (ultrasound-guided or surgical) revealing vacuolar degeneration of hepatocytes grouped in nodules surrounded by collapsed parenchyma (Gross et al., 1993; Allenspach et al., 2000, Outerbridge et al., 2002; Brenseke et al., 2011)
In SND cases with an unremarkable ultrasound further imaging modalities like CT might be considered.	b) Unremarkable or pancreatic mass or its metastases (rare) (Miller, 1992, Bond et al., 1995).

commonly seen with endocrine, metabolic or nutritional diseases (Miller, 1992; Gross et al., 1993; Outerbridge et al., 2002, Turek 2003). Above all, dogs with acute and chronic hepatopathies show increased plasma amino acid concentrations (Outerbridge et al., 2002). Thus, the etiopathogenesis in hepatic-related SND remains poorly understood.

Some SND cases have been shown to be associated with hepatotoxicity, ranging from mycotoxins (Little, Mc Neil and Robb, 1991) or anticonvulsant drugs (Bloom, Rosser and Dunstan, 1992; March, Hillier and Weisbrode, 2004), to (as in people) severe gastrointestinal disease (Florant et al., 2000). The skin lesions of 'toxin'-related cases resolved completely upon withdrawal of the offending agent (Little et al., 1991; Bloom et al., 1992; March et al., 2004).

Some authors have speculated that decreased skin or blood concentrations of essential fatty acids (Blackford et al., 1991; Outerbridge et al., 2002), zinc (Gross et al., 1993), and vitamin B (van Beek et al., 2004) may contribute to the cutaneous lesions, but supplementation with these nutrients has inconsistent effects. A single case report in the human literature describes the successful use of intravenous amino acids and intralipids (source of essential fatty acids) in the treatment of necrolytic migratory erythema in the glucagonoma syndrome (Alexander et al., 2002).

Very recently, Bach and Glasser (2013) reported one dog with SND, showing enhanced improvement through reduced length of treatment intervals due to the additional use of essential fatty acids with the amino acid infusions.

Nutritional management

In cases of SND associated with hepatopathy, consideration should be given to possible reversible causes of hepatopathy (e.g., mycotoxins, anticonvulsant drugs), although commonly the specific hepatopathy cannot be reversed. Correction of hypoaminoacidemia is an important goal in the palliative care of these dogs. Dietary modifications or intravenous amino acid infusions may be utilized. Outerbridge et al. (2002) reported that some dogs respond preferentially to intravenously rather than orally administered amino acids. A possible explanation might include impaired enteral absorption of amino acids or increased hepatic metabolism before amino acids are available for the skin (Alexander et al., 2002). Different commercially available parenteral solutions of amino acids have been used in the literature via different protocols (Table 19.2).

These treatments appear to be well tolerated although the risk of thrombophlebitis dictates the use of a central venous catheter. It remains to be determined whether the commercially available infusions contain the optimal amounts of the relevant amino acids for individual animals (Outerbridge et al., 2002; Cave, 2007).

A high quality protein diet is an important adjunctive treatment in all cases of SND (Norton et al., 1979; Stacpoole, 1981; Shepherd et al., 1991). In cases where intravenous administration is not feasible, the diet can be supplemented with whey powder as a source of protein and amino acids. Convalescent diets can be useful palatable sources of such protein (Jacobson, Kirberger and Nesbit, 1995; Byrne, 1999; Koutinas and others 2001), while eggs are an alternative (Gross and others 1993, Jacobson et al., 1995, Byrne 1999, Koutinas et al., 2001; Scott et al., 2001; Bexfield and Watson, 2009). Oral supplementation of essential fatty acids appears to be of limited value (Bond et al., 1995; Jacobson et al., 1995; Outerbridge et al., 2002; Mizuno et al., 2009). Although, its intravenous administration via a central catheter together with the amino acid solution might be of benefit (Bach and Glasser, 2013; Dan Chan personal communication). The potential benefit of essential fatty acid or zinc supplementation is also unclear in the human patient, though in a particular 'pseudoglucagonoma syndrome' in patients with alcoholism, zinc supplementation (Delaporte et al., 1997) may resolve the skin lesions on its own, or in combination with essential fatty acids (Blackford et al., 1991).

Table 19.2 Examples of commercially available amino acids solutions for injection, their composition and proposed administration protocols for dogs with superficial necrolytic dermatitis.

	Ispol 12% (Daigo Eiyo Co. Tokyo, Japan)	Aminosyn 10% (Hispora, Inc., Lake Forest, IL, USA)	Aminoven 25 (Fresenius Kabi Ltd., Runcorn, UK)
	25 mL/kg twice weekly over 6–8 h for 3 weeks; effect evaluated thereafter (Mizuno et al., 2009)	3 mL/kg/h over 24h; effect evaluated 6 days following the infusion (Oberkirchner et al., 2010)	3–4 mL/kg/h (combined with 10 mL/kg Intralipid 20%, over 24–48 h, effect evaluated 6 days following the infusion (authors in communication with Dan Chan)
Amino acids	in mg/100 mL	in mg/100 mL	in mg/100 mL
L-isoleucin	845	760	520
L-leucin	1175	1200	890
Lysine HCl	1032	677	1110
L-methionine	540	180	380
L-phenylalanine	1280	427	550
L-threonine	596	512	860
L-tryptophan	218	180	160
L-valine	865	673	550
L-arginine HCl	1200	1227	2000
L-histidine HCl	600	312	730
L-aspartic acid	600	527	–
L-glutamic acid	180	820	–
L-alanine	480	698	2500
L-cystine	24	–	–
Glycine	1825	385	1850
L-proline	240	812	1700
L-serine	240	495	960
L-tyrosine	60	44	40
Taurine	–	70	200

Adjunct medical therapy

Glucocorticoid therapy will initially reduce skin inflammation and pruritus, but it can increase the risk of overt diabetes mellitus (Miller, 1992; Torres et al., 1997b) and is therefore not recommended. S-adenosylmethionine (Mizuno et al., 2009; Bexfield and Watson, 2009), ursodeoxycholic acid and glutathione (Mizuno et al., 2009), commonly used in hepatopathies (Flatland, 2009), have been used with minimal success in SND cases.

Systemic or topical antimicrobials can be used to reduce occurrence or treat existing secondary infections (bacteria and or *Malassezia* yeasts), depending on the nature of the organism present on cytology or microbial culture results. Topical treatment regimens may include chlorhexidine, miconazole / chlorhexidine combinations, and silver sulfadiazine.

Topical moisturizers may soften the hyperkeratotic skin of the footpads, nasal planum and lips and reduce frequency of fissuring and subsequent pain and secondary infection. The authors' group favors a product containing soybean-, palm- and cajuput oils and allantoine.[1]

Special considerations

In human medicine, SND associated with glucagonoma can be treated with surgical tumour de-bulking or resection and this has an important role in improving debilitating skin lesions, even if complete excision cannot be achieved (Stacpoole, 1981). In one canine case, pancreatic tumour removal led to resolution of skin lesions within 45 days, with no relapse over a further 6 weeks (Torres, Caywood and O'Brien, 1997a). Pre-existing metastases and post-surgical pancreatitis limit the potential for successful surgery (Koutinas et al., 2001).

Subcutaneous injections of octreotide, a long-acting somatostatin analogue that antagonizes the effects of glucagon, have been used with limited success in people with glucagonoma (Long et al., 1979; Shepherd et al., 1991). Recently, one dog with metastatic pancreatic glucagonoma showed a marked improvement after ten days of octreotide treatment (2 μg/kg twice daily as subcutaneous injections; Oberkirchner et al., 2010). Previously, a dog was also successfully treated with somatostatin (6 μg/kg subcutaneously every 8 h), but had been euthanized due to costs and renal dysfunction (Scott et al., 2001). Mizuno et al. (2009) observed only minimal improvement in one case where a somatostatin analogue (2 μg /kg Sandostatin (Novartis)) was used twice daily as subcutaneous injections for 2 weeks. Decreased appetite is a potential side effect in both dogs and people, which might be ameliorated by dose adjustment (1 μg/ kg 4 times daily, Oberkirchner et al., 2010), or use of appetite stimulants and anti-emetics (Lamberts, van der Lely and de Herder, 1996).

SND in dogs carries a poor prognosis, with a mean survival time of 6.4 months reported in a series of 36 dogs, with 18% surviving longer than 12 months (Outerbridge et al., 2002). Many dogs can be partially controlled for short periods with nutritional management although ultimately the lameness associated with footpad hyperkeratosis often leads to euthanasia before systemic signs significantly impact the quality of life. Surgical removal of pancreatic glucagonoma may be beneficial in rare early cases without metastases. Owners and attending veterinarians should constantly review the welfare of these dogs during treatment.

Summary

Superficial necrolytic dermatitis is a rare skin disease of dogs that has a characteristic symmetrical cutaneous pathology most commonly associated with a hepatopathy. Severe hyperkeratosis with fissuring of the footpads and similar lesions in nasal planum, muzzle and lips are characteristic dermal findings. Concurrent liver pathology is commonly encountered but this syndrome can occur in the absence of primary liver pathology, e.g., glucagonoma. Severe hypoaminoacidemia is a hallmark finding and nutritional management entails use of intravenous amino acid infusions and increased dietary protein intake. Although nutritional management can improve clinical signs temporarily, this disorder carries a poor prognosis.

KEY POINTS

- SND is a rare but often debilitating disease in dogs.
- This disorder has an incompletely understood etiopathogenesis but it is most commonly associated with a hepatopathy and rarely with glucagonoma.
- Skin histopathology and abdominal ultrasound are the most useful tests in dogs with compatible clinical signs as the lesions are very characteristic and typical of the disease.
- Although there are limited data available, intravenous amino acid supplementation, possibly with essential fatty acids and adjunct supplemental dietary intake provides temporary benefit to these patients.
- SND ultimately has a poor prognosis in the majority of cases.

Note

1 Dermoscent BioPalm Aventix, Laboratoire de Dermo-Cosmétiquie Animale, Technopôle Castres-Mazamet-Castres-France.

References

Allenspach, K., Arnold, P., Glaus, T. et al., (2000) Glucagon-producing neuroendocrine tumour associated with hypoaminoacidaemia and skin lesions. *Journal of Small Animal Practice*, **41**, 402–6.

Alexander, E.K., Robinson, M., Staniec, M. et al. (2002) Peripheral amino acid and fatty acid infusion for the treatment of necrolytic migratory erythema in the glucagonoma syndrome. *Clinical Endocrinology*, **57**, 827–31.

Asakawa, M.G., Cullen, J.M. and Linder, K.E. (2013) Necrolytic metabolic erythema associated with a glucagon-producing primary hepatic neuroendocrine carcinoma in a cat. *Veterinary Dermatology*, **24**, 466–469.

Bach, J.F. and Glasser, S.A. (2013) A case of necrolytic migratory erythema managed for 24 months with intravenous amino acids and lipid infusions. *Canadian Veterinary Journal*, **54**, 873–875.

Becker, S.W., Kahn, D. and Rothman, S. (1942) Cutaneous manifestations of internal malignant tumors. A.M.A. *Archives of Dermatology and Syphilology*, **45**, 1069–80.

Bexfield, N. and Watson, P. (2009) Treatment of canine liver disease 2. Managing clinical signs and specific liver disease, *Practice*, **31**, 172–180.

Blackford, S., Wright, S. and Roberts, D.L. (1991) Necrolytic migratory erythema without glucagonoma: the role of dietary essential fatty acids. *British Journal of Dermatology*, **125**, 460–462.

Bloom, P., Rosser, E.J. and Dunstan, R. (1992) Anti-convulsant hepatitis-induced necrolytic migratory erythema (Abstract). Proceedings of the Second World Congress of Veterinary Dermatology. May 13 to 16, Montreal, Canada. p. 56.

Bond, R., McNeil, P.E., Evans, H. et al., (1995) Metabolic epidermal necrosis in two dogs with different underlying diseases. *Veterinary Record*, **136**, 466–477.

Brenseke, B.M., Belz, K.M. and Saunders, G.K. (2011) Pathology in practice. *Journal of the American Veterinary Medical Association*, **238** (4), 445–447.

Byrne, K.P. (1999) Metabolic epidermal necrosis–hepatocutaneous syndrome. *Veterinary Clinics of North America Small Animal Practice*, **29**, 1337–1355.

Cave, T.A., Evans, H., Hargreaves, J. and Blunden, A.S. (2007) Metabolic epidermal nectosis in a dog associated with pancreatic adenocarcinoma, hyperglucagonaemia, hyperinsulinaemia and hypoaminoacidaemia. *Journal of Small Animal Practice*, **48**, 522–526.

Cellio, L.M. and Dennis, J. (2005) Canine superficial necrolytic dermatitis. *Compendium on Continuing Education for the Practicing Veterinarian*, **27**, 820–825.

Cerundolo, R., McEvoy, F. and McNeil, P.E. (1999) Ultrasonographic detection of a pancreatic glucagon-secreting multihormonal islet cell tumour in a dachshund with metabolic epidermal necrosis. *Veterinary Record*, **145**, 662–666.

Day, M.J. (1997) Review of thymic pathology in 30 cats and 36 dogs. *Journal of Small Animal Practice*, **38**, 393–403.

Delaporte, E., Catteau, B. and Piette, E. (1997) Necrolytic migratory erythema-like eruption in zink deficiency associated with alcoholic liver disease. *British Journal of Dermatology*, **137**, 1027–1028.

Dorsey, C.L., Dennis, P., Fascetti, A.J. et al. (2010) Hypoaminoacidemia is not associated with ulcerative lesions in Black Rhinoceroses, Diceros Bicornis. *Journal of Zoo and Wildlife Medicine*, **41** (1), 22–27.

Doyle, J.A., Schroeter, A.L. and Rogers, R.S. (1979) Hyperglucagonemia and necrolytic migratory erythema in cirrhosis – possible pseudoglucagonoma syndrome. *British Journal of Dermatolology*, **100**, 581–587.

Ehrlein, H.J., Loeffler K., and Trautwein, G. (1968) Ekzem und Leberererkrankung beim Hund (hepatodermales Syndrom) [eczema and liver disease in the dog (hepatodermal syndrome)]. *Kleintierpraxis*, **13**, 123–128.

Flatland B. (2009) Hepatic support therapy. in *Kirk's Current Veterinary Therapy XIV*, (sds J.D. Bonagura and D.C. Twedt) W.B. Saunders, Philadelphia, pp. 554–557.

Florant, E., Guillot, J., DeGorce-Rubialis, F. et al. (2000) Four cases of canine metabolic epidermal necrosis (Abstract). Free Communications of the Fourth World Congress of Veterinary Dermatology. Aug 30 to Sept 02, San Francisco, USA, p. 18.

Gleeson, M.H., Bloom, S.R., Polak, J.M. et al. (1970) An endocrine tumor in kidney affecting small bowel structure, motility, and function. *Gut*, **11**, 1060.

Godfrey, D.R. and Rest, J.R. (2000) Suspected necrolytic migratory erythema associated with chronic hepatopathy in a cat. *Journal of Small Animal Practice*, **41**, 324–328.

Goodenberger, D.M., Lawley and T.J., Strober, W. (1979) Necrolytic migratory erythema without glucagonoma. *Archive of Dermatology*, **115**, 1429–1432.

Gross, T.L., Ihrke P.J., Walder E.J. et al. (2005) Skin Diseases of the Dog and Cat, 2nd edn, Blackwell Publishing, pp. 86–91.

Gross, T.L., Song, M.D. and Havel, P.J. (1993) Superficial necrolytic dermatitis (Necrolytic Migratory Erythema) in dogs. *Veterinary Pathology*, **30**, 75–81.

Kimmel, S.E., Christiansen W., and Byrne, K.P. (2003) Clinicopathological, ultrasonographic, and histopathological findings of superficial necrolytic dermatitis with hepatopathy in a cat. *Journal of the American Animal Hospital Association*, **39**, 23–27.

Jacobson, L.S., Kirberger, R.M. and Nesbit, J.W. (1995) Hepatic ultrasonography and pathological findings in dogs with hepatocutaneous syndrome: new concepts. *Journal of Veterinary Internal Medicine*, **6**, 399–404.

Koutinas, C.K., Koutinas, A.F., Saridomichelakis, M.N. et al. (2001) Metabolic epidermal necrosis (hepatocutaneous syndrome) in the dog: A clinical and pathological review of 6 spontaneous cases. *European Journal of Companion Animal Practice*, **12** (2), 163–171.

Lamberts, S.W., van der Lely, A.J. and de Herder, W.W. (1996) Octreotide. *New England Journal of Medicine*, **334**, 246–254.

Little, C.J.L., McNeil, P.E. and Robb, J. (1991) Hepatopathy and dermatitis in a dog associated with the ingestion of mycotoxins. *Journal of Small Animal Practice*, **32**, 23–26.

Long, R.G., Adrian, T.E., Brown, M.R. et al. (1979) Suppression of pancreatic endocrine tumour secretion by long-acting somatostatin analogue. *Lancet*, **2**, 764.

March, P.A., Hillier, A. and Weisbrode, S.E. (2004) Superficial necrolytic dermatitis in 11 dogs with a history of phenobarbital administration (1995–2002). *Journal of Veterinary Internal Medicine*, **18**, 65–74.

Mauldin, E.A., Morris, D.O. and Goldschmidt, M.H. (2002) Retrospective study: the presence of Malassezia in feline skin biopsies. A clinicopathological study. *Veterinary Dermatology*, **13**, 7–14.

Miller, W.H. (1992) Necrolytic migratory erythema in dogs: A cutaneous marker for gastrointestinal disease. in *Current Veterinary Therapy XI*, (eds R.W. Kirk and J.D. Bonagura) W.B. Saunders, Philadelphia, pp. 561–562.

Miller, W.H., Scott, D.W., Buerger, R.G. et al., (1990) Necrolytic migratory erythema in dogs: A hepatocutaneous syndrome. *Journal of the American Animal Hospital Association*, **26**,573–581.

Mizuno, T., Hiraoka, H. and Yoshioka, C. (2009) Superficial necrolytic dermatitis associated with extrapancreatic glucagonoma in a dog. *Veterinary Dermatology*, **20**, 72–79.

Munson, L., Koehler, J.W., Wilkinson, J.E. et al. (1998) Vesicular and ulcerative dermatopathy resembling superficial necrolytic dermatitis in captive black rhinoceroses (Diceros bicornis). *Veterinary Pathology*, **35**, 31–42.

Norton, J.A., Kahn, C.R., Scheibinger, R. et al. (1979) Amino acid deficiency and the skin rash associated with glucagonoma. *Annals of Internal Medicine*, **91**, 213–215.

Nyland, T.G., Barthez, P.Y., Ortega, T.M. et al. (1996) Hepatic ultrasonographic and pathologic findings in dogs with canine superficial necrolytic dermatitis. *Veterinary Radiology and Ultrasound*, **37** (3), 200–205.

Oberkirchner, U., Linder, K.E., Zadrozny, L. et al. (2010) Successful treatment of canine necrolytic migratory erythema (superficial necrolytic dermatitis) due to metastatic glucagonoma with octreotide. *Veterinary Dermatology*, **21**(5), 510–516.

Outerbridge, C.A., Marks, S.L. and Rogers, Q.R. (2002) Plasma amino acid concentrations in 36 dogs with histologically confirmed superficial necrolytic dermatitis. *Veterinary Dermatology*, **13**, 177–186.

Outerbridge, C.A. (2013) Cutaneous manifestations of internal disease. *Veterinary Clinics of North American Small Animal Practice*, **43**, 135–152.

Papadogiannakis, E., Frangia, K. and Matralis, D. (2009) Superficial necrolytic dermatitis in a dog associated with hyperplasia of pancreatic neuroendocrine cells. *Journal of Small Animal Practice*, **50**, 318.

Patel, A., Whitbread, T.J. and McNeil, P.E. (1995) A case of metabolic epidermal necrosis in a cat. *Veterinary Dermatology*, **7**, 221–226.

Peterson, L.L., Shaw, J.C., Acott, K.M. et al. (1984) Glucagonoma syndrome: in vitro evidence that glucagon increases epidermal arachidonic acid. *Journal of the American Academy of Dermatology*, **11**, 468–73.

Roggli, V.L., Judge, D.M. and McGavran M.H. (1979) Duodenal glucagonoma: A case report. *Human Pathology*, **10** (3), 350–353.

Scott, D.W., Miller, W.H. and Griffin, C.E. (2001) Necrolytic migratory erythema. in *Muller & Kirk's Small Animal Dermatology*. 6th edn. W.B. Saunders, Philadelphia. pp. 868–873.

Shepherd, M.E., Raimer, S.S., Tyring, S.K. et al. (1991) Treatment of necrolytic migratory erythema in glucagonoma syndrome. *Journal of the American Academy of Dermatology*, **25** (5), 925–928.

Stacpoole, P.W. (1981). The glucagonoma syndrome: clinical features, diagnosis and treatment. *Endocrine Review*, **2** (3), 347–361.

Torres, S.M.F., Caywood, D.D. and O'Brien, T.D. (1997a) Resolution of superficial necrolytic dermatitis following excision of a glucagon – secreting pancreatic neoplasm in a dog. *Journal of the American Animal Hospital Association*, **33**, 313–319.

Torres, S., Johnson, K. and McKeever, P. (1997b) Superficial necrolytic dermatitis and a pancreatic endocrine tumor in a dog. *Journal of Small Animal Practice*, **38**, 246–50.

Turek, M.M. (2003) Cutaneous paraneoplastic syndromes in dogs and cats: a review of the literature. *Veterinary Dermatology*, **14**, 279–296.

Van Beek, A.P., de Haas, E.R., van Vloten, W.A. et al. (2004) The glucagonoma syndrome and necrolytic migratory erythema: a clinical review. *European Journal of Endocrinology*, **151**, 531–537.

Van Poucke, S. and Rest, J.R. (2005) Superficial necroytic dermatitis associated with hepatic lipidosis in a red fox (Vulpes vulpes). *Veterinary Record*, **156**, 54–55.

Walton, D.K., Center, S.A. and Scott, D.W. (1986) Ulcerative dermatosis associated with diabetes mellitus in the dog: a report of four cases. *Journal of the American Animal Hospital Association*, **22**, 79–88.

CHAPTER 20

Nutritional support in acute kidney injury in dogs and cats

Denise A. Elliott

Waltham Centre for Pet Nutrition, Waltham on the Wolds, Leicestershire, UK

Introduction

Acute kidney injury (AKI) is a clinical syndrome characterized by a sudden reduction of renal function with rapid development of azotemia and failure to regulate fluid, electrolyte and acid–base balance. The etiology of intrinsic AKI is multifactorial and can include hemodynamic, infectious, immune-mediated, neoplastic or nephrotoxic damage to the vasculature, glomeruli, tubular epithelium or interstitium of the kidney. AKI frequently complicates other surgical or medical diseases and may be identified as a bystander of a generalized systemic inflammatory response causing multiple-organ dysfunction.

The clinical presentation of acute uremia depends on its cause, severity and concurrent diseases provoking the renal injury. The diagnosis is established from a comprehensive data base integrating history, physical examination, laboratory testing, diagnostic imaging and, in some instances, histopathology. AKI is associated with variable hyperkalemia and hypocalcemia, moderate to severe metabolic acidosis and hyperphosphatemia in addition to azotemia. Classically the syndrome of AKI has been characterized by oliguria and anuria; however, non-oliguric forms of AKI also occur. With timely diagnosis and appropriately administered therapy, AKI can be reversible. Delays or failure to initiate specific and supportive therapy may result in irreversible renal damage or death. The management of the acute uremia encompasses reversing the underlying cause(s) and ongoing risk factors (e.g., drugs, inadequate hemodynamics and concurrent diseases) for the renal injury, correcting the uremic intoxications and the fluid, electrolyte and acid–base imbalances, establishing adequate urine production and providing nutritional support until renal function has recovered.

Nutritional management strategies

The uremic manifestations of AKI compromise the appetite and contribute to nausea and vomiting. In addition, recovery from AKI may require a prolonged convalescence during which animals are at risk of protein calorie malnutrition

Nutritional Management of Hospitalized Small Animals, First Edition. Edited by Daniel L. Chan.

© 2015 John Wiley & Sons, Ltd. Published 2015 by John Wiley & Sons, Ltd.

due to poor dietary intake. Therefore, early nutritional assessment and institution of nutritional support is crucial in the management of patients with AKI. Nutritional supplementation should be individually tailored to patient needs to compensate for the specific abnormalities in protein, carbohydrate and lipid metabolism, and the marked alterations in fluid, electrolyte and acid–base balance characteristic of AKI. Nutritional management of the AKI patient is complex and can be significantly complicated by oliguria/anuria.

The metabolic status of the patient with AKI varies according to the variation of the disease (Fiaccadori, Parenti and Maggiore, 2008). However, most patients have some degree of protein catabolism and negative nitrogen balance (Mitch, May and Maroni, 1989a). Endocrine factors contributing to protein catabolism in uremia include insulin resistance, secondary hyperparathyroidism and increased circulating concentrations of catecholamines, glucagon and corticosteroids (Fiaccadori et al., 2008). Inflammatory mediators, including neutrophil-derived circulating proteases, interleukins and tumour necrosis factor, have also been shown to mediate hypercatabolism. Metabolic acidosis acting via a glucocorticoid-dependent pathway is also a major cause of muscle protein breakdown in AKI (Mitch et al., 1989b). Collectively, these mechanisms of catabolism and marked protein breakdown contribute to the uremic syndrome by exacerbating hyper-kalemia, hyperphosphatemia, acidosis and azotemia.

Therefore, the first step in managing the patient with AKI is to ensure that sufficient energy is provided to prevent endogenous protein catabolism. Energy metabolism in AKI varies and depends on the presence of underlying or concur-rent disease. However, it is generally considered that there is a decrease rather than an increase in energy expenditure (Kreymann et al., 2006). The energy expenditure of an individual patient may be assessed by indirect calorimetry, however, this technique is not widely available in veterinary hospitals (O'Toole et al., 2001). The amount of energy to provide for the patient can be calculated from the resting energy requirement (RER) $70(Wt_{kg})^{0.75}$ with intake subsequently adjusted according to individual patient needs, based on serial clinical assess-ment of body weight and body condition score. Excessive energy intake should be avoided, particularly in animals with compromised respiratory function (e.g. uremic pneumonitis) as the increased carbohydrate and fat metabolism generates CO_2. Carbohydrate and fat provide the non-protein sources of energy in the diet. Diets designed for the management of renal failure are usually formulated with a relatively high fat content because fat provides approximately twice the energy per gram than carbohydrate, increasing the energy density of the diet and thereby allowing the patient to obtain its nutritional requirements from a smaller volume of food.

Azotemia and uremia are due to the accumulation of protein metabolites (nitrogenous waste products) derived from dietary protein and degradation of endogenous protein. Ideally protein intake should be matched with catabolism to promote a positive nitrogen balance and thereby avoid protein calorie malnutrition while simultaneously reducing the production of uremic toxins to ameliorate the clinical signs of uremia. Nitrogen balance studies to estimate dietary protein requirements are not applicable in the critical care setting of AKI. Logically, every animal with AKI should be fed at least the minimal protein requirements (4 g/100 kcal for cats; 2 g/100 kcal for dogs) (NRC, 2006). However, this degree of restriction is necessary only in animals with profound uremia and, in most cases, the protein intake can be gradually adjusted to reach the recommended daily requirement (5 g/100 kcal for cats; 2.5 g/100 kcal for dogs) (NRC 2006) to ensure adequate protein intake while minimizing uremia. High quality protein sources must be used in the formulation of restricted protein diets to minimize the risks of essential amino acid deficiency.

Dietary phosphorus intake should be restricted to help manage hyperphosphatemia. Most dietary phosphate is contained within protein, hence dietary protein restriction will simultaneously reduce phosphate intake. Unfortunately, dietary protein restriction alone is unlikely to prevent hyperphosphatemia in AKI, and the administration of intestinal phosphate binding agents with the food is typically required. The potassium status of the patient with AKI is highly variable and can fluctuate on a day to day basis according to the urine output (anuria vs oliguria vs polyuria), emphasizing the need to monitor potassium status and adjust intake on an individual basis. Severe metabolic acidosis is a common complication of AKI, but variable primary or mixed acid–base disturbances may develop, depending on the underlying etiology and extent of the vomiting, diarrhea and respiratory components. While citrate supplemented diets can be selected to assist the management of metabolic acidosis, medical treatment is often necessary. Water soluble vitamins are excreted in urine and hence deficiency may develop due to polyuria associated with the recovery phase of AKI. Long chain omega 3 fatty acids, such as eicosapentaenoic acid and docosahexaenoic acid, compete with arachadonic acid and alter eicosanoid production. To be effective, they must be incorporated into cell membranes, therefore, it is not clear if supplementation with omega-3 fatty acids will be effective in modulating inflammation in the acute setting. Supplementation with exogenous antioxidants appears logical to combat oxidative stress and free radical damage.

Diets designed for the management of chronic kidney disease are widely available and typically contain appropriate nutrient modifications for patients with acute kidney disease. Therefore the challenges in managing the AKI patient are not with diet selection but rather with anorexia and food refusal that accompanies their critical illness, the management of which is further complicated by oliguria/anuria. Food intake can be encouraged by using odorous foods, warming the foods prior to feeding, and stimulating eating by positive reinforcement with petting and stroking behaviour. Appetite stimulants can be considered (see Chapter 13) but, in most cases, adequate daily food intake can only be achieved by enteral or parenteral interventional nutrition.

Enteral nutrition, facilitated by the placement of nasoesophageal or esophagostomy tubes, is a highly effective management devices to achieve dietary administration to animals reluctant to eat appropriate amounts of food ad libitum (see Chapters 4 and 5). Enteral tube feeding is recommended in all patients who can tolerate it as enteral feeding helps to maintain the gastrointestinal barrier and prevent the translocation of bacteria and systemic infections (Deitch, Winterton and Berg, 1987). The appropriate renal diet can be blended with water and the feeding solution administered intermittently or continuously using a syringe pump. To decreased the risk of refeeding syndrome the amount of the nutrient solution is gradually increased over two to three days until the nutritional requirements are met (Justin and Hohenhaus, 1995). The stomach should be aspirated every 2 to 4 hours to ensure gastric emptying and intestinal peristalsis are established, thereby prevent vomiting and aspiration. Fluid balance in the acute kidney injury patient is precarious, especially in the oliguric/anuric patient. Care should be taken to minimize the volume of water used to blend the commercial diet. In especially delicate cases, the water to blend the diet can be replaced with an appropriate commercial liquid; note that in this situation, a veterinary nutritionist should be consulted to ensure the combination of the two commercial products will still meet the nutrient needs of the patient. Several human enteral formulations for renal disease are available; however, these products often contain inadequate amounts of protein and essential nutrients, such as taurine, arginine and arachidonic acid, and hence should be used cautiously in dogs and cats.

Parenteral nutrition is indicated if the nutrient requirements cannot be met by the enteral route and the patient can tolerate the additional fluid load (Cano et al., 2009). Peripheral parenteral nutrition (PPN) involves the administration of isotonic nutritional solutions through a peripheral vein, thereby avoiding the requirement of a central vein. PPN cannot provide the complete nutrient requirements for the patient due to the isotonic nature of the solution that is specifically designed to avoid thrombophlebitis (see Chapter 11). PPN is rarely used in patients with AKI due to the difficulties with managing fluid balance.

Central parenteral nutrition (CPN), which can provide the appropriate nutrient requirements, necessitates administration into a central vein such as the vena cava due to the hyperosmolality of the solution. Fluid balance is still challenging using CPN, but clearly less so compared with the vast volumes required with PPN. Modified amino acid formulations for parenteral use in AKI are available, however, there are no studies to suggest that the modified amino acid solutions are any more effective than the standard amino acid solutions.

Special considerations

Fluid therapy is the cornerstone of medical management of patients with AKI. The goal is to normalize fluid balance, resolve any hemodynamic inadequacies and promote urine formation. Animals with AKI typically are dehydrated and hypovolemic because of anorexia, vomiting and diarrhea. The volume deficit should be corrected with the intravenous administration of saline or balanced polyionic replacement solutions within 2 to 4 hours. There is absolutely no indication for subcutaneous replacement of the fluid deficits. The rate of fluid administration may need to be tempered for patients with concurrent cardiovascular disease to prevent circulatory congestion and heart failure. Blood losses should be replaced with compatible blood transfusions to restore intravascular volume, blood pressure and haematocrit. If the estimated fluid deficit fails to induce a diuresis of at least 1 mL/kg/hr, the hydration status of the patient should be reassessed to ensure that the fluid deficits are indeed replete. Further fluid administration with balanced electrolyte solutions should be provided to achieve mild (3 to 5% of body weight) volume expansion. Maintenance fluid requirements must be provided after fluid deficits are restored and are predicated on assessment of ongoing fluid losses (urinary, vomitus, fecal) which are replaced with isonatric solutions and insensible fluid (free water 20–25 mL/kg/day) requirements which must be supplied orally or by parenteral administration of 5% dextrose in water.

Failure to induce adequate diuresis with fluid therapy predicts severe kidney injury. A number of therapeutic agents (e.g., mannitol, furosemide, dopamine) have been advocated to attenuate the severity of the renal injury or induce urine formation in the oliguric or anuric patient. Their efficacy remains controversial and should not supersede appropriate and timely administration of fluid therapy. It should be noted that conversion of an oliguric or anuric patient to a non-oliguric state may not necessarily equate with improvements in renal function or recovery but clearly facilitates the management of fluid, electrolyte, and acid–base disorders, in addition to alleviating the challenges associated with the administration of enteral or parenteral nutrition. If a diuretic response cannot be established or maintained within 4 to 6 hours following restoration of fluid deficits and administration of mannitol, furosemide and/or dopamine therapy, it is highly unlikely that additional administration of fluid or drugs will be safe or effective, and dialysis should be considered as an alternative.

Antiemetics should be used to control protracted vomiting. Gastrointestinal protective agents, such as histamine receptor blockers (e.g., cimetidine, ranitidine, famotidine) or proton pump blockers (e.g., omeprazole) may be used to prevent severe esophagitis and ulcerative gastritis during periods of uremia and persistent vomiting. Oral rinsing with 0.1% chlorhexidine solution is beneficial for uremic stomatitis and oral ulcerations. Systemic hypertension may require antihypertensive therapy to prevent retinal detachment and cerebral bleeding.

Monitoring and complications

AKI is a dynamic condition that has significant systemic effects. Regular monitoring and nutritional assessment is crucial to ensure that dietary and medical management remains optimal for the needs of the patient (Elliott, 2008). Complications are typically related to fluid, electrolyte and acid–base balance, and inadequate food intake. The likelihood for errors can be minimized by clear and concise treatment plans coupled with constant re-evaluation of the patient's status (Remillard et al., 2001). The amount of food eaten should be recorded in the medical record. It is equally important that all episodes of vomiting and diarrhoea be recorded in the medical record. The body weight should be monitored at least once daily and the amount of food delivered adjusted accordingly to prevent body weight loss. Body weight changes in the acute kidney patient can be misleading due to the concurrent fluid balance status. Therefore, in addition to changes in body weight, the clinician should also utilize changes in muscle mass to help guide their clinical decision-making. Fluid balance should be assessed regularly by changes in body weight and indices of hydration to direct ongoing fluid prescriptions. Oliguric or anuric animals are incapable of excreting an excessive fluid load, so care must be taken to avoid volume overload. Hypervolemia is a serious and potentially life-threatening complication of therapy that is difficult or impossible to correct.

Summary

Management of the patient with AKI is a complex medical challenge. The nutritional needs of the patient are likely to be ignored in the pursuit of diagnosis and management of the complex metabolic disturbances induced by acute uremia. Furthermore, most patients do not have a history of weight loss, nor do they present in poor body condition. However, it is extremely important to anticipate the need to feed the patient. The effects of uremia on appetite and metabolism are clear and devastating. Do not take a 'wait and see' attitude. To minimize catabolism and promote recovery nutritional therapy should be implemented within hours of admission to the hospital.

KEY POINTS

- Acute uremia is associated with fluid, electrolyte and acid–base abnormalities.
- The nutritional needs of the patient with acute kidney injury are often overlooked in the pursuit of diagnosis and treatment.
- Malnutrition and lean body wasting are common in acute kidney injury patients and will adversely affect outcome.
- Timely and appropriate nutritional therapy should be a fundamental component in the treatment plan of the hospitalized acute kidney injury patient.

References

Cano, N.J., Aparicio, M., Brunori, G. et al. (2009) ESPEN Guidelines on parenteral nutrition: adult renal failure. *Clinical Nutrition*, **28**, 401–414.

Deitch, E.A., Winterton, J. and Berg, R. (1987) Effect of starvation, malnutrition, and trauma on the gastrointestinal tract flora and bacterial translocation. *Archives of Surgery*, **122**, 1019–1024.

Elliott, D. A. (2008) Nutritional assessment. in *Small Animal Critical Care Medicine*. (eds D. Silverstein and K. Hoppe). Elsevier, St Louis, pp. 856–858.

Fiaccadori, E., Parenti, E. and Maggiore, U. (2008) Nutritional support in acute kidney injury. *Journal of Nephrology*, **21**, 645–656.

Justin, R.B. and Hohenhaus, A.E. (1995) Hypophosphatemia associated with enteral alimentation in cats. *Journal of Veterinary Internal Medicine*, **9**, 228–233.

Kreymann, K.G., Berger, M.M., Deutz, N.E. et al., (2006) ESPEN Guidelines on enteral nutrition: Intensive care. *Clinical Nutrition*, **25**, 210–223.

Mitch, W.E., May, R.C. and Maroni, B.J. (1989a) Review: mechanisms for abnormal protein metabolism in uremia. *Journal of the American College of Nutrition*, **8**, 305–309.

Mitch, W.E., May, R.C., Maroni, B.J. et al., (1989b) Protein and amino acid metabolism in uremia: influence of metabolic acidosis. *Kidney International, Supplement 27*, S205–S207.

National Research Council of the National Academies (2006) *Nutrient Requirements of Dogs and Cats*, National Academies Press, Washington DC.

O'Toole, E., McDonell, W.N., Wilson, B.A. et al. (2001) Evaluation of accuracy and reliability of indirect calorimetry for the measurement of resting energy expenditure in healthy dogs. *American Journal of Veterinary Research*, **62**, 1761–1767.

Remillard, R.L., Darden, D.E., Michel, K.E. et al. (2001) An investigation of the relationship between caloric intake and outcome in hospitalized dogs. *Veterinary Therapeutics*, **2**, 301–310.

CHAPTER 21

Nutritional support in hepatic failure in dogs and cats

Renee M. Streeter[1] and Joseph J. Wakshlag[2]

[1] Liverpool, NY, USA

[2] Cornell University College of Veterinary Medicine, Ithaca, NY, USA

Introduction

The liver is the primary organ regulating metabolism and detoxification processes. As such, when there is significant hepatic pathology present, the nutritional management for this patient is of critical importance. All nutritional approaches for the management of hospitalized canine and feline patients with various hepatopathies are not the same but can be generalized based on protein tolerance. Some hepatopathies, including early and chronic hepatic cirrhosis, cholangitis, triaditis and feline hepatic lipidosis do not generally require protein restriction, while congenital and acquired vascular shunting and end-stage cirrhosis may require significant protein restriction.

Acute liver disease: cirrhosis, hepatitis and cholestatic disease

The liver plays a central role in nutrient metabolism and because of this the requirements for specific nutrients may change following onset of liver failure. The liver's role in protein metabolism includes synthesis of albumin, globulins, ceruplasmin, ferritin, numerous serum enzymes and coagulation factors. Additionally the liver regulates amino acid metabolism, is involved in the detoxification of ammonia and is responsible for the subsequent synthesis of urea (Biourge, 1997; LaFlamme, 2000). Therefore, dietary protein concentrations should not be decreased in early liver disease, as protein restriction may cause catabolism of endogenous lean body mass, resulting in increased ammonia production and increased risk of hepatic encephalopathy (Biourge, 1997; LaFlamme, 2000). In hepatic disease the liver's regulatory role in amino acid homeostasis is altered and diminished glycogen stores may also be present. Supplying appropriate dietary protein enables a more rapid transition to glyconeogenesis from amino acids and can help fill the energy gap which results from

Nutritional Management of Hospitalized Small Animals, First Edition. Edited by Daniel L. Chan.

© 2015 John Wiley & Sons, Ltd. Published 2015 by John Wiley & Sons, Ltd.

Table 21.1 Calculation of protein content on a g/kg b.w. basis.

Assume a 10 kg dog's maintenance energy requirement (MER) is approximately 629 kcal.
A typical liver diet may contain 18% protein on an as-fed basis.
If product guide lists 4.2 g per 1000 kcal.
  Then, 42g × 0.629 Mcal = 26 g / 10 kg dog = 2.6 g per day.
If product guide lists 4.2 g/100 kcal;
  Then, 4.2 g × 6.29 Mcal = 26 g / 10 kg = 2.6 g per day

low glycogen stores in liver disease (Silk, O'Keefe and Wicks, 1991). Consequently, providing a diet with modestly increased protein content from high quality protein is essential in the management of chronic hepatopathies. If a reduced protein-content diet is necessary, the diet should contain no less than 2.1g protein/kg body weight for dogs and at least 4g protein/kg body weight for cats (Center, 1998; LaFlamme, 2000). While many clinicians prefer to think of nutrient content of foods on a dry matter or as fed basis, it is important to realize that calculating protein content on a gram per kg of body weight basis may be more appropriate when determining protein requirements for patients. Therefore it is preferable to calculate protein intake based on the caloric intake, which can be determined for most patients to maintain appropriate body condition, by using the information in product guides according to 100 kcal or 1000 kcal intake. Table 21.1 gives an example of how to calculate protein content of foods on a g/kg basis once the kilocalorie consumption is known.

Calories derived from fat increase the palatability of foods, which is beneficial in an otherwise inappetant patient and also helps prevent endogeneous protein catabolism. However, the fat content of foods should be limited in patients with potential cholelithiasis or cholestasis. Dietary fats stimulate cholecystokinin and motilin release from the duodenum, signalling contraction of the gall bladder which can be potentially detrimental in cases of bile duct obstruction (Center, 2009). Very high dietary cholesterol has also been found to have lithogenic properties in prairie dogs and in pigmented gall stones of dogs (Holzbach et al., 1976; Englert et al., 1977). Limiting fat intake in these patients may be necessary as lipid metabolism is compromised in hepatobiliary disease and long chain triglyceride digestion may decrease by as much as 30–50%. Thus, feeding excessive fat could contribute to diarrhea and lead to further nutrient depletion (LaFlamme, 2000). There have been reports in Shetland sheepdogs with gallbladder mucoceles which show improvement after management with a low fat diet (Aguirre et al., 2007; Walter et al., 2008). Although these reports do not give a recommended dietary fat value, a diet containing no more than 10% DM fat for dogs and less than 15% DM fat for cats would be considered a low fat diet and appropriate for cases of obstructive cholestasis.

Abnormal hepatic copper concentrations are often observed as a pathologic feature in hepatic disease. High copper concentration may be secondary to cholestatic liver disease or may be the result of a primary defect in hepatic copper excretion. Breeds associated with primary copper-associated hepatopathies include Skye terriers, West Highland white terriers, Doberman pinschers, Labrador retrievers and Bedlington terriers. Management of high hepatic copper concentrations will decrease hepatic mitochondrial damage and lipid peroxidation in hepatocytes (Sokol et al., 1989). Treatment has traditionally included decreasing total dietary copper content, increasing dietary zinc content, and chelation therapy (Hoffmann et al., 2009). Recommendations for chelation with zinc supplementation have varied widely from 1.5 mg/kg of elemental zinc to 100 mg/kg of elemental zinc (Brewer et al., 1992; Thornburg, 2000; Plumb, 2008). However, only one study has proven zinc to be efficacious at decreasing copper absorption at a dose of 100 mg/kg of elemental zinc for 3 months and then 50 mg/kg thereafter (Brewer et al., 1992). Although supplementation of zinc is advocated to decrease copper absorption, the use of a low copper diet may be equally, if not more effective. A recent investigation of Labrador Retrievers with copper hepatopathy suggests that additional zinc at a dose of 10 mg/kg did not diminish the effects of hepatic copper accumulation beyond what was observed with a low copper diet alone (Hoffmann et al., 2009). However, long term management was not evaluated and the use of 100 mg of elemental zinc supplementation was not examined in conjunction with dietary copper restriction therefore, in refractory cases it may still be beneficial to use supplemental zinc at high doses. The form of zinc is also an important concept, since sources such as zinc gluconate or zinc acetate have very different amounts of elemental zinc per milligram. The dosage of zinc should always be in elemental zinc content in the tablet or capsule which can be somewhat variable depending on the form of zinc being used.

Another goal with nutritional treatment of liver disease in early cirrhosis or triaditis is protection of the hepatocyte from apoptosis and fibrosis. Nutraceuticals, such as polyenylphosphatidylcholine (PEP), S-adenosylmethionine (SAMe), vitamin E and silymarin are often utilized for these functions. PEP is a compound made up of polyunsaturated phospholipids which work as antioxidants and collagenase stimulators to decrease hepatic fibrosis (Aleynik et al., 1997). PEP may also diminish oxidative mitochondrial and hepatocellular membrane injury by decreasing reactive oxygen species (ROS) generation thereby conserving hepatocyte glutathione (GSH), a potent endogenous antioxidant. Dosing in dogs and cats is extrapolated from human literature and is 25–50 mg/kg/day, not to exceed 3 g in large dogs (Center, 2004).

S-adenosylmethionine (SAMe) is made and utilized in hepatocytes for methylation reactions. Benefits of SAMe treatment in hepatic disorders include:decreased rate of liver disease progression, increased hepatic GSH stores, improved tolerance of free radicals and improvement of cholestatis and reperfusion injury and potentially improved regeneration and protein synthesis. Glutathione depletion has been observed in a variety of hepatopathies, particularly in cats, making the use of SAMe a standard therapeutic intervention (Center, 2004; Center et al., 2005). The recommended dosage in cats for cirrhosis (and hepatic lipidosis) is 20–55 mg/kg PO given on an empty stomach. In dogs, a dose of 17–20 mg/kg is used (Center, 2004; Center et al., 2005).

Vitamin E has also been used as adjunct therapy in early hepatic disorders. Vitamin E protects all cell membranes from lipid peroxidation and may suppress inflammatory cell activity and reduce free radical damage to hepatocytes (Cantürk et al., 1998; Center, 2004). Vitamin E also has anti-proliferative effects on vascular smooth muscle and suppresses hepatic collagen gene expression in the inflamed or injured liver (Chojkier et al., 1998; Center, 2004). Supplementation during hepatic disease is warranted not only due to the anti-inflammatory benefits, but also because hepatic concentrations of alpha-tocopherol in people with cirrhosis have been found to be three-fold lower than in control levels, even despite normal serum concentrations (Von Herbay et al., 1994). Currently a dose of 10 IU/kg per day of alpha-tocopherol has been suggested for treatment of patients with hepatic disorders (Center, 2004).

Silymarin is a complex of flavinolignans which are derived from milk thistle and include silybinin (or silybin), isosilibinin, silidianin and silicristin. Silymarin's mechanisms of action include providing antioxidant effects against relevant ROS and lipid peroxidation (Center, 2004.) Silymarin also accelerates hepatocellular regeneration as a result of increased gene transcription and translation and enhanced DNA biosynthesis. Inhibition of stellate cell activation and proliferation as well as signalling for type I collagen synthesis and production of metaloproteinase I tissue inhibitor may mitigate fibrosis. Silymarin may also induce a choleretic response associated with expansion of the endogenous pool of bile salts including the hepatoprotective bile acid urosodeoxycholic acid (Center, 2004). Although there are no studies on dogs and cats, a dose of 40–50 mg/kg/day of Silymarin-controlled fibrosis in rats with bile duct obstruction, and ample evidence exists showing that 50–150mg/kg is safe in dogs (Center, 2004). However, a commercial preparation of silybin compounds (Marin[1]), combined with phosphatidylcholine has been shown to have increased bioavailability in dogs (Filburn, Kettenacker and Griffin, 2007). Although this study used dosages of 14.6–17.3 mg/kg, the recommended dosage for Marin, which also contains zinc and vitamin E, is 1.3–2.8 mg/kg for dogs and 1.5–2.6 mg/kg for cats.

Ursodeoxycholic acid (Ursodiol) is a non-toxic hydrophilic dihydroxylated bile acid which was first identified in the gall bladder of Chinese Black Bear. Benefits of Ursodiol include: displacement of toxic bile acids with this less toxic form of bile acid, cytoprotection of hepatocytes and biliary epithelium, antioxidant effects, immunomodulatory effects, attenuation of bile acid secretion, enhanced biliary elimination of toxic substances and an inhibitory influence on fibrogenesis (Kumar and Tandon, 2001). It is used in the treatment of cirrhosis, cholangitis and non-obstructive forms of cholestasis (Kumar and Tandon, 2001). Assuming a biliary tree occlusion has been ruled out; the dose for treatment of necroinflammatory hepatic disorders is 10–15mg/kg/day in one or divided into two treatments, administered with food (Center, 2004).

Chronic liver diseases: chronic endstage cirrhosis, portosystemic shunts and vascular dysplasia

The goal with treatment of end-stage cirrhosis and shunt patients is to prevent hepatic encephalopathy while providing the appropriate nutrients to prevent wasting and capitalize on any existing hepatic function. In manipulating the diet for end-stage cirrhosis patients and patients with portosystemic shunts, it has been found that the use of vegetable or dairy proteins in place of meat proteins significantly decreased ammonia production (Bianchi et al., 1993). Recommendations include decreasing the total amount of protein in the diet (2–4 g/ kg body weight for dogs and 4–6 g/kg body weight for cats) (Tillson and Winkler, 2002) and increasing the overall quality of protein in the diet by choosing highly digestible sources that do not include excessive nitrogen or hemoglobin, both of which have been associated with worsening hepatic encephalopathy (Bianchi et al., 1993, Douglass, Mardini and Record, 2001). The minimum protein requirement should be titrated up until ammonium biurate crystals are seen in the urine or signs of hepatic encephalopathy become evident.

Water-soluble B vitamins are also supplemented in liver disease as vitamin B_{12}, folate, riboflavin, nicotinamide, thiamine, pantothenic acid and pyridoxine are stored in the liver and availability and storage patterns are altered with hepatic disease (Biourge, 1997). Vitamin B_{12} is essential for many metabolic activities in the liver and administration of vitamin B_{12} is recommended in patients with cholangitis and triaditis at a dose of 1mg SC every 7 to 28 days (Center, 1998). B complex vitamins at twice maintenance requirements are also recommended in severe cases of cirrhosis or late stage shunts (Center, 1998).

Vitamin K may be depleted in some forms of hepatic disease due to impaired hepatic synthesis, high turnover rate of clotting factors (i.e., consumptive coagulopathy) or the concurrent use of antibiotics which may cause a decrease in vitamin K producing bacteria in the intestine or interfere with hepatic enzymes which synthesize clotting factors (Peetermans and Verbist, 1990; Lisciandro, Hohenhaus and Brooks, 1998; Conly and Stein, 1994). Administration of 0.5–1.0 mg/kg SC every 12 hours for two days has proved useful in normalizing clotting times in animals with liver disease (Center, 1998).

The use of lactulose and soluble fibres, such as pectin, psyllium and inulin, is often instituted to decrease ammonia absorption from the colon and help prevent hepatic encephalopathy. Increased amounts of fermentable fiber encourage growth of acidophilic bacteria, such as *Lactobacillus,* which are less ammoniagenic and will reduce the pH of the colon (Crossley and Williams, 1984; Center, 1998). This decrease in pH causes a shift of ammonia to its ionic form (NH^{4+}) which is not absorbed from the gut and is excreted in the feces (Center 1998). In one study these effects have been demonstrated with ingestion of pectin (Herrmann, Shakoor and Weber, 1987) and a dose of 5–10 mL to about 150-200 kcal for dogs has been recommended (Center, 1998). Due to similar fermentative properties psyllium fiber or inulin may also be used at 1–2 teaspoons (3–6 g) per 10 kg body weight or 0.5–1 teaspoons (1.5–3.0 g) per day, respectively, for similar effects. Recommended lactulose dosages are 0.5–1.0 mL/kg PO every 6–8 hours titrated to produce 2–3 soft stools per day (Brent and Weise, 2010). Cats should receive 0.25–1 mL of lactulose PO titrating upwards to individualize the dose until semi-formed stools are produced (Scavelli, Hornbuckle and Roth, 1986).

SAMe may be used in the late stage cirrhotic and shunt patient as it plays a role in restoration of glutathione levels and is thus important in detoxification mechanisms of hepatocytes (Center et al., 2005). However, SAMe does provide an additional source of the amino acid methionine which can lead to hepatic encephalopathy and it should be used with caution in severe cases when hepatic encephalopathy is likely (Center, 2004). In chronic liver disease antioxidant therapies such as PEP, vitamin E, silamarin, SAMe and ursodiol are often used as described above for early hepatic disease.

Hepatic lipidosis and treatment in cats

Hepatic lipidosis is most commonly associated with cats. It is caused when there is an increase in peripheral lipolysis with decreased export of very low density lipoproteins (VLDL) from the liver. Current thoughts suggest that protein deficiency from decreased intake impairs synthesis of apolipoproteins, limiting transport. Intrahepatic fat accumulates and leads to distended canaliculi and pronounced intrahepatic cholestasis and hepatic failure if left untreated.

Primary nutritional therapy consists of rapid replenishment with a high protein (if there is no evidence of encephalopathy), moderate carbohydrate and moderate fat, to meet resting energy requirements. When examining substrate utilization, protein in the diet ameliorates this disease process making feeding a priority, particularly since most cats are severely jaundiced and anorexic at presentation (Biourge et al., 1994). Due to inappetance and clinician's unwillingness to induce food aversion, placement of a nasoesophageal tube until the cat is stable enough for an esophagotomy or gastrotomy tube placement is imperative. Enteral nutrition through tube placement may be necessary for 3–6 weeks or until the cat is willing to eat on its own.

The use of blenderized high protein recovery cat foods or veterinary formulated liquid enteral diets is recommended. Refeeding should be initiated slowly over 3 days giving $\frac{1}{3}$ of the RER on day one, $\frac{2}{3}$ of the RER on day two and full RER on day three. This gradual implementation will be less likely to lead to hyperammonemia and attenuate the potential for the possible refeeding syndrome. Hypophosphatemia has been observed during enteral feeding of cats with various hepatopathies including hepatic lipidosis which underscore the importance of monitoring electrolytes with this condition (Justin and Hohenhaus, 1995). If hyperammoniemia is suspected, as suggested by the presence of signs of encephalopathy or confirmed by measuring blood ammonia, then switching to a lower protein diet and beginning lactulose or soluble fibre therapy is recommended.

The use of L-carnitine is often implemented as it has been shown that it may improve whole body fat metabolism and help prevent hepatic lipidosis and ketosis even though liver and serum carnitine concentrations in hepatic lipidosis are not depleted (Jacobs et al., 2009; Center, 1998; Center, 2004; Blanchard et al., 2002). The mechanisms of action using carnitine supplementation are poorly understood, but current thought suggests it might help peripheral tissues utilize ketones and fatty acids for energy or decrease hepatic ketone production (Blanchard et al., 2002). Supplementation of L-carnitine is recommended at a dose of 250 mg/day (Center, 1998).

Since storage and utilization of water-soluble vitamins is distorted in hepatic lipidosis, vitamin B supplementation is also suggested at two times maintenance (Biourge, 1997). If clinical signs of thiamine deficiency, such as neck ventroflexion, are present, supplementation at a dose of 50–100 mg/cat each day in the food for one week is recommended. Testing for serum folate and vitamin B_{12} is commonly performed and should be considered for most lipidotic patients as they are often low or low normal. Vitamin B_{12} at 1mg every 7–28 days has been successfully used to replenish B_{12} serum concentrations in cats (Center, 1998).

The liver produces vitamin K dependent clotting factors which become depleted in chronic hepatic disease (Center, 1998). Thus, vitamin K administration to compensate for poor production of clotting factors in hepatic lipidosis may also be warranted. Dosages of 0.5–1.5 mg/kg IM or SC every 12 hours for 3 doses and then once weekly for two weeks is recommended (Center, 1998).

Acute hepatotoxicosis

Hepatic insult can be caused by many toxins. Two of the more common causes of acute hepatitis are caused by acetaminophen toxicity and *Amanita phalloides* ingestion. Acetominophen toxicosis is often treated with N-acetylcysteine as the antidote with a loading dose of 140 mg/kg as a 5% dilution given IV and then 70 mg/kg given for 7 more doses. In severe cases a dose of 280 mg/kg with a 70 mg/kg maintenance dose administered for 14 days. SAMEe has also been shown to be a useful antidote therapy for acetaminophen toxicosis with a loading dose of 40 mg/kg and a follow-up maintenance dose of 20 mg/kg q 24 h for 7 days P.O (Wallace et al., 2002). *Amanita phalloides* is a mushroom which when ingested causes fulminant hepatic necrosis. Proven effective treatment includes silybinin, which at a dose of 50 mg/kg decreased hepatic necro-inflammatory lesions and increased survival rates in beagles (Vogel and et al., 1984). A treatment flow chart illustrates therapeutic options for various hepatopathies (Figure 21.1 and Tables 21.2 and 21.3 list dosages for important nutritional therapies in dogs and cats.

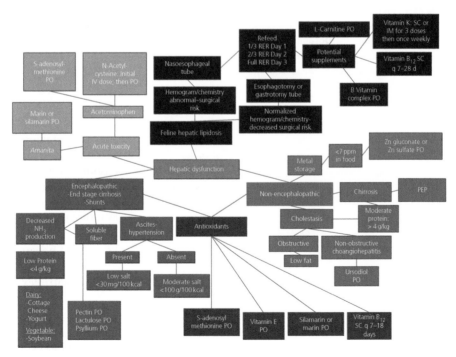

Figure 21.1 Treatment options.

Table 21.2 Dosages for important nutritional therapies in dogs.

Supplement/Drug	Dosage	Dosage Frequency	Indications
Elemental zinc	100 mg/kg for 3 months then 50mg/kg PO	SID	Copper storage
Polyenylphosphitidyl choline (PEP)	25–50mg/kg/day, not to exceed 3g PO	each day	Chirrhosis/ Hepatitis
S-adenosylmethionine (SAMe)	17–20mg/kg PO	each day	Chirrosis/Hepatitis, Cholestasis
Vitamin E	10 IU/kg PO	each day	Chirrosis/Hepatitis, Cholestasis
Silybin A & B in Marin	1.3–2.8 mg/kg/day PO	each day	Chirrosis/Hepatitis, Cholestasis
Ursodiol - dogs	10–15mg/kg PO	SID	Non-obstructive cholangitis
Vitamin K	0.5–1mg/kg IM or SC	3 doses BID then once weekly	Chirrosis/ Hepatits, Portosystemic Shunts
Pectin - dogs	5–10mL to 150–200kcal PO	each day	Hyperammonemia
Psyllium	1–3 tsp. PO	each day	Hyperammonemia
Lactulose	15–30mL PO titrated to effect	QID	Hyperammonemia

Table 21.3 Dosages for important nutritional therapies in cats.

Supplement/Drug	Dosage	Dosage Frequency	Indications
Polyenylphosphitidyl choline (PEP)	25–50mg/kg/day	each day	Chirrhosis/Hepatitis
S-adenosylmethionine (SAMe)	20–40mg/kg PO	each day	Chirrosis/Hepatitis, Cholestasis
Vitamin E	10 IU/kg PO	each day	Chirrosis/Hepatitis Cholestasis
Silybin A & B in Marin	1.5–2.6mg/kg/day PO	each day	Chirrosis/Hepatitis, Cholestasis
Vitamin K	0.5–1.5mg/kg IM or SC	3 doses BID then once weekly	Chirrosis/Hepatitis, Hepatic Lipidosis
Pectin	5–10mL to 150–200kcal PO	each day	Hyperammonemia
Psyllium	1–3 tsp. PO	each day	Hyperammonemia
Lactulose	0.25–1mL PO titrated to effect	SID	Hyperammonemia
Vitamin B12	1mg SC	every 7–28 days	Cholangitis, Hepatitis, Portosystemic Shunts
Vitamin B Complex	50–100mg PO	each day	Hepatic Lipidosis
L-Carnitine - cats	250 mg PO	each day	Hepatic Lipidosis

Summary

Nutritional management of hepatic diseases is often considered a primary therapeutic intervention. Manipulation of macronutrients such as protein and fiber plays an integral role in controlling hepatic encephalopathy, while the fat content of a diet plays an important role in management of obstructive cholangiohepatopathies. Minerals such as iron and copper can cause serious hepatic damage, while others such as zinc are considered therapeutic in some cases. Antioxidants appear to play a role in reversing membrane peroxidation damage and collagenase activity, effectively reducing fibrosis. Supplementation of hepatic-dependent micronutrients also prevents depletion, preventing systemic consequences. Regardless of what hepatopathy is present, nutritional intervention can be used to improve the clinical signs and potentially recovery.

KEY POINTS

- The liver plays a central role in nutrient metabolism and because of this, the requirements for specific nutrients may change following onset of liver failure.
- The nutritional approaches for the management of hospitalized canine and feline patients with various hepatopathies are not all the same but can be generalized based on protein tolerance.
- Some hepatopathies, including early and chronic hepatic cirrhosis, cholangitis, triaditis and feline hepatic lipidosis, do not generally require protein restriction while congenital and acquired vascular shunting and end-stage cirrhosis may require significant protein restriction.
- Manipulation of macronutrients such as protein and fibre may play an important role in controlling or preventing hepatic encephalopathy.
- If reduced protein-content diet is necessary, the diet should contain no less than 2.1 g protein/kg of body weight for dogs, and at least 4 g protein/kg of body weight for cats.
- Nutraceuticals, such as polyenylphosphatidyl choline, S-Adenosyl-methionine, vitamin E and silamarin, are used for hepatoprotective properties, although evidence of clinical benefit is limited.

Note

1 Marin: Nutramax Labratories, Inc. Edgewood, MD.

References

Aguirre, A.L., Center, S.A., Randolph, J.F. et al. (2007) Gallbladder disease in Shetland Sheepdogs: 38 cases (1995-2005). *Journal of the American Veterinary Medical Association*, **231**, 79–88.
Aleynik, S.I., Leo, M.A., Ma, X. et al. (1997) Polyenylphosphatidylcholine prevents carbon tetrachloride-induced lipid peroxidation while it attenuates liver fibrosis. *Journal of Hepatology*, **27**, 554–561.
Bianchi, G.P., Marchesini, G., Fabbri, A. et al. (1993) Vegetable versus animal protein in diet in cirrhotic patients with chronic encephalopathy. A randomized cross-over comparison. *Journal of Internal Medicine*, **233**, 385–392.

Biourge VC. (1997) Nutrition and Liver Disease. *Seminars in Veterinary Medicine and Surgery: Small Animal*, **12**, 34–44.

Biourge V.C., Massat, B., Groff, J.M. et al. (1994) Effects of protein, lipid, or carbohydrate supplementation on hepatic lipid accumulation during rapid weight loss in obese cats. *American Journal of Veterinary Research*, **10**, 1406–1415.

Blanchard, G., Paragon, B.M., Milliat, F. et al. (2002) Dietary L-carnitine supplementation in obese cats alters carnitine metabolism and decreases ketosis during fasting and induced hepatic lipidosis. *Journal of Nutrition*, **132**, 204–210.

Brent, A.C. and Weisse, C. (2010) Hepatic vascular anomalies. in *Textbook of Veterinary Internal Medicine*, 7th edn (eds S.J. Ettinger and E.C. Feldman) W.B. Saunders, Philadelphia. pp. 1649–1672.

Brewer, G.J., Dick, R.D., Schall, W. et al. (1992) Use of zinc acetate to treat copper toxicosis in dogs. *Journal of the American Veterinary Medical Association*, **201**, 564–568.

Canturk, N.Z., Canturk, Z., Utkan, N.Z. et al. (1998) Cytoprotective effects of alpha tocopherol against liver injury induced by extrahepatic biliary obstruction. *East African Medicine*, **75**, 77–80.

Center, S.A. (1998) Nutritional support for dogs and cats with hepatobiliary disease. *American Society for Nutritional Sciences*, 2733S–2746S.

Center, S.A. (2004) Metabolic, antioxidant, nutraceutical, probiotic and herbal therapies relating to the management of hepatobiliary disorders. *Veterinary Clinics of North America: Small Animal Practice*, **34**, 67–172.

Center, S.A. (2009) Diseases of the gallbladder and biliary tree. *Veterinary Clinics of North American: Small Animal Practice*, **39**, 543–598.

Center, S.A., Randolph, K.L., Warner, J. et al. (2005) The effects of S-Adenosylmethionine on clinical pathology and redox potential in the red blood cell, liver, and bile of clinically normal cats. *Journal of Veterinary Internal Medicine*, **19**,303–314.

Chojkier, M., Houglum, K., Lee, K.S. et al. (1998) Long- and short-term D-alpha-tocopherol supplementation inhibits liver collagen alpha1(l) gene expression. *American Journal of Physiology*, **275**, G1480–G1485.

Conly, J. and Stein, K. (1994) Reduction of vitamin K2 concentrations in human liver associated with the use of broad spectrum antimicrobials. *Clinical and Investigative Medicine*, **17**, 531–539.

Crossley, I.R. and Williams, R. (1984) Progress in the treatment of chronic portosystemic encephalopathy. *Gut*, **25**, 85–98.

Douglass, A., Mardini, H.A. and Record, C. (2001) Amino acid challenge in patients with cirrhosis: a model for the assessment of treatments for hepatic encephalopathy. *Journal of Hepatology*, **34**, 658–664.

Englert, E,, Harman, C.G., Freston, J.W. et al. (1977) Studies on the pathogenesis of diet-induced dog gallstones. *Digestive Diseases*, **22**, 305–314.

Filburn, C.R., Kettenacker, R. and Griffin, D.W. (2007) Bioavailability of a silybin-phosphatidylcholine complex in dogs. *Journal of Veterinary Pharmacology and Therapeutics*, **30**, 132–188.

Herrmann, R., Shakoor, T. and Weber, F.L. (1987) Beneficial effects of pectin in chronic hepatic encephalopathy. *Gastroenterology*, **92**,1795 (abs.)

Hoffman, G., Jones, P.G., Biourge, V. et al. (2009) Dietary management of hepatic copper accumulation in Labrador retrievers. *Journal of Veterinary Internal Medicine*, **23**, 957–963.

Holzbach, R.T., Corbusier, C., Marsh, M. et al. (1976) The process of cholesterol cholelithiasis induced by diet in the prarie dog: a physiochemical characterization. *Journal of Labratory Clinical Medicine*, **87**, 987–998.

Jacobs, G., Cornelius, K., Keene, B. et al. (1990) Comparison of plasma, liver, and skeletal muscle carnitine concentrations in cats with idiopathic hepatic lipidosis and in healthy cats. *American Journal of Veterinary Research*, **51**, 1349–1351.

Justin, R.B. and Hohenhaus, A.E. (1995) Hypophosphatemia associated with enteral alimentation in cats. *Journal of Veterinary Internal Medicine*, **9**, 228–233.

Kumar, D. and Tandon, R.K. (2001) Use of ursodeoxycholic acid in liver disease. *Journal of Gastroenterology and Hepatology*, **16**, 3–14.

LaFlamme, D.P. (2000) Nutritional management of liver disease. in *Kirk's Current Veterinary Therapy XIII: Small Animal Practice*. (ed. J.D. Bonagura) Saunders, Philadelphia, pp. 693–697.

Lisciandro, S.C., Hohenhaus, A. and Brooks, M. (1998) Coagulation abnormalities in 22 cats with naturally occurring liver disease. *Journal of Veterinary Internal Medicine*, **12**, 71–75.

Peetermans, W. and Verbist, L. (1990) Coagulation disorders cuased by cephalosporins containing methylthiotetrazole side chains. *Acta Clinica Belgica*, **45**, 327–333.

Plumb D.C. (2008) Zinc. in *Plumb's Veterinary Handbook*, 6th edn (ed. D. C. Plumb) PharmaVet Inc, Stockholm, WI, pp. 1261–1263.

Scavelli, T.D., Hornbuckle, W.E. and Roth, L. (1986) Portosystemic shunts in cats: seven cases (1976-1984). *Journal of the American Veterinary Medical Association*, **189**, 317–325.

Silk, D.B.A., O'Keefe, S.J.D. and Wicks, C. (1991) Nutritional support in liver disease. *Gut* Supplement, S29–S33.

Sokol, R.J., Devereaux, M.W., Traber, M.G. et al. (1989) Copper toxicity and lipid peroxidation in isolated rate hepatocytes: effect of vitamin E. *Pediatric Research*, **25**, 55–62.

Tillson D.M. and Winkler, J.T. (2002) Diagnosis and treatment of portosystemic shunts in the cat. *Veterinary Clinics of North America: Small Animal Practice*, **32**, 881–899.

Thornburg, L.P. (2000) A perspective on copper and liver disease in the dog. *Journal of Veterinary Diagostic Investigation*, **12**, 101–110.

Vogel, G,, Tuchweber, B., Trost, W. et al. (1984) Protection by silibinin against Amanita phalloides intoxication in beagles. *Toxicology and Applied Pharmacology*, **72**, 355–362.

Von Herbay A, de Groot H,Hegi U, et al. (1994) Low vitamin E content in plasma of patients with alcoholic liver disease, hemochromatosis and Wilson's disease. *Journal of Hepatology*. **20**, 41–46.

Wallace, K.P., Center, S.A., Hickford, F.H. et al. (2002) S-adenosyl-L-methionine (SAMe) for the treatment of acetaminophen toxicity in a dog. *Journal of theAmerican Animal Hospital Association*, **38**, 246–254.

Walter, R., Dunn, M.E., d'Anjou M.A. et al. (2008) Nonsurgical resolution of gallbladder mucocele in two dogs. *Journal of the American Veterinary Medical Association*, **232**,1688–1693.

CHAPTER 22

Nutritional management of the septic patient

Daniel L. Chan

Department of Veterinary Clinical Sciences and Services, The Royal Veterinary College, University of London, UK

Introduction

Sepsis is typified by an exaggerated inflammatory response by the host to a pathogen. The condition is driven by a storm of cytokines and this also has implications for energy and substrate metabolism. Given the serious sequelae of sepsis, preservation or reversal of deteriorating nutritional status via nutritional support should be considered an important aspect in the treatment of septic patients. However, studies specifically evaluating nutritional interventions in septic patients are very limited and many of the recommendations for this population have been extrapolated from other critically ill populations. Nutritional support for the septic patient should be aimed at minimising the impact of malnutrition and enhancing the rate of recovery. To this end, designing the optimal nutritional approach for septic patients has proven difficult. Many of the challenges in designing an optimal approach centre on three areas: the mode of nutritional support, the timing of initiating nutritional support and the composition of the diet used. The evidence appears to suggest that feeding the patient enterally whenever possible should be the preferred approach. Initiation of enteral nutrition early (within 48 hours) appears to be preferable compared with delayed initiation. Although there are promising breakthroughs in enhancing the composition of nutritional support (e.g., inclusion of glutamine, fish oils and antioxidants), these strategies remain controversial and are largely untried in veterinary medicine.

Metabolic derangements in sepsis

Sepsis is one of the most serious disease processes encountered in animals and results in a complex sequence of metabolic derangements. In some cases, the body's response can be exaggerated with several important effects on metabolism. The initial stress response may be characterized by a hypermetabolic phase where there is increased oxygen consumption, hyperglycemia, hyperlactatemia

---

Nutritional Management of Hospitalized Small Animals, First Edition. Edited by Daniel L. Chan.
© 2015 John Wiley & Sons, Ltd. Published 2015 by John Wiley & Sons, Ltd.

and accelerated protein catabolism (Biolo et al., 1997; Marik, 2005). These metabolic alterations occur as a result of inflammatory cytokines and regulatory and counter-regulatory hormones and this has also been demonstrated in a canine model of sepsis (Shaw and Wolfe, 1984).

Accelerated loss of skeletal muscle can occur in just a few days of critical illness. In people, this rapid loss of lean body mass is a predictor of mortality (Biolo et al., 1997; Marik, 2005). During critical illness the initial metabolic response is to utilize liver and muscle glycogen stores for energy. Following rapid exhaustion of glycogen stores, new glucose is derived from gluconeogenesis and results in muscle protein breakdown. Along with changes in protein metabolism there are also alterations in carbohydrate metabolism. These alterations include enhanced peripheral glucose uptake and utilization, hyperlactatemia, increased glucose production, depressed glycogenesis, glucose intolerance and insulin resistance (Biolo et al., 1997). The most important mechanism of "stress hyperglycemia" is likely to be excessive glucose production relative to glucose clearance (Krenitsky, 2011). In sepsis, hyperglycemia is mainly caused by increased hepatic output of glucose, more so than impaired tissue glucose extraction. The implications of this hyperglycemia in critically ill patients are quite controversial. Hyperglycemia related to diabetes is well known to decrease neutrophil and macrophage function, increase risk of infection and increase overall morbidity and mortality. However, the effects of non-diabetic hyperglycemia are not well understood. The use of insulin to control hyperglycemia in critically ill patients is quite controversial as the outcome is sometimes worse with insulin therapy (Song et al., 2014).

Although stress is typically associated with increased gluconeogenesis, there is evidence that septic patients may be distinguished by a biphasic response; lethal models of sepsis in animals demonstrate an initial phase of hyperglycemia during which gluconeogenesis is increased, followed by a subsequent phase during which glucose production is suppressed and hypoglycemia occurs (Polk and Schwab, 2011). Endotoxin-induced hypoglycemia in rats is associated with a decrease in activity of a rate-limiting enzyme in gluconeogenesis. There are also suggestions that cytokines may also play a role in hypoglycemia associated with sepsis. Increased peripheral utilization of glucose also plays a role in the pathogenesis of hypoglycemia; animal models of sepsis have demonstrated hypoglycemia despite increased hepatic glucose production (Polk and Schwab, 2011). Although hypoglycemia in animals is common, this is considered to be rare in people.

Interestingly, fat is the preferred fuel for oxidation in patients with sepsis and this oxidation cannot be suppressed to the same level with glucose infusion as it can in healthy patients (Biolo et al., 1997; Leyba and others 2011, Cohen and Chin 2013). In sepsis, hypertriglyceridemia and increased fat oxidation are the main features of altered fat metabolism (Biolo and others 1997, Marik 2005, Leyba, Gonzalez and Alonso, 2011; Cohen and Chin, 2013). Some of the derangements are caused by failure of specific organs, while others are part of the host response. Again, the role of TNF-α and altered fat metabolism are closely related. TNF-α can increase lipolysis directly, or via other hormones (Biolo et al., 1997; Marik, 2005). Catecholamines and cortisol also stimulate lipolysis. The increased hypertriglyceridemia in sepsis is thought to occur through increased very low density lipoprotein (VLDL) concentrations. Another feature of sepsis is suppression of lipoprotein lipase activity (also mediated by endotoxin and TNF-α), and this may also lead to decreased clearance of plasma VLDL. Under the influence of cytokines, there is a rise in hepatic triglyceride production. Normally, non-esterified fatty acids (NEFAs) are only released by peripheral adipose tissue to provide metabolic fuel and plasma levels of NEFAs are regulated by lipolysis and adipose tissue blood flow. These regulatory mechanisms seem to be altered in sepsis. Endotoxin increases plasma NEFA concentration via its effects on cytokines and hormones (Biolo et al., 1997, Marik, 2005).

Given the complexity of the many metabolic and hormonal derangements during sepsis, it would seem logical to try to modulate these derangements via providing nutritional support. Indeed, the treatment of critically ill human patients has recently focused on nutritional interventions, including early enteral nutrition and immune-modulating nutrition (Yuan et al., 2011; Kaur, Gupta and Minocha, 2005; Galban and others 2000: Leyba et al., 2011). So while there is a growing body of evidence supporting the use of these approaches in people with serious diseases, including sepsis, careful consideration is required before similar approaches are adopted in veterinary medicine.

Differences between abdominal sepsis in people and dogs

One important distinction worth mentioning is that the majority of studies in people identifying the benefit of critical care nutrition relate to "septic" patients and not specifically to "septic peritonitis" patients. The reason to highlight this difference is that the vast majority of "sepsis" in people is not related to "septic peritonitis" and, as such, these patient populations are not interchangeable. In contrast, septic peritonitis happens to be the most common, if not the most serious, example of sepsis in the dog; however, this is not true in people, where pneumonia is far more common. Therefore, although there may be very positive results related to providing nutritional support to critically ill, septic human patients, there are actually only limited studies especially evaluating the use of nutrition in septic peritonitis in people. In fact, the closest disease processes in people are enterocutaneous fistulas and non-traumatic perforating peritonitis. Studies evaluating the impact of nutritional support in these patients are relative small (Kaur et al., 2005; Yuan et al., 2011). Measured benefits in these studies include earlier closure times of the abdominal wall, fewer infectious complications, reduction of post-operative ileus and improved nitrogen balance (Kaur et al., 2005; Yuan et al., 2011).

Nutritional management strategies of septic patients

The optimal nutritional approach to the septic patient is still evolving but likely centres on the form of nutritional support, the timing of initiation and the composition of the diet. Unless there is complete intolerance to enteral feeding, the

Table 22.1 Comparison of the benefits of enteral nutrition (EN) with the consequence of withholding enteral nutrition in critically ill septic patients.

Physiological benefit of initiating EN	Consequences of withholding EN
Stimulates splanchnic blood flow and perfusion	Decreases splanchnic perfusion leading to ischemia, devitalization
Stimulates release of secretory IgA, inhibits pathogenic bacteria adherence to epithelial cells	Encourages pathogenic bacterial adherence and invasion leading to barrier defense disruption
Supports commensal bacterial flora that degrades bacterial toxins and inhibits colonization by pathogenic organisms	Encourages bacterial overgrowth of pathogenic bacteria
Stimulates intestinal contractility, sweeping bacteria downstream, controlling overall bacterial flora	Promotes gastrointestinal dysmotility, promotes bacterial overgrowth
Maintains functional and structural integrity of intestinal epithelium	Compromises paracellular channels between epithelial cells, increasing gastrointestinal permeability, allowing influx of bacterial toxins

preferred mode of nutritional support in septic patients is the enteral form (Table 22.1). As for timing, initiation of EN in septic patients should start early, within 48 hours but only after resuscitation of the patient. Splanchnic perfusion may be compromised in hypotensive patients and, therefore, there have been concerns about EN inducing intestinal ischemia; however, this risk is very low (Zaloga, Roberts and Marik, 2003; Leyba et al., 2011). Current recommendations are to initiate EN after patient resuscitation, or at least when the cardiovascular system is stable (e.g., when the dosage of vasoactive substances, such as dopamine and norepinephrine, have stabilized). In critically ill animals there should be an aim to initiate early enteral feeding as soon as it is feasible. Some veterinary studies have implemented enteral nutrition as early as within 10 hours of admission (Mohr et al., 2003). Although it is difficult to assess whether these measures actually influence outcome, one thing that has been established is that many patients previously assumed to require "bowel rest," actually tolerated early enteral feeding. The most notable studies demonstrating this tolerance to feeding evaluated puppies with parvoenteritis, cats with acute pancreatitis and, most recently, dogs with severe and acute pancreatitis (Mohr et al., 2003; Klaus, Rudloff and Kirby, 2009; Mansfield et al., 2011). It is therefore reasonable to pursue enteral feeding in septic animals, even in cases believed to have significant gastrointestinal dysfunction.

Results support the notion that employing early EN is achievable in many patients and, therefore, this should be pursued in virtually every patient. Although an early veterinary abstract found no advantage in instituting early nutritional support in canine septic peritonitis, a more recent study has demonstrated that instituting early enteral feeding can be associated with decreased length of hospitalization in dogs with septic peritonitis (Hackndahl and Hill, 2007; Liu, Brown and Silverstein, 2012). Unfortunately, this study was not designed to evaluate the effect of early enteral nutrition on outcome but it did demonstrate that this approach is feasible and not associated with any negative effects. When the currently available evidence is considered, effective nutritional support strategies do appear to have a positive effect on septic patients and unless additional studies contravene these results, early enteral nutrition should be instituted in septic patients (Mohr et al., 2003; Campbell et al., 2010; Brunetto et al., 2010; Liu et al., 2012).

In animals that fail to tolerate provision of EN, there should be consideration given to using parenteral nutritional (PN) support. The optimal timing for initiating PN is very controversial, however, even in people. Recent publications specifically evaluating timing of initiating PN support have suggested that early initiation of PN (i.e., within 48 h of admission to ICU) was associated with higher morbidity and mortality (Casaer et al., 2011). Other studies have found no detrimental impact of initiating PN within 36 hours of admission to ICU when compared with EN and in fact demonstrated decreased rates of hypoglycemia and vomiting (Harvey et al., 2014). However, there should be considerable caution in extrapolating results in critically ill human patients to companion animals. First, the differences were rather modest (6% increase in likelihood of being discharged alive, $P = 0.04$) and the clinical relevance of such modest differences needs to be considered (Casaer et al., 2011).

A perhaps more important distinction in the provision of nutritional support, is the optimal calorie target. There is ample evidence in both the human and veterinary literature demonstrating the deleterious effects of over-feeding in both morbidity and perhaps mortality (O'Toole et al., 2004; Pyle et al., 2004; Marik, 2005; Stappleton, Jones and Heyland, 2007; Dickerson, 2011).

For these reasons, recent veterinary recommendations have centered on simply targeting the resting energy requirement (RER) (see Chapter 2). Although there are similar recommendations in human ICUs, an analysis of the caloric target in the recent studies, which demonstrated longer hospitalization times with longer ICU stays, shows that patients who did worse were essentially "aggressively fed" and likely overfed. Patients that received enteral feeding only for the first 8 days, basically received hypocaloric nutrition (previously shown to be beneficial) and only received PN if they failed to consume 50% of targeted calories after day 8 (Marik, 2005, Casaer et al., 2011). This was in contrast to the PN group which were fed a much greater number of calories (within 48 hours) and, therefore, it is reasonable to question whether complications weren't simply a reflection of problems with overfeeding rather than related to the timing of PN implementation. Future studies implementing an iso-caloric component to these trials are needed to confirm or refute initial findings. In animals, where a combination of enteral and parenteral nutrition was associated with better outcome, the total target was less than RER (Chan et al., 2002). It is therefore possible that positive outcomes can be achieved with supplemental PN, as long as the total caloric target is set very conservatively at RER.

The final aspect of optimal nutritional support in septic patients relates to nutrient composition of the diet. In respect to metabolic changes associated with sepsis, fats should be considered the preferred source of energy (Biolo et al., 1997). However, gastrointestinal dysmotility disorders are common in septic patients (see Chapter 17) and high fat diets will delay gastric emptying which

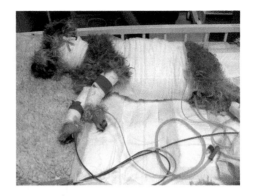

Figure 22.1 Dogs with septic peritonitis managed with open peritoneal drainage have particularly high protein requirements due to exudative losses of protein. Nutritional support of these patients will require additional protein provision.

could lead to patient discomfort, supress appetite, increase vomiting and regurgitation and increase risk for development of aspiration pneumonia. From a practical point of view, enteral diets designed for convalescence in dogs and cats tend to be high in fat to increase caloric density and this could make feeding septic animals problematic. Clinicians must balance the potential benefits and risks associated with feeding septic patients diets with high fat content.

Protein requirements in septic patients may be particularly high due to rapid turnover of lean muscle catabolism combined with excessive protein losses (e.g., open peritoneal drainage, draining wounds) (Biolo et al., 1997) (Figure 22.1). Although data on protein requirements of dogs and cats with sepsis are scarce, the most up-to-date guidelines list 6 g/100 kcal (25% of total energy requirements) for dogs and 8 g/100 kcal (35% of total energy requirements) for cats (Michel and Eirmann, 2014). Fortunately, most diets designed for convalescence are high in protein.

Carbohydrate content may also be important in the management of septic patients. Carbohydrates are a convenient and easily assimilated energy source. The problem that must be carefully monitored is the propensity for development of hyperglycemia. Although intensive insulin therapy for management of septic human patients has been studied, this remains a very controversial topic as there appear to be high complication rates without benefits on outcome (Song et al., 2014). Thus far, there have been no studies in dogs or cats that have evaluated the use or merits of intensive insulin therapy and, therefore, it cannot be recommended. However, avoidance of hyperglycemia may be desirable and so carbohydrate content should be considered when formulating the nutritional plan.

In people, the use of immunomodulating nutrients (e.g, glutamine, omega-3 fatty acids, nucleotides and antioxidants) (see Chapter 18) in septic populations has been evaluated to a very limited extent with mixed results. In most cases, the septic sub-groups have been so small that no conclusions could be formulated in regards to potential beneficial or detrimental effects (Kieft et al., 2005; Heyland et al., 2001; Montejo et al., 2003). A meta-analysis that included the results of these studies concluded that the use of immunomodulating nutrients was associated with decreased mortality, secondary infections and length of intensive care unit stay in septic patients, however, further prospective studies are warranted before this approach should be adopted (Marik and Zaloga, 2008).

The most promising result to date is a small prospective study that evaluated omega-3 fatty acids and antioxidants in early sepsis and found that such a diet was associated with reducing respiratory and cardiovascular complications (Pontes-Arruda et al., 2011). Currently, the use of immunomodulatory nutrients has not been studied in clinical veterinary populations and recommendations for their use cannot be made.

Summary

Nutritional support of septic patients continues to be a challenging topic in veterinary critical care, mostly due to lack of specific evidence. Extrapolation from other populations suggests that early enteral feeding, conservative energy targets and sufficient protein content are the most sensible recommendation at this time for dogs and cats with sepsis. Further research focusing on energy and nutrient requirements and the role of immunomodulating nutrients in the management of animals with sepsis is urgently warranted.

KEY POINTS

- Sepsis is a serious, often life-threatening condition typified by an exaggerated inflammatory response with significant implications for energy and substrate metabolism.

- Preservation or reversal of deteriorating nutritional status via nutritional support should be considered an important aspect in the treatment of septic patients.

- The optimal nutritional approach to the septic patient is still evolving but likely centers on the form of nutritional support, the timing of initiation and the composition of the diet.

- Current recommendations are to initiate enteral nutrition when the patient is cardiovascularly stable.

- The ideal composition of diets for septic dogs and cats has not been identified but current evidence suggests that diets that are limited (although not restricted) in fat, with a protein content of 6 g/100 kcal for dogs and 8 g/100 kcal for cats may be beneficial.

- Future evaluations of diets with immunomodulatory nutrients in dogs and cats with sepsis may be warranted but cannot be currently recommended.

References

Biolo, G., Toigo, G., Ciocchi, B. et al. (1997) Metabolic response to injury and sepsis: changes in protein metabolism. *Nutrition*, **13**, 52S–57S.

Brunetto, M.A., Gomes, M.O., Andre, M.R. et al. (2010) Effects of nutritional support on hospital outcome in dogs and cats. *Journal of Veterinary Emergency Critical Care*, **20**, 224–231.

Campbell, J.A., Jutkowitz, L.A., Santoro, K.A.,et al. (2010) Continuous versus intermittent delivery of nutrition via nasoenteric feeding tubes in hospitalized canine and feline patients: 91 patients (2002-2007). *Journal of Veterinary Emergency Critical Care*, **20**, 232–236.

Casaer, M.P., Mesotten, D., Hermans, G. et al. (2011) Early versus late parenteral nutrition in critically ill adults. *New England Journal of Medicine*, **365**, 506–517.

Chan, D.L., Freeman, L.M., Labato, M.A. et al. (2002) Retrospective evaluation of partial parenteral nutrition in dogs and cats. *Journal of Veterinary Internal Medicine*, **16**, 440–445.

Cohen, J. and Chin, W.D.M. (2013) Nutrition and Sepsis. *World Review of Nutrition Dietetics*, **105**, 116–25.

Dickerson, R.N. (2011) Optimal caloric intake for critically ill patients: First, do no harm. *Nutrition in Clinical Practice*, **26**, 48–54.

Galbán, C., Montejo, J.C., Mesejo, A., et al. (2000) An immune-enhancing enteral diet reduces mortality rate and episodes of bacteremia in septic intensive care unit patients. *Critical Care Medicine*, **28**, 643–648.

Hackndahl, N.H. and Hill, R.C. (2007) Enteral feeding in dogs with septic peritonitis (Abstract). *Journal of Veterinary Internal Medicine*, **21**, 356.

Harvey, S.E., Parrott, F., Harrison, D.A., et al. (2014) Trial of the route of early nutritional support in critically ill adults. *The New England Journal of Medicine*, **371**(18), 1673–1684.

Heyland, D.K., Novak, F., Drover, J.W. et al. (2001) Should immunonutrition become routine in critically ill patients: a systematic review of the evidence. *Journal of the American Medical Association*, **286**, 944–53.

Kaur, N., Gupta, M.K. and Minocha, V.R. (2005) Early enteral feeding by nasoenteric tubes in patients with perforation peritonitis. *World Journal of Surgery*, **29**, 1023–1027.

Kieft, H., Roos, A.N., Van Drunen, J.D. et al. (2005) Clinical outcome of immunonutrition in a heterogeneous intensive care population. *Intensive Care Medicine*, **31**, 524–532.

Klaus, J.A., Rudloff, E. and Kirby, R. (2009) Nasogastric tube feeding in cats with suspected acute pancreatitis: 55 cases (2001-2006). *Journal of Veterinary Emergency and Critical Care*, **19**, 327–346.

Krenitsky, J. (2011) Glucose control in the intensive care unit: a nutrition support perspective. *Nutrition in Clinical Practice*, **26**, 31–43.

Leyba, C. O., Gonzalez, J.C.M. and Alonso, C.V. (2011) Guidelines for specialized nutritional and metabolic support in the critically-ill patient. Update. Consensus SEMICYUC-SENPE: Septic patient. *Nutricion Hospitalaria*, **26**, S67–S71.

Liu, D.T., Brown, D.C. and Silverstein, D.C. (2012) Early nutritional support is associated with decreased length of hospitalization in dogs with septic peritonitis: A retrospective study of 45 cases (2000-2009). *Journal of Veterinary Emergency Critical Care*, **22**, 453–459.

Mansfield, C.S., James, F.E., Steiner, J.M. et al. (2011) A pilot study to assess tolerability of early enteral nutrition via esophagostomy tube feeding in dogs with severe acute pancreatitis. *Journal of Veterinary Internal Medicine*, **25**, 419–425.

Marik, P.E. (2005) Nutritional support in patients with sepsis. in (eds R.H. Rolandelli, R. Bankhead, J.I. Boullata, J.I. et al.) *Clinical Nutrition: Enteral and Tube Feeding*. 4th edn, Elsevier Saunders, Philadelphia, pp. 373–380.

Marik, P.E. and Zaloga, G.P. (2008) Immunonutrition in critically ill patients: a systematic review and analysis of the literature. *Intensive Care Medicine*, **34**, 1980–90.

Michel, K.E. and Eirmann, L. (2014) Parenteral nutrition. in *Small Animal Critical Care Medicine*, 2nd edn, (eds D.C. Silverstein and K. Hopper) Elsevier Saunders, St Louis, pp. 687–690.

Mohr, A.J., Leisewitz, A.L., Jacobson, A.S. et al. (2003) Effect of early enteral nutrition on intestinal permeability, intestinal protein loss, and outcome in dogs with severe parvoviral enteritis. *Journal of Veterinary Internal Medicine*, **17**, 791–798.

Montejo, J.C., Zarazaga, A., Lopez-Martinez, J. et al. (2003) Spanish society of Intensive Care Medicine and Coronary Units. Immunonutrition in the intensive care unit. A systematic review and consensus statement. *Clinical Nutrition*, **2**, 221–233.

O'Toole, E., Miller, C.W., Wilson, B.A. et al. (2004) Comparison of the standard predictive equation for calculation of resting energy expenditure with indirect calorimetry in hospitalized and healthy dogs. *Journal of American Veterinary Medical Association*, **225**, 58–64.

Pontes-Arruda, A., Martins, L. F., de Lima, S.M. et al. (2011) Enteral nutrition with eicosapentaenoic acid, gamma-linolenic acid and antioxidants in the early treatment of sepsis: results from a multicenter, prospective, randomized, double-blinded, controlled study: The INTERSEPT study. *Critical Care*, **15**, R144. doi: 10.1186/cc10267.

Polk, T.M. and Schwab, C.W. (2011) Metabolic and nutritional support of the enterocutaneous fistula patient: a three-phased approach. *World Journal of Surgery*, **36**, 524–533.

Pyle, S.C., Marks, S.L., Kass, P.H. et al. (2004) Evaluation of complication and prognostic factors associated with administration of parenteral nutrition in cats: 75 cases (1994-2001). *Journal of the American Veterinary Medical Association*, **225**, 242–250.

Shaw, J.H. and Wolfe, R.R. (1984) A conscious septic dog model with hemodynamic and metabolic responses similar to responses of humans. *Surgery*, **95**, 553–561.

Song, F., Zhong, L.J., Han, L. et al. (2014) Intensive insulin therapy for septic patients: a meta-analysis of randomized controlled trials. *Biomedical Research International*, 698265.

Stappleton, R.D., Jones, N. and Heyland, D.K. (2007) Feeding critically ill patients: What is the optimal amount of energy? *Critical Care Medicine*, **35**, S535–S540.

Yuan, Y., Ren, J., Gu, G. et al. (2011) Early enteral nutrition improves outcomes of open abdomen in gastrointestinal fistula patients complicated with severe sepsis. *Nutrition in Clinical Practice*, **26**, 688–694.

Zaloga, G.P., Roberts, P.R. and Marik, P. (2003) Feeding the hemodynamically unstable patient: a critical evaluation of the evidence. *Nutrition in Clinical Practice*, **18**, 285–293.

CHAPTER 23

Nutritional support during acute pancreatitis

Kristine B. Jensen[1] and Daniel L. Chan[2]

[1] Djursjukhuset Malmö, Cypressvägen Malmö, Sweden

[2] Department of Veterinary Clinical Sciences and Services, The Royal Veterinary College, University of London, UK

Introduction

Acute pancreatitis (AP) is a frequently encountered illness in both dogs and cats. Although most cases are mild and self-limiting, some cases develop systemic complications that can result in death. Establishing a diagnosis is commonly complex, especially in cats, and the successful management may depend on a number of factors. Experimental and clinical data strongly support that nutritional management plays an important therapeutic role in both veterinary and human patients suffering from AP (Mansfield et al., 2011; Qin et al., 2007; Petrov, Kukosh and Emelyanov, 2006). While the optimal nutritional management of AP in dogs and cats remains unclear and warrants further research, consensus is growing that enteral nutrition (EN) should be implemented in most cases, and earlier than previously thought. Parenteral nutritional (PN) support, although no longer considered necessary, may be required in cases when EN is not tolerated.

Pathophysiology

The underlying pathophysiology of AP is incompletely understood, but is thought to involve two key events: dysfunctional lysosomal function leading to intracellular accumulation of vacuoles in acinar cells and to abnormal intra-acinar activation of digestive enzymes, such as trypsinogen (Gukovskaya and Gukovsky 2012; Gukovsky, Pandol and Gukovskaya, 2011). The result of these events leads to interactions between inert pancreatic zymogens and lysosomal proteases within the acinar cells. Trypsin is then activated and leads to activation of the other pancreatic zymogens to active enzymes. Activated pancreatic enzymes are then released in the pancreatic tissue and inflammation ensues.

Nutritional Management of Hospitalized Small Animals, First Edition. Edited by Daniel L. Chan.

© 2015 John Wiley & Sons, Ltd. Published 2015 by John Wiley & Sons, Ltd.

Nutritional management strategies

The traditional nutritional approach to AP centered on the premise that withholding food would reduce pancreatic auto-digestion by decreasing pancreatic stimulation and enzyme release (Simpson and Lamb, 1995; Williams, 1995). However, it is now clear that the trigger for pancreatitis involves intracellular premature activation of proteolytic enzymes rather than pancreatic stimulation. Avoidance of feeding as a means to decrease pancreatic stimulation may be unwarranted as this could not only lead to malnutrition, but also complicate the disease by potentially impairing gastrointestinal barrier function. (Nathens et al., 2004; Ioannidis, Lavrentieva and Botsios, 2008; Curtis and Kudsk, 2007) It also has been demonstrated in experimental rodent models and in people with naturally occurring disease that exocrine pancreatic secretion actually decreases during pancreatitis and that the decrease is more pronounced with increasing severity of inflammation (Niederau et al., 1990; O'Keefe et al., 2005). For these reasons it is becoming clear that there should be particular consideration for implementing nutritional support in this patient population.

Enteral nutrition during acute pancreatitis
Nutritional support during AP has been well-documented to play a central role in the management of AP in people. Parenteral nutrition had been the standard therapy for many years based on the theory that EN stimulated pancreatic secretion, potentially exacerbating the inflammatory response and delaying recovery. However, recent data suggest that EN in people is not only well tolerated but is safer and associated with fewer complications than with PN, and is even associated with improved survival in some studies (Petrov et al., 2006; Spanier, Bruno and Mathus-Vliegen, 2011; Guptaa et al., 2003). In recent years EN has become the new gold standard of nutritional therapy in managing AP in people (Petrov et al., 2006; Spanier et al., 2011; Guptaa et al., 2003; McClave, 2004; Gianotti et al., 2009). The current consensus is also that EN should be initiated as early as possible (ideally within the first 48 hours of diagnosis) (Nathens et al., 2004, Gionotti et al., 2009).

Although studies prospectively evaluating tolerance of EN in dogs and cats with AP are limited, there is growing evidence supporting this approach in dogs and cats with AP. Experimental studies in dogs with induced AP have compared the effects of early intrajejunal feedings and PN and showed no effect on serum concentrations of amylase and lysosomal enzyme activities relative to the PN group (Qin and other 2007; Qin and others 2002). In addition, circulating plasma endotoxin activity and bacterial translocation was reduced significantly in the intrajejunal fed group versus the PN group (Qin et al., 2007; Qin et al., 2002). The intrajejunal fed group also displayed improved gut barrier when assessed histopathologically by enteral villi height, thickness of mucosa and bowel wall in the ileum and transverse colon. Additional studies by the same group of investigators assessed pancreatic activation in response to a number of enteric hormones. They found that increased concentrations of gastrointestinal hormones did not induce increased release of pancreatic enzymes, which previously have been assumed to be the reason for induction of pancreatic autodigestion in AP (Qin et al., 2003).

A recent small pilot study evaluating the tolerability of prepyloric EN in dogs with AP showed promising results with no exacerbation of pain or vomiting in the enteral fed group when compared to the parenterally fed group (Mansfield et al., 2011). The frequency of vomiting or regurgitation episodes was higher in the group of dogs receiving PN and it was hypothesized that EN may improve gut health and thereby reduce ileus and vomiting. Additionally, no evidence of exacerbation of abdominal pain was found in the enteral fed group. However, due to the study's very small sample size (i.e., 5 dogs in each group) further studies are warranted to confirm these findings.

Nasogastric (NG) tube feeding has been assessed retrospectively in 55 cats with AP. Administration of bolus feeding or continuous rate infusion were compared in addition to whether or not the cats had received an amino acid-dextrose solution (Klaus, Rudloff and Kirby, 2009). In the study, NG feeding was well tolerated and there was no significant difference between groups with respect to the clinical variables assessed before or after feeding (including frequency of vomiting, incidence of diarrhea and hypersalivation). Complications were considered mild and the overall rate of complications was considered low. Based on the broad evidence in human studies and the preliminary results of experimental and clinical studies in animals, EN, when possible, should be considered as the mode of choice for feeding patients with AP.

Feeding tubes and routes

Given the importance of EN in the management of patients with AP and the poor reliability of simply offering or enticing food to animals suffering from AP, more effective means of nutritional support is often required. Feeding tubes can provide an effective means of facilitating nutritional support and several options are available. Selection and placement of various feeding tubes are discussed elsewhere (see Chapters 4–6).

Nasoesophageal feeding tubes are easily placed with a local anesthetic and do not require general anesthesia. They are, therefore, an appropriate choice for short-term nutritional support of the severely debilitated patient, where a general anesthetic is contra-indicated. The major disadvantage is their small diameter, which means they may clog more frequently and limits feeding to liquid enteral diets. Moreover, currently available liquid veterinary diets have a relatively high fat content (e.g., 45% of total calorie content) to increase calorie density, which may not be ideal for dogs with hyperlipidemia-associated pancreatitis. Although human liquid diets with a lower fat content are available, they are not complete with respect to amino acid composition and therefore may be inappropriate for use in veterinary patients, especially cats, unless supplemented with various amino acids (e.g., arginine).

Esophagostomy tubes require a short general anesthetic for placement but are an excellent option for cats and dogs of most sizes and have the advantage that a liquidized complete diet can be fed, permitting better individualized diet selection (e.g., lower fat content) (Figure 23.1). A recent study demonstrated good results when dogs with acute AP where fed a commercial low-fat diet via esophagostomy tubes (Mansfield et al., 2011). In cases when surgery is required (e.g., pancreatic abscess), placement of gastrostomy or jejunostomy feeding tubes

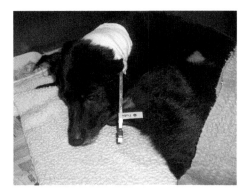

Figure 23.1 A dog with acute pancreatitis being nutritionally managed with an esophagostomy feeding tube. Previous recommendations for 'bowel rest' in patients with pancreatitis are now replaced with recommendations for early enteral feeding.

ensures access for enteral feeding (See chapter 7). Two retrospective veterinary studies described the application of jejunostomy tubes in dogs and cats with AP undergoing surgical management for pancreatitis (Son et al., 2010; Thompson, Seshadri and Raffe, 2009). These studies evaluated complications and potential prognostic factors but did not describe the complications encountered in relation to jejunostomy tubes in detail.

Minimally invasive techniques for placement of nasojejunal tubes using fluoroscopy or endoscopy in dogs have been described but have not yet been widely adopted (Papa at al., 2009; Beal and Brown, 2011). Feeding tubes were successfully placed in the jejunum in 74 to 78% of cases, however, in one study the success rate increased over time to 100%, indicating that technical proficiency improves over time. The major complication was oral tube migration (less than a third of cases). Acute pancreatitis was the primary diagnosis of dogs undergoing fluoroscopic wire-guided placement of nasojejunal tubes in one study (Beal and Brown, 2011). Slow constant rate infusion of a liquid diet ("trickle feeding") is recommended and jejunostomy tubes are therefore only suitable for hospitalized patients.

Parenteral nutrition

In patients with severe AP and intractable vomiting who do not tolerate EN, parenteral nutrition can be a valuable treatment modality to prevent malnutrition and is covered in detail elsewhere (see Chapter 11). Although compounding PN solutions requires specialized expertise and is limited to referral centers, ready-made amino acid/glucose solutions for PN can be used in general practice as interim solutions until the animal can tolerate either placement of a feeding tube or is voluntarily eating (Gajanayake, Wylie and Chan, 2013). The sole use of PN in experimental animal models of AP has been associated with a high risk of infection and gut atrophy, with subsequent increased risk of bacterial translocation and sepsis (Alverly, Ayos and Moss, 1988). However, there are no studies on PN in dogs or cats that indicate a high risk for infection or sepsis and, in the single veterinary study that specifically evaluated PN nutritional support in dogs with AP, no septic complications were identified (Freeman et al., 1995). Although most patients fed parenterally had to have demonstrated intolerance to EN initially, many may tolerate provision of trickle feeding and gradual weaning onto EN, which may help to maintain intestinal integrity and function. This introduction of enteral feeding should start as soon as possible and maybe within 24 hours of initiating PN. This approach is supported by the fact that early enteral feeding has been associated with earlier return of gastrointestinal motility and cessation of vomiting (Wernerman, 2005). The time for initiation of PN is controversial in the light of recent findings that initiation of PN in critically ill human patients in the first 7 days of ICU hospitalization could be harmful (Casaer et al., 2011). The effect of time to PN initiation or combination of PN with EN in veterinary patients has not been studied so it is uncertain but in most studies detailing PN, the time to initiation is usually in the first 3 days of hospitalization (Chan et al., 2002; Gajanayake et al., 2013).

Selection or formulation of an appropriate nutritional solution is critical when using PN and it necessitates consideration of the caloric requirement of the patient and comorbidities present. Commercially available PN solutions for people are not designed to meet the needs of animals and may not provide adequate nutritional support (Campbell, Karriker and Fascetti, 2006). Although, a great proportion of energy in 3-in-1 PN solutions is derived from fat, there is currently no evidence to suggest that the lipid content in PN solutions is detrimental in the management of canine or feline pancreatitis. High lipid formulations appear to be well-tolerated in non-hyperlipidemic acute pancreatitis (Campbell et al., 2006). The optimal solution for dogs with pancreatitis and hypertriglyceridemia is not known.

Dietary considerations

When implementing enteral feeding, an appropriate diet should be selected. Although there is a paucity of veterinary studies evaluating the influence of diet type on disease course, a highly digestible diet designed for patients with gastro-intestinal disease is generally recommended. Avoidance of a diet high in fat has been the general recommendation for years although, in naturally occurring disease, the link between a high dietary fat content and pancreatitis is not very clear. The presence of hypertriglyceridemia in certain dog breeds has been shown to act as a predisposing factor and fat-restricted diets will therefore serve a benefit in management of pancreatitis in these cases (Verkest et al., 2008; Fleeman, 2010). Although fat restriction is considered an important component of the management of chronic pancreatitis in dogs, the role in non-hypertriglyceridemic acute pancreatitis is not well understood.

Cats have specialized dietary requirements that differ considerably from dogs with respect to dietary fat and protein requirements and may be more prone to carbohydrate-intolerance. The high dietary protein requirement makes cats more susceptible to protein-energy malnutrition and lean muscle loss during stressed starvation. Cats have the ability to digest and use high levels of dietary fat and there is no current evidence supporting restricting fat in the diet of cats with pancreatitis. In a retrospective study evaluating nasogastric tube feeding in cats with AP, feeding of a liquid enteral high lipid diet (45% of total calories fed) was well tolerated (Klaus et al., 2009).

Emerging role of immunonutrition

In human medicine there is increasing evidence supporting the idea that certain nutrients, such as glutamine, arginine and fatty acids, play a significant role in metabolic, inflammatory and immune processes in AP and the use of these specific nutrients in the care of critically ill human patients, including those with AP, is becoming quite common, with increasing evidence of their benefits with little risk of complications (Cetinbas, Yelken and Gulbas, 2010; Ockenga et al., 2002). The role of immunonutrition is covered elsewhere (see Chapter 18) but because glutamine supplementation has particular applications to the management of AP a brief discussion is warranted.

Glutamine is the most abundant amino acid in the plasma and is essential for a wide variety of physiological processes. The pancreas has a high protein turnover and glutamine supplementation in animals has resulted in the prevention of atrophy of pancreatic acinar cells, improvement in pancreatic exocrine function and improved outcomes following critical illness (Fan et al., 1997; Helton et al., 1990; Zou et al., 2010; Belmonte et al., 2007). Human patients with AP treated with glutamine-enriched PN solutions demonstrated significant improvement in C-reactive protein (CRP) concentrations, as well as decreased dependence on PN, reduced infectious complications and reduced length of hospitalization (Ockenga et al., 2002). Glutamine-supplemented PN is challenged by the fact that glutamine is relatively unstable in solution and generally has to be provided as di-peptides to maintain stability (Khan et al., 1991). Glutamine is currently not supplemented routinely to PN formulations in veterinary medicine and no clinical trials evaluating its use in pancreatitis have been published. As many meta-analyses of the use of immune-enhancing diets in critically ill patients have shown a reduction of hospital stay and infection rate, but no adverse effect on mortality rate, this was deemed a safe therapeutic option (Galban et al., 2003). However, most recently, a large multicentred prospective placebo-controlled trial unexpectedly demonstrated a statistical trend for higher mortality risk in critically ill patients treated with glutamine and antioxidants. (Heyland et al.,2013). It is worth noting that the target population in this trial (i.e., mechanically ventilated patients in shock) is quite different than patients with pancreatitis. Nevertheless, this significant finding, especially given the high quality of this latest trial, raises questions over the appropriateness of this approach in all patient populations. The exact causal relationship for increased risk of death was not determined.

Monitoring and complications

Monitoring patients with AP receiving nutritional support will depend on the mode of feeding employed. Aspects common to all modes of nutritional support include monitoring for tolerance of feeding, metabolic, mechanical and septic complications. It is currently unknown if serial monitoring of canine pancreatic lipase immunoreactivity (cPLI) is indicated or useful to monitor resolution of pancreatitis. Specific monitoring of techniques can be found in specific chapters devoted to these techniques.

Summary

There is increasing evidence supporting the important role of early EN (within 48 hours of diagnosis of pancreatitis) in positively impacting outcome beyond simply proving energy and nutrients in AP. Nutritional support is now considered an integral and key aspect of the successful management of AP. Even in veterinary medicine the use of enteral feeding is considered to be safe, effective and well tolerated in severe AP. Use of feeding tubes has been shown to be effective and safe in dogs and cats and they should be used unless specific contra-indications are identified. The exact composition of the diet has not been identified but diets commonly used for convalescent dogs and cats have been used successfully. Avoidance of high fat content does not appear to be necessary in the majority of patients. Despite the growing evidence that EN can be used effectively in management of patients with AP, there may still be patients requiring some form of PN until EN can be tolerated.

KEY POINTS

- Nutritional support is considered a key part of the management of patients with acute pancreatitis.

- Feeding should be attempted in all patients if cardiovascularly stable and PN should not be considered unless enteral feeding is not tolerated.

- Placement of feeding tubes should be considered the standard for providing nutritional support in patients with acute pancreatitis.

- Parenteral nutrition still has a place in the management of patients with acute pancreatitis, but it is to be reserved for patients who fail to tolerate enteral nutrition.

References

Alverdy, J., Ayos, E, and Moss, G. (1988) Total parenteral nutrition promotes bacterial translocation from the gut. *Surgery*, **104**, 185–190.

Beal, M.W. and Brown, A.J. (2011) Clinical experience utilizing a novel fluoroscopic technique for wire-guided nasojejunal tube placement in the dog: 26 cases (2006–2010). *Journal of Veterinary Emergency and Critical Care*, **21**, 151–157.

Belmonte, L., Coëffier, M, Le Pessot, F. et al. (2007) Effects of glutamine supplementation on gut barrier, glutathione content and acute phase response in malnourished rats during inflammatory shock. *World Journal of Gastroenterology* **13**, 2833–2840.

Casaer, M.P., Mesotten, D., Hermans, G. et al. (2011) Early versus Late Parenteral Nutrition in Critically Ill Adults. *New England Journal of Medicine*, **365**, 506–517.

Campbell, S.J., Karriker, M.J. and Fascetti, A.J. (2006) Central and peripheral parenteral nutrition. *Waltham Focus*, **16**, 22–30.

Cetinbas, F., Yelken, B. and Gulbas, Z. (2010) Role of glutamine administration on cellular immunity after total parenteral nutrition enriched with glutamine in patients with systemic inflammatory response syndrome. *Journal of Critical Care*, **25**, 61.e1–e6.

Chan, D.L., Freeman, L.M., Labato, M. et al. (2002) Retrospective evaluation of partial parenteral nutrition in dogs and cats. *Journal of Veterinary Internal Medicine*, **16**, 440–445.

Curtis, C.S. and Kudsk, K.A. (2007) Nutrition Support in Pancreatitis. *Surgical Clinics of North America*, **87**, 1403–1415.

Fan, B., Salehi, A., Sternby, B. et al. (1997) Total parenteral nutrition influences both endocrine and exocrine function of rat pancreas. *Pancreas*, **15**, 147–153.

Fleeman, L.M. (2010) Is hyperlipidemia clinically important in dogs? *Veterinary Journal*, **183**,10.

Freeman, L., Labato, M., Rush, J. et al. (1995) Nutritional support in pancreatitis: a retrospective study. *Journal of Veterinary Emergency Critical Care*, **5**, 32–41.

Gajanayake, I., Wylie, C.E. and Chan, D.L. (2013) Clinical experience with a lipid-free, ready-made parenteral nutrition solution in dogs: 70 cases (2006–2012). *Journal of Veterinary Emergency Critical Care*, **23**. doi: 10.1111/vec.12029.

Galbán, C., Montejo, J., Mesejo, A. et al. (2003) An immune-enhancing enteral diet reduces mortality rate and episodes of bacteremia in septic intensive care unit patients. *Critial Care Medicine*, **28**, 643–648.

Gianotti, L,, Meier, R,, Lobo, D.N. et al. (2009) ESPEN Guidelines on Parenteral Nutrition: Pancreas. *Clinical Nutrition*, **28**, 428–435.

Gukovskaya AS, Gukovsky I. (2012) Autophagy and pancreatitis. *American Journal of Physiology, Gastrointestinal Liver Physiology*, **303**, 993–1003.

Gukovsky, I,, Pandol, S.J., Gukovskaya, A.S. (2011) Organellar dysfunction in the pathogenesis of pancreatitis. *Antioxidant Redox Signalling*, **15**, 2699–2710.

Guptaa, R., Patela, K,, Calderb, P.C. et al. (2003) A randomised clinical trial to assess the effect of total enteral and total parenteral nutritional support on metabolic, inflammatory and oxidative markers in patients with predicted severe acute pancreatitis (APACHE II ≥6). *Pancreatology*, **3**, 406–413.

Helton, W., Jacobs, D., Bonner-Weir, S., et al. (1990) Effects of glutamine-enriched parenteral nutrition on the exocrine pancreas. *Journal of Parenteral Enteral Nutrition*, **14**, 344–352.

Heyland, D., Muscedere, J., Wischmeyer, P.E. et al. (2013) A randomized trial of glutamine and antioxidants in critically ill patients. *New England Journal of Medicine*, **368**, 1489–1497.

Ioannidis, O,, Lavrentieva, A. and Botsios, D. (2008) Nutrition support in acute pancreatitis. *Journal of the Pancreas*, **9**, 375–390.

Khan, K,, Hardy, G,, McElroy, B, et al. (1991) The stability of L-glutamine in total parenteral nutrition solutions. *Clinical Nutrition*, **10**, 193–198.

Klaus, J., Rudloff, E. and Kirby, R. (2009) Nasogastric tube feeding in cats with suspected acute pancreatitis: 55 cases (2001-2006). *Journal of Veterinary Emergency Critical Care*, **19**, 337–346.

Mansfield, C.S., James, F.E., Steiner, J.M. et al. (2011) A pilot study to assess tolerability of early enteral nutrition via esophagostomy tube feeding in dogs with severe acute pancreatitis. *Journal of Veterinary Internal Medicine* **25**, 419–425.

McClave, S.A. (2004) Defining the new gold standard for nutritional support in acute pancreatitis. *Nutrition Clinical Practice*, **19**,1–4.

Nathens, A.B., Curtis, J.R., Beale, R.L. et al. (2004) Management of the critically ill patient with severe acute pancreatitis. *Critical Care Medicine*, **32**, 2524–2536.

Niederau, C., Niederau, M., Lüthen, R., et al. (1990) Pancreatic exocrine secretion in acute experimental pancreatitis. *Gastroenterology*, **99**, 1120–1127.

O'Keefe, S.J.D., Lee, R.B., Li, J. et al. (2005) Trypsin secretion and turnover in patients with acute pancreatitis. *American Journal Physiology, Gastrointestinal Liver Physiology*, **289**, 181–187.

Ockenga, J,, Borchert, K., Rifai, K. et al. (2002) Effect of glutamine-enriched total parenteral nutrition in patients with acute pancreatitis. *Clinical Nutrition*, **21**, 409–416.

Pápa, K., Psáder, R., Sterczer. A. et al. (2009) Endoscopically guided nasojejunal tube placement in dogs for short-term postduodenal feeding. *Journal of Veterinary Emergency Critical Care*, **19**, 554–563.

Petrov, M., Kukosh, M. and Emelyanov, N. (2006) A Randomized controlled trial of enteral versus parenteral feeding in patients with predicted severe acute pancreatitis shows a significant reduction in mortality and in infected pancreatic complications with total enteral nutrition. *Digestive Surgery*, **23**, 336–345.

Qin, H.L., Su, Z.D., Gao, Q., et al. (2002) Early intrajejunal nutrition: bacterial translocation and gut barrier function of severe acute pancreatitis in dogs. *Hepatobiliary Pancreatic Disease International*, **1**, 150–154.

Qin, H.L., Su, Z.D., Hu, L.G., et al. (2007) Effect of parenteral and early intrajejunal nutrition on pancreatic digestive enzyme synthesis, storage and discharge in dog models of acute pancreatitis. *World Journal of Gastroenterology*, **13**, 1123–1128.

Qin, H.L., Su, Z.D., Hu, L.G. et al. (2003) Parenteral versus early intrajejunal nutrition: effect on pancreatitic natural course, entero-hormones release and its efficacy on dogs with acute pancreatitis. *World Journal of Gastroenterology*, **9**, 2270–2273.

Simpson, K, and Lamb, C. (1995) Acute pancreatitis. *In Practice*, **17**, 328–337.

Spanier, B.W.M., Bruno, M.J. and Mathus-Vliegen, E.M.H. (2011) Enteral nutrition and acute pancreatitis: a review. *Gastroenterology Research Practice*, **9**,10–12.

Son, T.T., Thompson, L., Serrano, S. et al. (2010) Surgical intervention in the management of severe acute pancreatitis in cats: 8 cases (2003–2007) *Journal of Veterinary Emergency Critical Care*, **20**, 426–435.

Thompson, L.J., Seshadri, R. and Raffe, M.R. (2009) Characteristics and outcomes in surgical management of severe acute pancreatitis: 37 dogs (2001–2007). *Journal of Veterinary Emergency Critical Care*, **19**, 165–173.

Verkest, K,, Fleeman, L,, Rand, J. et al. (2008) Subclinical pancreatitis is more common in overweight and obese dogs if peak postprandial triglyceridemia is >445 mg/dL. *Journal of Veterinary Internal Medicine*, **22**, 820.

Wernerman, J. (2005) Guidelines for nutritional support in intensive care unit patients: a critical analysis. *Current Opinion in Clinical Nutrition Metabolism Care*, **8**, 171–175.

Williams, D,A. (1995) Diagnosis and management of pancreatitis. *Journal of Small Animal Practice*, **35**, 445–454.

Zou, X., Chen, M., Wei, W. et al. (2010) Effects of enteral immunonutrition on the maintenance of gut barrier function and immune function in pigs with severe acute pancreatitis. *Journal of Parenteral and Enteral Nutrition*, **34**, 554–566.

CHAPTER 24

Nutritional support in the mechanically ventilated small animal patient

Daniel L. Chan

Department of Veterinary Clinical Sciences and Services, The Royal Veterinary College, University of London, UK

Introduction

Small animal patients receiving long-term mechanical ventilation (i.e., > 24 hours) require a host of supportive measures including nutritional support to ensure successful management and resolution of the underlying disease. Preservation of nutritional status has important implications for immune function, wound healing and muscle function to enable the patient to be weaned successfully from mechanical ventilation. Respiratory muscles, much like skeletal muscles, are negatively impacted by malnutrition. In the context of the long-term mechanically ventilated patient, malnutrition will result in muscle weakness, fatigability, and decreased endurance, which makes weaning patients off ventilation more difficult. Decrease in respiratory function results in increased respiratory muscle work, with increased energy demands, which further exacerbate the catabolic state (Ravasco and Camilo, 2003; Doley, Mallampalli and Sandberg, 2011).

Patients receiving early nutritional support (i.e., within 2 days of admission) have lower risks of developing nosocomial infections, require fewer days of mechanical ventilation and have overall better patient outcomes (Artinian, Krayem and Di Giovine, 2006; Strack van Schijndel et al., 2009; Reignier, 2013). However, provision of nutrition in this patient population is particularly challenging and measures must be taken to decrease the risk of complications. Aspects of nutritional support that require special consideration include the timing when nutrition should be initiated, the route of feeding, the composition of the diet and other aspects of management that may impact nutritional management. The biggest obstacles for provision of nutrition support in the ventilated patient include intolerance to enteral feeding, difficulties with airway management and the reality that many of these patients may be cardiovascularly unstable, and therefore priority is given to interventions with immediate patient benefits. Cardiovascular instability is regarded as a relative contraindication to enteral feeding and therefore many ventilated patients are not assessed as ready to

Nutritional Management of Hospitalized Small Animals, First Edition. Edited by Daniel L. Chan.

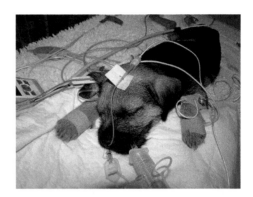

Figure 24.1 Nutritional support in mechanically ventilated patients often receives a low priority, however, early institution of enteral nutrition may be beneficial in these patients.

receive nutritional support (Figure 24.1). Protocols in human medicine indicate that ventilated patients should receive enteral feeding on day 3 of mechanical ventilation, however, recent studies have emphasized initiating feeding after 24 hours of mechanical ventilation (Parrish and McCray, 2003; Doley et al., 2011).

During critical illness, patients often develop gastrointestinal dysmotility problems that require a host of medical and nutritional strategies to manage these complications (see Chapter 17). Patients receiving mechanical ventilation have additional challenges that make provision of nutrition difficult. For example, in patients requiring mechanical ventilation, the frequency, amplitude, and percentage of propulsive contractions of the esophagus are reduced (Kölbel et al. 2000). This may explain the propensity for fluid to accumulate within the esophagus and result in regurgitation. The most pressing clinical concerns with esophageal dysmotility disorders center on the development of gastroesophageal reflux, esophagitis, and subsequent aspiration (Nind et al., 2005).

Human critically ill patients often have gastrointestinal intolerance that is manifested by an increased gastric residual volume (GRV) (Mentec et al., 2001). Published human feeding protocols have tried to define the threshold volume above which feeding should be withheld as well as to recommend the frequency of GRV assessment (Barr et al., 2004). The GRVs considered to be excessive in ventilated patients have ranged from 120 to 500 mL per aspiration (1.7 to 7.1 mL/kg assuming a 70 kg person) (Soroksky et al., 2010). A low GRV threshold results in multiple interruptions in EN provision due to frequent assessments of GRV, discarding checked volumes, and withholding feeding or reducing the rate of feeding due to presumed high GRV result in overall decrease in caloric intake, failure to achieve caloric targets, increased use of parenteral nutrition, which may all negatively impact outcome (Mentec et al., 2001; McClave et al., 1999). More recent data have questioned the relationship between increased GRV and higher risk of aspiration pneumonia as well as the need to check GRV more than once daily (McClave et al., 2005; Soroksky et al., 2010; Marik, 2014). In the light of these findings, some authors recommend against adjusting enteral feeding unless the GRV exceeds 500 mL and to reduce checking GRV to only once daily or not at all (Soroksy et al., 2010; Reignier et al., 2013). Unfortunately, there is virtually no information available in ventilated veterinary patients in regards to GRV and risk of feeding. While some authors (Haskins and King, 2004) recommended checking GRV before every feed, and that GRV should not be allowed to exceed 10 mL/kg, there are currently no data to corroborate whether such guidelines are necessary, although such recommendations may be sensible. Holahan et al. (2010) could not relate GRV and gastrointestinal complications in dogs fed via nasogastric tubes and some of these dogs had > 200 mL/kg of GRV, however, it is unknown if any of the dogs evaluated were mechanically ventilated. The median (range) GRV in this population of critically ill dogs was 4.5 mL/kg (0 to 213 mL/kg) (Holahan et al., 2010). As current human guidelines (Bankhead et al., 2009) state that enteral feedings should not be with held unless GRV are >500 mL (approximately 7 ml/kg based on 70 kg person), it may be prudent to use a similar approach and so animals with GRV with >10 mL/kg should be treated with pro-kinetic agents (see Chapter 17) and their feed reduced temporarily.

Nutritional management strategies

In people, the provision of enteral nutrition can be delivered via nasogastric or nasojejunal feeding tubes. Nasojejunal feeding has been recommended as the preferred route in patients with a high risk of aspiration as well as in those patients for whom gastric feeding is not tolerated, or who have repeated high gastric residual volumes (McClave et al., 2009). Unfortunately, there are little veterinary data regarding nutritional support of small animal patients receiving mechanical ventilation. Upon reviewing available veterinary clinical studies on mechanical ventilation, as well as veterinary studies on assisted feeding and parenteral nutrition, there are only brief mentions of patients that were venti-lated and received some form of nutritional support (King and Hendricks, 1994; Reuter et al., 1998; Beal et al., 2001; Chan et al., 2002; Pyle et al., 2004; Lee et al., 2005; Armitage-Chan, O'Toole and Chan, 2006; Crabb et al., 2006; Hopper et al., 2007;Campbell et al., 2010; Holahan et al., 2010; Hoareau, Mellems and Silverstein, 2011; Rutter et al., 2011; Gajanayake, Wylie and Chan, 2013; Queau et al., 2013; Yu et al., 2013; Edwards et al., 2014). From the information avail-able, it is clear that, in some studies, only a proportion of ventilated patients (40 to 50%) receive any form of nutritional support, that a high proportion receive parenteral nutrition (up to 38%) and in those that have enteral nutrition, it was stopped in up to 60% of patients due to regurgitation, high GRV and aspi-ration (Hopper et al., 2007; Rutter et al., 2011). Therefore formulation of feeding recommendations in ventilated small animals must be mostly extrapolated from information available in other populations and species.

The first question relates to optimal timing of nutritional support initiation. The urgency of initiating nutritional support will depend on the nutritional assessment (see Chapter 1) and nutritional status of the patient. As in other critically ill small animals, nutritional support should only be considered in cardiovascularly stable patients, but should generally be initiated within 48 to 72 hours of mechanical ventilation. Although avoidance of enteral feeding in mechanically ventilated patients may seem reasonable, parenteral nutrition should only be used if there are contraindications to enteral feedings, such as persistent vomiting or regurgitation (see Chapter 11). Enteral access devices for ventilated patients include nasogastric (Chapter 4), esophageal (Chapter 5), gastric (Chapter 6), and nasojejunal feeding tubes (Chapters 8). Nasogastric may be most appropriate for most ventilated patients, although some may benefit from post-pyloric placement of feeding tubes. Enteral feed may be delivered continuously or intermittently as there appears to be little difference in complication rates (Holahan et al., 2010; Campbell et al., 2010; Yu et al., 2013).

In terms of optimal caloric intake and composition of the diet for ventilated small animals, there are little data available. Overfeeding, particularly of carbohydrates, can result in a number of complications that may have important implications for ventilated patients, such as excess carbon dioxide production, which increases respiratory work (complicating weaning off the ventilator), and hyperglycemia (which can lead to gastrointestinal dysmotility). As in other critically ill populations, a caloric target of 80–100 % resting energy requirements (RER) may be appropriate, with the first day not exceeding 50% RER.

In people, there are encouraging results for patients with acute lung injury and acute respiratory distress syndrome that were fed enteral diets that were enriched with omega-3 fatty acids and antioxidants (Gadek et al., 1999;, Singer et al., 2006: Pontes-Arruda, Aragao and Albuquerque, 2006). No data are available in veterinary patients regarding the benefits of such an approach, but further research is warranted. A calorically dense, liquid diet appears appropriate for most cases.

Monitoring and complications

Ventilated patients are routinely monitored very closely. In regards to nutritional support, patients should be assessed for worsening nutritional status, tolerance to enteral feeding (including evidence of regurgitation or vomiting), abdominal distension and excessive GRV. As in other critically ill patients, frequent assessment of biochemistry profiles and blood gases are indicated.

Summary

Patients requiring mechanical ventilation are often the most critical and complex cases in any given veterinary hospital and present the veterinary team with a number of challenges. Determining the ideal time for initiating nutritional support, the route of delivery, the caloric targets, diet composition and closely monitoring for tolerance of feeding, are essential components of the strategy to manage mechanically ventilated patients.

> **KEY POINTS**
>
> - Small animal patients receiving mechanical ventilation require a host of supportive measures including nutritional support to ensure successful management and resolution of the underlying disease.
> - Preservation of nutritional status has important implications for immune function, wound healing and muscle function to enable the patient to be weaned successfully from mechanical ventilation.

- Provision of nutrition in this patient population is particularly challenging and measures such as the use of prokinetic agents, nasogastric or nasojenunal feeding tubes may be necessary.
- Aspects of nutritional support that require special consideration include the timing that nutrition should be initiated, the route of feeding, the composition of the diet and other aspects of management that may impact nutritional management.
- Enteral nutritional support using liquid critical care diets should be initiated within 48 to 72 hours in most patients requiring long-term mechanical ventilation.
- Nutritional support may be a key component in the successful management of ventilated patients.

References

Armitage-Chan, E.A., O'Toole, T. and Chan, D.L. (2006) Management of prolonged food deprivation, hypothermia and refeeding syndrome in a cat. *Journal of Veterinary Emergency and Critical Care*, **16**, S34–S41.

Artinian, V., Krayem, H. and DiGiovine, B. Effects of early enteral feeding on the outcome of critically ill mechanically ventilated medical patients. *Chest*, **129**, 960–967.

Bankhead, R., Boullata, J., Brantley, S. et al. (2009) A.S.P.E.N. enteral nutrition practice recommendations. *Journal of Parenteral and Enteral Nutrition*, **33**, 122–167.

Barr, J., Hecht, M., Flavin, K.E. et al. (2004) Outcomes in critically ill patients before and after the implementation of an evidence-based nutritional management protocol. *Chest*, **125**, 1446–1457.

Beal, M.W., Paglia, D.T., Griffin, G.M. et al (2001) Ventilatory failure, ventilator management, and outcome in dogs with cervical spinal disorders: 14 cases (1991-1999). *Journal of theAmerican Veterinary Medical Association*, **218**,1598–1602.

Campbell, J.A., Jutkowitz, A.L., Santoro, K.A. et al. (2010) Continuous versus intermittent delivery of nutrition via nasoenteric feeding tubes in hospitalized canine and feline patients: 91 patients (2002- 2007). *Journal of Veterinary Emergency and Critical Care*, **20**, 232–236.

Chan, D.L., Freeman, L.M., Labato, M.A. et al. 2002. Retrospective evaluation of partial parenteral nutrition in dogs and cats. *Journal of Veterinary Internal Medicine*, **16**, 440–445.

Crabb, S.E., Chan, D.L., Freeman, L.M. et al. 2006. Retrospective evaluation of total parenteral nutrition in cats: 40 cases (1991-2003). *Journal of Veterinary Emergency and Critical Care*, **16**, S21–S26.

Doley, J.D., Mallampalli, A. and Sandberg, M. (2011). Nutrition management for the patient requiring prolonged mechanical ventilation. *Nutrition, Clinical Practice*, **26**, 232–241.

Edwards, T.H., Coleman, A., Brainard, B.M. et al. (2014) Outcome of positive-pressure ventilation in dogs and cats with congestive heart failure: 16 cases (1992-2012). *Journal of Veterinary Emergency and Critical Care*, **24**, 586–593.

Gadek, J.E., DeMichele, S.J., Karlstad, M.D. et al. (1999) Effect of enteral feeding with eicosapentaenoic acid, gamma-linolenic acid, and antioxidants on patients with acute respiratory distress syndrome. *Critical Care Medicine*, **27**, 1409–1420.

Gajanayake, I., Wylie, C.E. and Chan, D.L. 2013. Clinical Experience Using a Lipid-free, Readymade Parenteral Nutrition Solution in Dogs: 70 cases (2006-2012). *Journal of Veterinary Emergency and Critical Care*, **23**, 305–313.

Haskins, S.C. and King, L.G. (2004) Positive pressure ventilation. in Textbook of Respiratory Diseases in Dogs and Cats (ed. L.G. King) Elsevier, St Louis, MO, pp. 217–229.

Holahan, M., Abood, S., Hauptman, C. et al. (2010) Intermittent and continuous enteral nutrition in criticallu ill dogs: a prospective randomized trial. *Journal of Veterinary Emergency and Critical Care*, **24**, 520–526.

Hopper, K., Haskins, S.C., Kass, P.H. et al. (2007) Indications, management and outcome of long-term positive-pressure ventilation in dogs and cats: 148 cases (1990–2001). *Journal of the American Veterinary Medical Association*, **230**, 64–75.

Hoareau, G.L., Mellema, M.S. and Silverstein, D.C. (2011) Indications, management, and outcome of brachycephalic dogs requiring mechanical ventilation. *Journal of Veterinary Emergency and Critical Care*, **21**, 226–235.

Lee, J.A., Drobatz, K.J., Koch, M.W. et al. (2005) Indications for and outcome of positive-pressure ventilation in cats: 53 cases (1993–2002), *Journal of the American Veterinary Medical Association*, **226**, 924–31.

King, L.G. and Hendricks, J.C., (1994) Use of positive-pressure ventilation in dogs and cats: 41 cases (1990–1992). *Journal of the American Veterinary Medical Association*, **204**, 1045–1052.

Kölbel, C.B., Rippel, K., Klar, H. et al. (2000) Esophageal motility disorders in critically ill patients: a 24-hour manometric study. *Intensive Care Medicine*, **26**,1421–1427.

Marik, P.E. (2014) Enteral nutrition in the critically ill: myths and misconception. *Critical Care Medicine*, **42**, 962–969.

McClave, S.A., Lukan, J.K., Stefater, J.A. et al. (2005) Poor validity of residual volumes as a marker for risk of aspiration in critically ill patients. *Critical Care Medicine*, **33**, 324–330.

McClave, S.A., Martindale, R.G., Vanek, V.W. et al (2009) Guidelines for the provision and assessment of nutrition support in the adult critically ill patient: Society of Critical Care Medicine.

McClave, S.A., Sexton, L.K., Spain, D.A., et al. (1999) Enteral tube feeding in the intensive care unit: factors impeding adequate delivery. *Critical Care Medicine*, **27**, 1252–1256.

Mentec, H., Dupont, H., Bomlhetti, M. et al. (2001) Upper digestive intolerance during enteral nutrition in critically ill patients: frequency, risk factors, and complications. *Critical Care Medicine*, **29**, 1955–1961.

Nind, G., Chen, W-H., Protheroe, R. et al. (2005) Mechanisms of gastroesophageal reflux in critically ill mechanically ventilated patients. *Gastroenterology*, **128**, 600–606.

Parrish, C.R. and McCray, S.F. (2003) Nutrition support for the mechanically ventilated patient. *Critical Care Nurse*, **23**, 77–80.

Pontes-Arruda, A., Aragao, A.M. and Albuquerque, J.D. (2006) Effects of enteral feeding with eicosapentaenoic acid, gamma-linolenic acid, and antioxidants in mechanically ventilated patients with severe sepsis and septic shock. *Critical Care Medicine*, **34**, 2325–2333.

Pyle, S.C., Marks, S.L., Kass, P.H. et al. (2004) Evaluation of complication and prognostic factors associated with administration of parenteral nutrition in cats: 75 cases (1994–2001). *Journal of the American Veterinary Medical Association*, **225**, 242–250.

Queau, Y., Larsen, J.A., Kass, P.H. et al. (2013) Factors associated with adverse outcomes during parenteral nutrition administration in dogs and cats. *Journal of Veterinary Internal Medicine*, **25**, 446–452.

Ravasco, P. and Camilo, M.E. (2003) Tube feeding in mechanically ventilated critically ill patient: a prospective clinical audit. *Nutrition Clinical Practice*, **18**, 247–433.

Reignier, J. (2013) Feeding ICU patients on invasive mechanical ventilation: Designing the optiomal protocol. *Critical Care Medicine*, **41**, 2825–2826.

Reignier, J., Mercier, E., Le Gouge, A. et al. (2013) Effect of not monitoring residual gastric volume on risk of ventilator-associated pneumonia in adults receiving mechanical ventilation and early enteral feeding. *Journal of the American Medical Association*, **309**, 249–256.

Reuter, J.D., Marks, S.L., Rogers, Q. R. et al. (1998) Use of total parenteral nutrition in dogs: 209 cases (1988-1995). *Journal of Veterinary Emergency and Critical Care*, **8**, 201–213.

Rutter, C.R., Rozanski, E.A., Sharp, C.R. et al. (2011) Outcome and medical management in dogs with lower motor neuron disease undergoing mechanical ventilation: 14 cases (2003-2009) *Journal of Veterinary Emergency and Critical Care*, **21**, 531–541.

Singer, P., Theilla, M., Fisher, H. et al. (2006) Benefit of an enteral diet enriched with eicosapentaenoic acid and gamma-linolenic acid in ventilated patients with acute lung injury. *Critical Care Medicine*, **34**, 1033–1038.

Soroksky, A., Lober, J., Klinowski, E. et al. (2010) A simplified approach to the management of gastric residual volumes in crtically ill mechanically ventilated patients: a pilot prospective study. *Israel Medical Association Journal*, **12**, 543–548.

Strack van Schijndel, R.J., Weijs, R.J., Koopmans, R.H. et al. (2009) Optimal nutrition during the period of mechanical ventilation decreases mortality in critically-ill, long term acute female patients: A prospective observation cohort study. *Critical Care*, **13**, R132.

Yu, M.K., Freeman, L.M., Heinse, C.R., et al. (2013) Comparison of complication rates in dogs with nasoesophageal versus nasogastric feeding tubes. *Journal of Veterinary Emergency and Critical Care*, **23**, 300–304.

CHAPTER 25

Nutritional support in exotic pet species

Jeleen A. Briscoe[1], La'Toya Latney[2] and Cailin R. Heinze[3]

[1] Animal Care Program, United States Department of Agriculture Animal and Plant Health Service, Riverdale, MD, USA
[2] Exotic Companion Animal Medicine and Surgery, University of Pennsylvania School of Veterinary Medicine, Philadelphia, PA, USA
[3] Department of Clinical Sciences, Tufts Cummings School of Veterinary Medicine, North Grafton, MA, USA

Introduction

Providing nutritional support to exotic pet (EP) species[1] presents a unique challenge for the practitioner. Malnutrition in these types of animals is common due to misinformation and an overall lack of research into their nutrient requirements. Inadequate caloric and nutrient intake has long-term detrimental effects on the immune system, wound healing and overall well-being, thus influencing the outcome of any presentation, whether it be acute trauma or chronic infectious disease. There are multiple EPs commonly maintained in captivity, none of which are considered domesticated to the extent of dogs and cats. Limited research on nutritional requirements for these animals exists, with even less on species-specific differences within the same taxonomical orders or even genera. Common strategies to overcome this challenge include extrapolation from known requirements in similar species with comparable gastrointestinal morphology to that of the target species, application of research on diet specializations of free-living members of that species, extrapolation from the specie's wild diets and natural history, and experience gained by veterinarians (Koutsos, Matsos and Klasing, 2001), zoologists, curators and other animal caretakers.

With the exception of ferrets and some reptiles, most EPs are prey species, thus they hide clinical signs of disease until they are comparatively more ill than dogs or cats on presentation. EPs may also alter their behavior when in a new environment, particularly when people are observing them (Pollock, 2002), making imperative training of staff to recognize subtle changes in demeanor for multiple species. The practitioner must constantly weigh the pros and cons of aggressive treatment with the risk of stressing the animal with handling. Aside from providing warmth, supplemental oxygen if required, a low stress environment and restoring hydration, addressing nutritional needs is one of the

---

Nutritional Management of Hospitalized Small Animals, First Edition. Edited by Daniel L. Chan.
© 2015 John Wiley & Sons, Ltd. Published 2015 by John Wiley & Sons, Ltd.

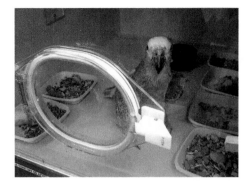

Figure 25.1 Blue-fronted Amazon parrot (*Amazona aestiva*) in hospital oxygen cage with assortment of foods. Addressing nutritional needs is a high priority for exotic pet species, especially those with high metabolic rates, such as birds and small mammals.

major keys to treatment success for most presentations (Figure 25.1), often far beyond any medication protocol. For birds and small mammals, metabolic rates are higher than those for cats and dogs, and the animals have fewer reserves, requiring the practitioner to place nutrition needs high on the list of treatment priorities. Basic guidelines for avian and mammalian exotic pets are to feed early and often, and to get the animal eating a nutritionally complete diet on its own, without assistance, as soon as possible. In addition to monitoring food intake, routine and accurate weighing (at least daily) of the animal using proper scales (i.e. gram scales for animals less than 1 kg, scales designed for human infants for animals over a kg) will provide a good indication of the need to apply or adjust assisted feeding strategies to the patient. Assisted feeding should be considered when the patient loses 5% or more of its weight, and should be mandatory when that loss reaches 10%, or the animal is completely anorexic (Pollock, 2002) for more than half a day.

The most common methods used for assisted feeding of EPs, based on ease of administration and limited stress on the animal, are syringe feeding for small mammals and gavaging for birds and reptiles. Other more invasive methods, such as nasogastric or pharyngostomy tubes, should be weighed in the light of the effect they may have on natural behaviors of the species, as some may not tolerate them. For example, nasogastric tubes may require placement of an Elizabethan collar on rabbits to prevent them from pulling them out; this will impair their ability to ingest caecotrophs and may interfere with their eating habits, thus resulting in anorexia and altering gastrointestinal flora, leading to dysbiosis and even death (Figure 25.2).

Basic guidelines across species for syringe- or gavage-feeding are the same: customize the diet to the normal feeding strategy of the animal (i.e., meat diets for carnivores, vegetarian diets for herbivores), make sure that the consistency of the diet administered will pass easily through the syringe or tube without clogging (test on a spare tube if unfamiliar with the diet), and calculate the initial caloric dose based on the animal's resting energy requirement (RER), taking into account the health state of the animal (Donoghue, 1998). For severely malnourished animals, start with 10–20% of the RER the first day; gradually increase over the next few days by increments of 10–25% until 100% RER is reached. This approach is intended to decrease the chance of "refeeding syndrome," a condition that occurs when a severely malnourished animal is fed too many calories

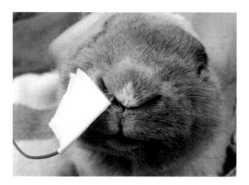

Figure 25.2 Nasoesophageal tube placement in a rabbit (*Oryctolagus cuniculus*). Indications and protocols for such procedures in exotic pet species are similar for domestic pets, but may not be tolerated as well. NE tubes in rabbits may impair ingestion of caecotrophs and normal eating habits, leading to dysbiosis and even death.

too quickly, leading to an insulin spike and resulting phosphorus and potassium uptake into cells along with glucose, causing hypophosphatemia, hypokalemia, and even death (de la Navarre, 2006, Martinez-Jimenez and Hernandez-Divers, 2007). Animals that have been anorexic for short durations may tolerate 25–100% of the RER the first day. It is generally safest to feed less initially until tolerance can be determined. The calorie intake should slowly be increased from the RER as necessary to maintain a steady body weight or slow weight gain if appropriate.

Special considerations: equipping the hospital to accommodate nutritional needs of exotic pets

It is the variety of EPs that require care and nutritional support in the hospital that dictates the need for a dedicated storage and food preparation area. Ideally, there should be separate food preparation areas for meat and produce, and sanitation protocols for these areas, storage containers, and food receptacles (Crissey et al., 2001; Schmidt, Travis and Williams, 2006). To increase client education, compliance and, potentially, revenue, the practitioner may consider offering certain commercial EP diets for sale (Fisher, 2005). Prior to stocking commercial foods for patients or offering them for purchase, thorough investigation into the quality of the food is important for patient health and hospital credibility. Minimally, manufacturer knowledge, quality control and validity of any marketing claims should be assessed (Schmidt et al., 2006).

Setting up a practice to accommodate the nutritional needs of hospitalized exotic pets requires detailed planning. First, the types of feeding strategies and basic foods that will be kept in stock to meet those feeding strategies should be identified (Table 25.1). Storage needs for those foods include a pest-proof cabinet for dry goods (Figure 25.3), a refrigerator for fresh produce dedicated to animal food only, and a freezer for storage of frozen foods and dry goods (Figure 25.4) to prolong viability of nutrient content. As the nutrient quality of food decreases over time (Schmidt et al., 2006), a schedule for replacement of those foods and a protocol for monitoring expiration dates, checking viability of frozen prey (Crissey et al., 2001), and discarding spoiled or expired foods should be determined. For example, a year after cutting hay, half of its vitamin A activity from beta carotene is diminished (Donoghue, 1998).

Table 25.1 Suggested foods to stock in a hospital for zoological companion animals. Dry goods should be kept in air-tight, resealable containers, away from extreme temperatures and moisture. Foods requiring refrigeration or freezing should be kept separate from food intended for human use. In addition to the below, powdered convalescent or hand-feeding diets designed for a range of species (e.g. Oxbow Critical Care for herbivores and Carnivore Care)[a] should also be in stock, along with a high-calorie cat and human liquid diets (e.g. Clinicare[b] and TwoCal[b]).

Feeding strategy	Suggested foods to stock
Herbivorous, including rabbits, guinea pigs, parrots, iguanas, tortoises.	• Commercial pelleted diets designed in type and size for a range of species (e.g. Mazuri Tortoise Diet[c] , Zupreem Nature's Promise™ Premium small mammal line[d]) • Dried hay in long-stem and cubed forms: timothy, alfalfa, and wild grasses • Fresh produce: dark leafy greens (e.g. kale, chard and parsley); and palatable, brightly colored fruits and vegetables to stimulate eating (e.g. strawberries, mango, and blueberries)[e]
Carnivorous/Insectivorous, including ferrets, raptors, and turtles	• Appropriate commercial diets (pelleted and canned) designed for range of species (e.g. Mazuri Insectivore Diet[c] and Marshall Premium Ferret Diet[f]) • Insects in ventilated containers with appropriate nutritional substrate • Frozen prey[g]
Granivorous, including passerines and small rodents	• Commercial extruded/pelleted diets and seed mixes designed for a range of species (e.g. ZuPreem FruitBlend™ Flavor Premium Daily Bird Food line[e,d] and Kaytee Fiesta line[h]) • Palatable seeds and nuts to stimulate eating in anorexic hospitalized birds, e.g. sunflower, safflower seeds and spray millet for smaller birds and bird treats, such as Lafeber's Nutri-Berry line[i]

[a] Oxbow Animal Health, Murdock, NE, USA.
[b] Abbott Laboratories, Abbott Park, IL, USA.
[c] PMI Nutrition, Henderson, CO, USA (Mazuri products are distributed under the tradename "Nutrazu" in the European Union).
[d] ZuPreem, Shownee, KS, USA.
[e] The following website has a searchable database on nutritional content for fresh produce: http://www.nal.usda.gov/fnic/foodcomp/search/.
[f] Marshall Pet Products Inc., NY, USA.
[g] Improper thawing can increase microbial content, lipid peroxidation, and decrease nutrient quality and palatability. Thawing under refrigeration is recommended (Crissey et al., 2001).
[h] Kaytee Products, Inc., Chilton, WI, USA.
[i] Lafeber Company, Cornell, IL, USA.

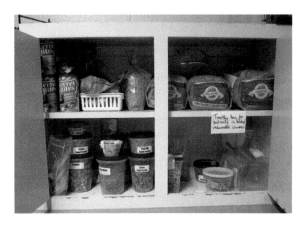

Figure 25.3 Dry goods storage of hospital foods for exotic pet species. Addressing the nutritional needs in hospitalized exotic pets require protocols for proper storage and product replacement.

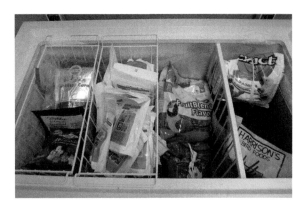

Figure 25.4 Frozen goods storage of hospital foods for exotic pet species. Addressing the nutritional needs in hospitalized exotic pets require protocols for proper storage and product replacement.

For the less common species with specialized diets, owners should be told when they call for an appointment that may require hospitalization to bring in their pet's food with instructions for feeding.

Nutritional management strategies

Reptiles

Reptiles are ectothermic and thus are dependent on environmental sources to maintain body temperature. Unlike birds and mammals whose generation of heat and energy is highly dependent on physiologic processes, reptilian mechanisms for regulation are dictated by complex neuroendocrine processes and are for the most part behavioral. They must physically move into and out of different thermal zones to maintain their body temperature. Reptiles move to warmer thermal zones only for the periods that require more energy, for example, mating, territorial defence, predator avoidance and feeding. This strategy allows reptiles to have 3% of the daily energy requirements of similarly-sized mammals. As such, they have a decreased need for food and are more efficient at transforming food energy into body tissue, provided they can remain within their set point temperature range – or set body temperature – around which thermoregulation occurs. This range of temperatures is called the preferred body

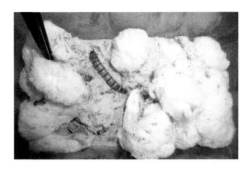

Figure 25.5 Nutritional substrate and moisture for superworms (*Zophobas molitor*) intended for the insectivorous diet. Invertebrate prey for insectivorous exotic pet species must be maintained on a nutritious substrate, such as an avian hand-feeding formula, with a source of moisture (e.g. moistened cotton material, seen here).

temperature (PBT) or preferred optimum temperature zone (POTZ) (Donoghue, 1998; Pough, 2004; Rossi, 2006).

Hospitalized reptiles should be stabilized and maintained within the upper end of their PBT, with the option to move through a range of temperatures, prior to addressing nutritional needs. Although reptiles can go longer without food due to their physiology, deciding when to offer food or assist feed should be one of the top treatment priorities and will depend on a variety of factors, including body condition, duration in time from the last meal, thermoregulatory behaviour of the animal and hydration status.

Carnivorous reptiles (e.g. snakes) have a relatively short, simple gastrointestinal tract with limited fermentative activity. Diets consumed by strict carnivores should consist of 30–60% protein on a metabolizable energy (ME) basis, with fat making up the remainder of the daily calories with little to no carbohydrate (Donoghue, 1998). Whole prey, either vertebrate or invertebrate, is considered the ideal diet for carnivores. Although there are processed diets available commercially, acceptance may be poor. Invertebrate prey must be gut loaded (fed) by maintaining them on a nutritious substrate prior to feeding (Figure 25.5) (Donoghue, 1998, Mitchell, 2004). Nutritional analyses are available for many commonly reared insects used as prey for insectivorous species and the calcium content of some insects has been shown to be influenced by the type of substrate available to them (Latney et al., 2009; Finke,Dunham and Kwabi, 2005).

Like other herbivores, herbivorous reptiles (e.g. *Iguana iguana* and *Uromastyx* spp.) have a longer small intestine where hydrolytic digestion takes place and a large, specialized lower bowel for fermentative digestion. Diets consumed by herbivorous reptiles are relatively high in carbohydrates and low in dietary fat (<10% DM) (Donoghue, 1998).

Omnivorous reptiles (e.g. *Pogona vitticeps*) consume a mixture of diets utilized by carnivorous and herbivorous reptiles, with intermediate levels of carbohydrate and protein. Feeding strategies can change over time for some species that undergo an ontogenetic diet shift (e.g., aquatic turtles) and consume a more carnivorous diet during development while becoming primarily omnivorous or herbivorous at maturity (Donoghue, 1998).

Assisted feeding in reptiles

Options for assisted feeding include syringe feeding, orogastric feeding using gavage needles or red rubber tubes attached to a syringe, or a pharyngostomy (Figure 25.6) or gastrostomy tube. Indications and techniques for these procedures

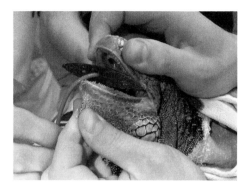

Figure 25.6 Green iguana (*Iguana iguana*) receiving a tube feeding. Assisted gavage feeding through a tube in reptiles requires proper handling and secure restraint of the jaw. Herbivorous reptiles, such as this iguana, can be fed an herbivorous convalescent diet (see Table 25.1) diluted enough to be administered through a feeding tube.

are well described elsewhere (de la Navarre, 2006; Martinez-Jimenez and Hernandez-Divers, 2007; Sykes and Greenacre, 2006).

One equation for estimating RER for reptiles is kcal/day = 10(body weight in kg)$^{0.75}$ (Martinez-Jimenez and Hernandez-Divers, 2007). The daily volume of food to administer is RER ÷ kcal/mL divided into the number of meals per day (Martinez-Jimenez and Hernandez-Divers, 2007). Note that these calculations represent an artificial generalization across numerous species, and thus should be considered basic guidelines until further research on bioenergetics of individual species becomes available. All animals should be fed enough while hospitalized to at least maintain body weight.

Birds

The anatomy of the avian gastrointestinal tract varies depending on the feeding strategy of the species. This section will focus on the species more commonly kept as pets, such as psittacines and passerines. The feeding strategies of these species range from mostly granivorous (e.g. finches, cockatiels and budgerigar parakeets) to omnivorous (e.g. Grey and Amazon parrots), with some tending more towards frugivorous (e.g. macaws) or nectivorous (e.g. lorikeets) (Klasing, 1999). Although many parrot species will often accept meat as part of a captive diet, this practice has not been well-evaluated.

Information on nutrient requirements for commonly kept avian species is limited, particularly when considering the vast range of species kept in captivity. For example, a study of Grey parrots (*Psittacus erithacus*) suggested a protein requirement of 10–15% DM, while that of a budgerigar parakeet (*Melopsittacus undulatus*) is 6.8% (McDonald, 2006). Duplicating the wild diet is often impossible, as domestic fruits are higher in sugar and water and lower in nutrients while seeds from domestic plants are higher in fat and lower in protein and nutrients than those found in the natural environments of many companion species' wild counterparts. Additionally, companion birds generally have lower energy requirements than free-living birds due to decreased activity. Based on similarities between the gastrointestinal morphology of psittacines and passerines and domestic poultry (e.g. chickens and turkeys), it is assumed, however erroneously, that many of the nutritional requirements may be the same across these species. Although commonly fed, commercially available seed diets have been found to be deficient in numerous essential nutrients including amino acids, calcium, phosphorus, sodium, manganese, zinc, iron, vitamins A, D, and K, B-vitamins,

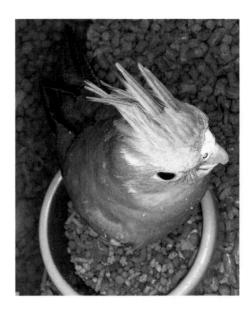

Figure 25.7 Cockatiel (*Nymphicus hollandicus*) perched on a food bowl containing a commercial extruded-pelleted diet. Commercially available extruded-pelleted diets have been shown to be higher in vitamins and minerals and lower in fat than seed diets.

choline, iodine, and selenium (Ullrey, Allen and Baer, 1991). Fat often provides more than 50% of the calories in nut and seed diets (Stahl and Kronfeld, 1998) and can contribute to obesity. Commercial "complete" extruded-pellet diets (Figure 25.7) for psittacines and passerines (initially based on poultry requirements) have been available for decades and while these diets are not perfect, they are usually an improvement over seed or seed plus fruit and vegetable diets. One study showed improved fledgling success in a variety of parrot species fed an extruded-pelleted diet versus seeds (90% success for extruded-pellets versus 66% for seeds) (Ullrey et al., 1991). In another study, a variety of commercially-available extruded-pelleted diets were found to contain much less fat than seed mixtures (8.6% in pelleted feeds vs. 31.7% in seed mixtures), as carbohydrate, rather than fat, is the main energy source in pelleted diets (Werquin, De Cock and Ghysels, 2005). Despite their nutritional inferiority, seed diets are very palatable and may be more eagerly consumed by hospitalized birds.

Assisted feeding in birds

Options for assisted feeding include syringe feeding, gavage feeding into the crop using a gavage needle (Figure 25.8) or, more rarely, esophagostomy or duodenostomy tubes. Indications and techniques for these procedures are well described elsewhere (Powers, 2006a; de Matos and Morrisey, 2005; Lennox, 2006). Powdered convalescent diets made for psittacines or chick hand-feeding diets can be reconstituted with a liquid human enteral product to increase calorie content, but the overall mixture may need to be diluted with enough water for the solution to pass through the tube being used. Convalescent and hand-feeding diets are not meant to be fed to healthy adult birds long-term (Lennox, 2006).

The energy requirement of birds depends on the environmental climate of the species' natural environment. A proposed RER calculation for tropical psittacines is $73.6(\text{body weight in kg})^{0.73}$ while species from temperate climates

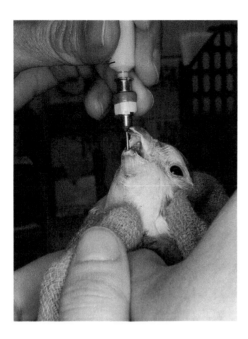

Figure 25.8 Gavage feeding of a cockatiel (*Nymphicus hollandicus*). Assisted feeding into the crop through a specialized metal gavage tube takes proper handling and expertise but is a convenient, expedient way to meet nutritional requirements in hospitalized, anorexic birds.

(e.g., Australia) have 21% higher energy requirements due to greater environmental temperature variation (Koutsos et al., 2001). As these equations can be quite complex, many practitioners rely on the more general range of 20–50 mL/ kg per feeding, depending on the amount the bird is eating on its own and how much food the crop can accommodate (Powers, 2006b); this does not take into consideration the caloric density of the diet provided. Regardless of the initial feeding amount chosen, close monitoring of body weight and adjustment of intake are essential to ensure that adequate calories are being provided.

Small mammals

Herbivorous mammals primarily eat plant material, the digestion of which requires a specialized microbial population and large bowel in which to break down fiber and extract nutrients from the diet. Fiber is essential to the herbivorous diet of monogastric hind-gut fermenters, such as rabbits, guinea pigs and chinchillas. Low-fiber diets have been linked to caecocolonic hypomotility, which can lead to over-population of *Clostridia* and *E. coli* (Cheeke, 1987) and dysbiosis. Because of this, a common recommendation is to offer all species free-choice timothy or other grass hays, with limited to no pellets for rabbits. At least some pellets should be offered to guinea pigs and chinchillas since they have been shown to eat hay more slowly than rabbits and may not be able to meet their nutritional requirements on hay alone (Donnelly and Brown, 2004). Similar to non-human primates, guinea pigs must have a dietary source of vitamin C (Donnelly and Brown, 2004). The daily vitamin C dose range is from 10 mg/kg body weight to 50 mg daily for any size guinea pig.

Published nutritional requirements are available for small rodents such as rats, mice, and gerbils, due to their extensive use in biomedical research

(National Research Council, 1995). However, these guidelines were designed for laboratory animals and may not be applicable to companion animals with their different nutrition end-goals. Laboratory animal guidelines are often designed to optimize lactation or reproduction, rather than health and longevity. Commercial "rodent chow" and other formulated diets are readily available and contain a minimum of 16% protein and 4–5% fat on a DM basis (Kupersmith, 1998). These diets can be supplemented for enrichment and variety with small amounts of seed and nuts as well as fresh produce. Specialized rodent blocks with plant-based protein sources are available and, with more research, may be proven to be more appropriate for overweight or growing animals or those with certain disease conditions

Ferrets are obligate carnivores and thus have a relatively short intestinal tract and colon (approximately half the length of that of a cat), and lack a caecum and ileocolic valve. Ferret diets should be highly digestible (i.e., low in fiber), as the gastrointestinal transit time is only 3–4 hours (Kupersmith, 1998, Bixler and Ellis, 2004). Ferrets require at least 30% high quality protein on a dry matter basis in their diets (Kupersmith, 1998) and should be fed minimal carbohydrates.

Assisted feeding in small mammals

Because hindgut fermenters need to maintain constant food intake to stimulate proper motility (Cheeke, 1987), and ferrets have such a rapid gut transit time, in cases of hyporexia or anorexia, assisted feeding must be instituted as soon as the animal is stabilized. Options for assisted feeding of small mammals include syringe feeding (Figure 25.9), nasogastric, or esophagostomy tubes. Indications and techniques are well described elsewhere (Bixler and Ellis, 2004; Brown, 1997a,b; de Matos and Morrisey, 2006; Graham, 2006; Klaphake, 2006; Paul-Murphy, 2007; Powers 2006c). Canned convalescent diets designed for cats can be fed to ferrets, either offered for free-feeding (Figure 25.10) or mixed with water or a commercial liquid cat enteral formulation as needed to pass through a syringe or tube. Commercially available powdered convalescent diets designed for mammalian carnivores may also be used. Similar products are available for mammalian herbivores that can also be diluted with water or a liquid human enteral formulation as needed to obtain the consistency that can fit through a feeding syringe or tube (Bixler and Ellis, 2004; Powers 2006c). Further study is needed to address the impact simple sugars in human enteral formulations have on these species, but such products have been used extensively by exotic pet veterinarians with no obvious ill-effects.

Resting energy requirements for most mammals can be estimated by the equation RER = 70(body weight in kg)$^{0.75}$. Calories administered should be adjusted to maintain body weight during hospitalization. Many practitioners rely on more general guidelines, focusing on maintaining food intake to stimulate gut motility rather than meeting precise caloric requirement. Ferrets can be fed as much as they will take in a feeding (usually 12–25 ml per 2–4 feedings a day) (Bixler and Ellis, 2004), and the herbivorous/omnivorous mammals can be fed 20 ml/kg in each feeding up to 4 times a day, depending on how much they are eating on their own. Daily weighing is critical to ensure that the appropriate amount of calories is provided.

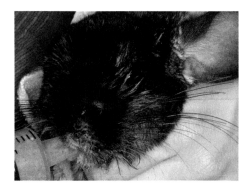

Figure 25.9 Syringe feeding of a chinchilla (*Chinchilla laniger*). Anorexic monogastric hind-gut fermenters, such as rabbits, chinchillas and guinea pigs, should be syringe fed a convalescent diet designed for herbivores to stimulate gut motility and restoration to health.

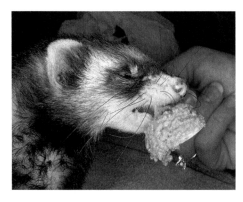

Figure 25.10 Assisted feeding of a ferret (*Mustela putorius furo*) with a canned convalescent diet. Unlike herbivorous small mammals, ferrets are less likely to tolerate restraint for syringe feeding, thus encouraging them to eat a canned diet without restraint is ideal.

Summary

Addressing the nutritional needs of exotic pets in practice need not be difficult, as long as protocols are in place for stocking, safe food preparation, expiration date monitoring, and product replacement as needed. It is imperative for hospital staff to have an appreciation for (i) different feeding strategies for exotic pets and how to address them, (ii) species-specific behaviour patterns and food intake and (iii) subtle changes in body condition and weight across the range of commonly kept exotic pets. Currently much of the approach to nutrition for exotic pets is based on extrapolation from domestic animals, but as more research is performed and the understanding of ethology and comparative gastrointestinal morphology expands, our ability to address nutritional needs at the species level will improve.

KEY POINTS

- Species-specific research on which to rely for nutritional guidance in exotic pets is ideal but limited.
- Addressing the nutritional needs of exotic pets in practice need not be difficult, as long as protocols are in place for stocking, safe food preparation, expiration date monitoring and product replacement as needed.
- It is imperative for hospital staff to have an appreciation for (i) different feeding strategies for exotic pets and how to address them, (ii) species-specific behaviour

patterns and food intake, and (iii) subtle changes in body condition and weight across the range of commonly kept exotic pets.

- One of the goals for successful treatment of hospitalized exotic pets is to have them consume the appropriate diet without assistance. If they are anorexic, nutritional supplementation is imperative, especially for those species with high metabolic rates, such as birds and small mammals. Gavage and syringe feeding are preferred for ease of administration and lower stress on the animal, as compared to more invasive methods such as nasoesophageal or pharyngostomy tube placement.

- Taking into account the feeding strategy and ethology of the species in the wild is ideal for determining which diets to feed in hospital. Convalescent diets tailored to carnivorous and herbivorous species are readily available and easy to administer.

Note

1 Exotic pet species include small animals, other than dogs and cats, which are commonly kept as pets, including birds, such as canaries and parrots, reptiles, amphibians and small mammals, such as rabbits, guinea pigs, ferrets, chinchillas, and rats.

References

Bixler, H. and Ellis, C. (2004) Ferret care and husbandry. *Veterinary Clinics Exotic Animal Practice*, **7**, 227–255.

Brown, S. A. (1997a) Clinical techniques in rabbits. *Seminars Avian and Exotic Pet Medicine*, **6**, 86–95.

Brown, S. A. (1997b) Clinical techniques in domestic ferrets. *Seminars Avian and Exotic Pet Medicine*, **6**, 75–85.

Cheeke, P. R. (1987) *Rabbit Feeding and Nutrition*. Harcourt Brace Jovanovich Publishers (Academic Press), Orlando.

Crissey, S. D., Slifka, K. A., Shumway, P. and Spencer, S. B. (2001) *Handling Frozen/Thawed Meat and Prey Items Fed to Captive Exotic Animals: A Manual of Standard Operating Procedures*. U. S. D. A. AWIC, Beltsville, MD.

de la Navarre, B. J. S. (2006) Common procedures in reptiles and amphibians. *Veterinary Clinics Exotic Animal Practice*, **9**, 237–267.

de Matos, R. and Morrisey, J. K. (2005) Emergency and critical care of small psittacines and passerines. *Seminars Avian and Exotic Pet Medicine*, **14**, 90–105.

de Matos, R. and Morrisey, J. K. (2006) Common procedures in the pet ferret. *Veterinary Clinics Exotic Animal Practice*, **9**, 347–365.

Donnelly, T. M. and Brown, C. J. (2004) Guinea pig and chinchilla care and husbandry. *Veterinary Clinics Exotic Animal Practice*, **7**, 351–373.

Donoghue, S. (1998) Nutrition of pet amphibians and reptiles. *Seminars Avian and Exotic Pet Medicine*, **7**, 148–153.

Finke, M. D., Dunham, S. and Kwabi, C. (2005) Evaluation of four dry commercial gut loading products for improving the calcium content of crickets, *Acheta domesticus. Journal of Herpetological Medicine and Surgery*, **15**, 7–12.

Fisher, P. G. (2005) Equipping the exotic mammal practice. *Veterinary Clinics Exotic Animal Practice*, **8**, 405–426.

Graham, J. (2006) Common procedures in rabbits. *Veterinary Clinics Exotic Animal Practice*, **9**, 367–388.

Klaphake, E. (2006) Common rodent procedures. *Veterinary Clinics Exotic Animal Practice*, **9**, 389–413.

Klasing, K. C. (1999) Avian gastrointestinal anatomy and physiology. *Seminars Avian and Exotic Pet Medicine*, **8**, 42–50.

Koutsos, E. A., Matson, K. D. and Klasing, K. C. (2001) Nutrition of birds in the order Psittaciformes: A review. *Journal of Avian Medicine and Surgery*, **15**, 257–275.

Kupersmith, D. S. (1998) A practical overview of small animal nutrition. *Seminars Avian and Exotic Pet Medicine*, **7**, 141–147.

Latney, L. V., Toddes, B. T., Wyre et al., (2009) Improving the nutrition of insectivorous animals: evaluation of the nutrient content of Tenebrio molitor and Zophobas morio fed four different diets. Proceedings of the Association of Zoo Veterinarians Nutritional Advisory Group. October 24 to 28, Tulsa, OK, USA. pp. 22–23.

Lennox, A. M. (2006) Common procedures in other avian species. *Veterinary Clinics Exotic Animal Practice*, **9**, 303–319.

Martinez-Jimenez, D. and Hernandez-Divers, S. J. (2007) Emergency care of reptiles. *Veterinary Clinics Exotic Animal Practice*, **10**, 557–585.

McDonald, D. (2006) Nutritional considerations: nutrition and dietary supplementation. in *Clinical Avian Medicine* (eds G. J. Harrison and T. L. Lightfoot) Spix Publishing, Inc., Palm Beach, pp. 86–107.

Mitchell, M. A. (2004) Snake care and husbandry. *Veterinary Clinics Exotic Animal Practice*, **7**, 421–466.

National Research Council, B. o. A. C. o. L. N., Subcommittee on Laboratory Animal Nutrition (1995) *Nutrient Requirements of Laboratory Animals*, National Academy Press, Washington, D.C.

Paul-Murphy, J. (2007) Critical care of rabbit, *Veterinary Clinics Exotic Animal Practice*, **10**, 437–461.

Pollock, C. (2002) Postoperative management of the exotic animal patient. *Veterinary Clinics Exotic Animal Practice*, **5**, 183–211.

Pough, F. H. (2004) Herpetology as a field of study. in *Herpetology*, 3rd edn, (eds F. H. Pough, R. M. Andrews, J. E. Cadle et al., Pearson Education, Inc., Upper Saddle River, pp. 1–228.

Powers, L. V. (2006a)Techniques for drug delivery in psittacine birds. *Journal of Exotic Pet Medicine*, **15**, 193–200.

Powers, L. V. (2006b) Common procedures in psittacines. *Veterinary Clinics Exotic Animal Practice*, **9**, 287–302.

Powers, L. V. (2006c) Techniques for drug delivery in small mammals. *Journal of Exotic Pet Medicine*, **15**, 201–209.

Rossi, J. V. (2006) General husbandry and management. in *Reptile Medicine and Surgery*, 2nd edn, (eds S.J. Divers and D.R. Madar) Elsevier, St. Louis. pp. 25–41.

Schmidt, D. A., Travis, D. A. and Williams, J. J. (2006) Guidelines for creating a food safety HACCP program in zoos or aquaria. *Zoo Biology*, **25**, 125–135.

Stahl, S. and Kronfeld, D. (1998) Veterinary nutrition of large psittacines. *Seminars Avian and Exotic Pet Medicine*, **7**, 128–134.

Sykes, J. M. and Greenacre, C. B. (2006) Techniques for drug delivery in reptiles and amphibians. *Journal of Exotic Pet Medicine*, **15**, 210–217.

Ullrey, D. E., Allen, M. E. and Baer, D. J. (1991) Formulated diets versus seed mixtures for psittacines. *Journal of Nutrition*, **121**, S193–S205.

Werquin, G. J., De Cock, K. J. and Ghysels, P. G. (2005) Comparison of the nutrient analysis and caloric density of 30 commercial seed mixtures (in toto and dehuled) with 27 commercial diets for parrots. *Journal of Animal Physiology and Animal Nutrition*, **89**, 215–221.

Index

Note: Page numbers in *italics* refer to Figures; those in **bold** to Tables.

Nutritional Management of Hospitalized Small Animals, First Edition. Edited by Daniel L. Chan.
© 2015 John Wiley & Sons, Ltd. Published 2015 by John Wiley & Sons, Ltd.

Printed and bound by CPI Group (UK) Ltd, Croydon, CR0 4YY

27/10/2024

14580164-0001